PHYSICIAN GROUP MANAGEMENT AT THE CROSSROADS

Developing, Operating & Growing Physician and Dental Groups

PHYSICIAN GROUP MANAGEMENT AT THE CROSSROADS

Developing, Operating & Growing Physician and Dental Groups

PRICEWATERHOUSECOOPERS, LLP
SANDY LUTZ

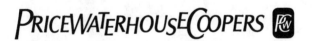

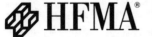 HFMA® Healthcare Financial Management Association

Educational Foundation

McGraw-Hill
New York   San Francisco   Washington, D.C.   Auckland   Bogotá
Caracas   Lisbon   London   Madrid   Mexico City   Milan
Montreal   New Delhi   San Juan   Singapore
Sydney   Tokyo   Toronto

Library of Congress Cataloging-in-Publication Data
Physician group management at the crossroads : developing, operating &
    growing physician and dental groups / PricewaterhouseCoopers, LLP ;
    Sandy Lutz.
       p.   cm.
    Includes bibliographical references and index.
    ISBN 0-07-135085-3
    1. Group medical practice—United States.   2. Group dental practice—
United States.   3. Physician management companies—United States.
I. Lutz, Sandy.   II. PricewaterhouseCoopers, LLP.
    [DNLM: 1. Group Practice—United States.   2. Group Practice, Dental—
United States.   W 92 P578   1999]
R729.5.G6P478   1999
610′.65′0973—dc21
DNLM/DLC
for Library of Congress   98-14166
                                                                                CIP

McGraw-Hill

A Division of The McGraw·Hill Companies

    2 3 4 5 6 7 8 9 0 BKM / BKM   9 0 9

ISBN 007-135085-3

Printed and bound by Book-Mart Press, Inc.

Cover illustration by Steve Dininno.

This book was typeset using 10 point Times.

This publication is designed to provide accurate and authoritative information
in regard to the subject matter covered. It is sold with the understanding that
neither the author nor the publisher is engaged in rendering legal, accounting,
or other professional service. If legal advice or other expert assistance is
required, the services of a competent professional person should be sought.

*—From a Declaration of Principles jointly adopted by a Committee of
    the American Bar Association and a Committee of Publishers.*

INTRODUCTION

Wall Street viewed physicians as a fragmented industry, lush with cash flow, but in need of capital to invest in infrastructure, information systems, and marketing. Health expenditures directly attributable to physician care are estimated at $246 billion annually. What's more, physicians control more than 80% of the overall healthcare industry expenditures of $1 trillion annually. In a report on the practice management industry, (Larry) Marsh declared that "physician groups, if properly motivated, can meaningfully reduce costs in the U.S. healthcare delivery system." The potential is awesome.

> From Chapter 1 of *Physician Group Management at the Crossroads.*

How true. Perhaps at no other time in our history have physicians, dentists, and their group practices been at such an important crossroads. The potential is awesome. But the risks are just as awesome. Physicians, dentists, and their business advisors need to think carefully through the maze of issues and options they must consider to develop, operate, and grow their practices. To do this, they need resources to help frame the issues and explore the options. This book is an important resource in that effort.

In this book, the authors carefully set the stage for this framework by describing the impetus behind physicians' and dentists' actions related to consolidation and answering the questions most asked. One such question is "Are practice management organizations the higher ground that physicians are looking for—is it really relieving them of the hassles and allowing them to practice good medicine and find good outcomes?" In answering this question, the authors also review the options by examining the different organizational models available.

Additionally, issues of importance to group practices at the crossroads include operational and billing and reimbursement issues. Here, the authors examine cost saving strategies and essential tools for billing and reimbursement guidelines and procedures. The information technology discussion focuses on moving the practice into the 21st century by identifying the questions that should be answered before investing in information technology infrastructure.

Compensation, contracting, and compliance are three words that are similar because they begin with the letter "c," and because they cause considerable concern. These issues cause concern because of the impact on cash flow and risk management. Effective compensation programs, managed care contracting processes, and compliance programs are fundamental to successful practice management of revenues, costs, and risks.

Valuation and raising capital are topics covered by the authors to help physicians and dentists understand what is important to potential acquirers or lenders. The amount that an individual or organization will pay for a practice is based on key drivers, tax implications, compensation arrangements, managed care contracts, and so on. Or, if sale of the practice is not in the immediate future, what are the sources of capital that can be tapped by a practice to meet its strategic goals? How would a potential lender view the credit-worthiness of a practice? What security can be offered?

Finally, common wisdom states that if we don't learn from the past we will be condemned to relive it. Taking this wisdom to heart, the authors conclude the book with "Turnarounds, Unforced Errors, and Lessons Learned." What happens if the whole thing blows up? How do you repair damage to relationships within the group and others? What have we learned from the past five years? The answers to these questions and many more are vital to any practice.

The potential for group practices is indeed awesome. Achieving that potential, however, requires that physicians, dentists, and their business advisors take action based on a well thought out plan. That plan must consider the issues and options raised in this book and chart a course for practice management at the crossroads.

Richard L. Clarke, FHFMA
President
Healthcare Financial Management Association
February 1999

FOREWORD

Healthcare is a highly personal enterprise that begins in an exam room where a relationship is forged between a physician and a patient.

While this relationship is the foundation of our healthcare system, physicians and health organizations are learning that physicians' domains must expand beyond the exam room. Physicians must be included in solving the fundamental business problems that face this industry. Our nation's best hospitals, health plans, and physician groups are swamped by clinical, regulatory, and financial changes. To succeed, these medical entities must work with physicians to understand the underlying business principles that dictate today's market realities.

Too often physicians and their leaders have ignored the basics of business and gotten bogged down in the traditions, culture, and glories of our vocation. Unfortunately the glories are waning. The pride and optimism once shared among physicians has dissolved, and many physicians believe themselves to be victims of a runaway health system.

Only those organizations that can figure out how to lead, inspire, and manage physician groups can bring critical change and rejuvenate the profession and industry we work in. Yet, harnessing the power of physician groups is an enigma that confounds hospitals, health systems, and even physicians themselves.

This book is an answer to that enigma, providing guidelines and stepstones for physician groups and health systems in working with physicians. It describes many of the fundamentals of business that are essential and interlocking. With these fundamentals, physicians can be leaders in the changes under way, rather than swept away by those changes.

RAPID EVOLUTION

The fundamental and personal relationship between a physician and a patient has been threatened in recent years by the onset of managed care. Managed care was a response to the double-digit healthcare inflation that spun wildly out of control in the 1980s.

In the truly American tradition of the middleman, medical inflation was tempered by the entry of managed care organizations. Managed care's commitment to scrutinize care and cap the cost was hailed by employers.

While managed care gleaned most of the credit for the abatement of double-digit medical inflation, an outgrowth of managed care was equally responsible. Healthcare providers learned that size matters in the managed care world. They began to amalgamate into large health systems that could wield greater power at the negotiating table with managed care organizations. As hospitals, physicians, and other providers banded together to negotiate with health plans, the plans themselves grew larger so they could gain economies of scale and dictate reimbursement terms back to providers.

As systems and plans grew larger, clear lines of competition developed in individual markets. Market-based competition brought price competition and prices started driving costs. Systems began to develop cost structures based on the prices they received in the market—a 180-degree turn from the previous economic model in which costs drove prices.

Another key factor in this evolution of managed care was the move from a guild-based system to a free market-based system. Again, this change demanded that practitioners understand how market forces work and how business discipline is required. Like other businesses, healthcare enterprises are finding that they must focus on the customer. Lose that focus and you will not succeed.

Hospitals and health plans were more adept than physicians at playing—and winning—in this new marketplace of medicine. Because of a lack of leadership, physicians began to see themselves as victims, and even today, many are in the middle of a grief cycle brought on by that development. As the industry adopted marketplace economics, physicians found they lacked the clout and the business savvy to compete. Physicians are often reactionary and autonomous—two attributes that worked against them in a world that was consolidating and focused on market-based strategies.

The void of physician leadership meant that consolidating healthcare organizations also lacked the key ingredient to make their systems work more efficiently and effectively. Because physicians are the locus of control in healthcare, the lack of their proactive participation hampered the efforts of the organizations that strived to work with them.

Physicians have phenomenal leverage to effect change in the system but often don't have the business knowledge base and culture to exert it. Healthcare organizations found that they can only progress so far without physicians as change partners.

FANTASTIC OPPORTUNITY

Therein lies the opportunity. Physician leaders must step up to exert cost control by bringing real business discipline to their endeavors.

At Lovelace Health Systems, we have seen the successful effects when business discipline is brought to bear on a healthcare organization. Lovelace is owned by Cigna, a large national insurance company. However, the health system is and always has been physician-led and directed. The CEO has always been a local physician, and the board is dominated by physicians who make up seven of the nine members.

In Albuquerque, New Mexico, we compete in a difficult environment in which premiums fell so low that expenses outpaced revenues. Even though we had a national reputation for disease management and reengineering care, we found that wasn't enough. We had to understand the business issues. Further, we had to develop a system of financial accountability.

By empowering physicians with fundamental business skills and discipline, we achieved a $34 million financial turnaround—remarkable in today's environment. The total system—including the hospitals, physician groups, and health plan—went from a $22 million loss in 1997 to a $12 million profit in 1998. PricewaterhouseCoopers' knowledge, in both financial and operational matters, helped us make this turnaround.

While Lovelace is somewhat unique as an integrated system, other hospitals and health organizations that work with physicians similarly need to educate their physicians to put their institutions on solid financial ground.

The business principles described in this book are applicable to medical groups, hospitals, and health systems. Physicians need to have the information so they can see how their old behavior contributes to nonviability, and how new behaviors have to be adhered to.

PHYSICIANS LEADING PHYSICIANS

To be credible, this educational process must begin with strong physician leadership. Why? Physicians traditionally don't trust nonphysicians. Physicians will embrace thoughts and actions of competent physician leaders.

Again, communicating the information is not enough. Physicians must understand the financial fundamentals that underlie the data and make the analysis possible.

Why are physicians so necessary to leading change? As I described earlier, our industry is built on the foundation of a physician's relationship with a patient. Each physician eventually has to look his or her patient in the eye. The hospital administrator doesn't have to do that. The Wall Street banker doesn't have to do that. The health plan doesn't have to do that. The physician does.

Physicians have a fiduciary responsibility to maintain quality of care for their patients.

As the industry moves forward, all physicians, not just physician leaders, must learn to grasp the business issues driving the industry.

I understand that this will cause physicians additional stress. Some may want to delay that stress, saying, "I want to see how this all shakes out." Don't be lulled by that argument. That leaves somebody else to shake the rug and physicians will be left out of control.

If physicians are boxed in as strictly clinicians, this industry will be run by people who see it first as a financial endeavor. Those people are never in the exam room and they never look the patient in the eye.

We, as physicians, know medicine today.

However, for the future, we must learn business.

We have the ability to make medicine a wonderful vocation, but to do that we have to understand how the business works. This book will bring physicians, their leaders, and the organizations that work with them closer to understanding these business issues and using them for progress.

Martin Hickey, M.D., is president and chief executive officer of Lovelace Health Systems, which comprises about 300 employed physicians, 2,500 physician network partners, a 265-bed medical center, regional and local primary care centers, and a health plan with more than 250,000 members. Dr. Hickey also teaches at the University of New Mexico as an adjunct associate professor of medicine.

Martin Hickey, M.D.
President and CEO,
Lovelace Health Systems

ACKNOWLEDGMENTS

This book drew upon the experience and wisdom of dozens of professionals working in the practice management industry. I'd like to thank the following individuals and their organizations for giving their time, expertise, and insight to this project.

John Allen
Corda Medical Care

William Altman
FemPartners

Ronald Anspaugh
PricewaterhouseCoopers

Bill Appling
MediSphere Health Partners

Leslie Barringer
PricewaterhouseCoopers

Christi Bennett
PricewaterhouseCoopers

Mary A. Bennett
MedPartners

Robert Boyle, Jr.
First Physician Care

Bruce Broussard
Harbor Dental

Gary Cage
Monarch Dental Group

Blake Carter
Tejas Securities

John Casey
Physician Reliance Network

Jack Castle, Jr.
Castle Dental Centers

Frank Cavanaugh
PricewaterhouseCoopers

Rob Cepielik
PricewaterhouseCoopers

Steven Cooley, M.D.
USCardiovascular

Jonathan Coslet
Texas Pacific Group

Rosemary Davis
Fleet Capital

John Deane
MedPartners

John Diebold
PricewaterhouseCoopers

Paul DeMuro
Latham & Watkins

Tim Domain
PricewaterhouseCoopers

Michelle Durham
*National CPA Healthcare Advisors
  Association*

Cynthia Dotson
MediSphere Health Partners

Thomas Erickson
CareSelect

Michael Fiore
Gentle Dental

Bart Fleming
PricewaterhouseCoopers

Joseph Frank
Valley Forge Dental

Cynthia Fry
PricewaterhouseCoopers

Gary Garbrecht
PricewaterhouseCoopers

Martha Garner
PricewaterhouseCoopers

Sarah Garvin
Physicians Health Corp.

William Gil
UniMed

Michael Goffinet
PricewaterhouseCoopers

Charles Goldberg
PricewaterhouseCoopers

Jonathan Goldstein
TA Associates

Arthur Greenberg, M.D.
Innova

Woody Grossman
PricewaterhouseCoopers

Peter Gyorgy
PricewaterhouseCoopers

Patrick Haggerty
PricewaterhouseCoopers

William Hanlon III
Shattuck Hammond

Allen Hahn
PricewaterhouseCoopers

David Hellerstein, M.D.
PricewaterhouseCoopers

Al Holloway
The IPA Association of America

Mel Hope
PricewaterhouseCoopers

Joseph Hutts
PhyCor

John Hunkeler, M.D.
Hunkeler Eye Clinic

Christopher Ideker
Medaphis

Jo Ann Jany
PricewaterhouseCoopers

Kathryn Johnston
MediSphere Health Partners

Ira Korman, Ph.D.
IntraMed

Tim Knutson
CareSelect

Mitchell Kornblit
Shattuck Hammond

John Lacy
USCardiovascular

Christopher Laurent
Fleet Capital

Michael Linn
UniMed

Robert Lunbeck
Hambrecht & Quist

Larry Marsh
Salomon Smith Barney

Diane Nobles
MedPartners

Jeff Perkins
PricewaterhouseCoopers

Wayne Posey
ProMedCo

Fred Pounds
American Oncology Resources

Steve Puckett
MedCath

Robin Rhoden
PricewaterhouseCoopers

Bert Robles
PricewaterhouseCoopers

Gary Roland
PricewaterhouseCoopers

A.J. Rosmarin
IMACS

R. Dale Ross
American Oncology Resources

John Runningen
Cordova Capital

Leo Sands
American Oncology Resources

Jane Sarra
PricewaterhouseCoopers

Jim Sillman
CareSelect

Jerry Sokol
McDermott, Will & Emery

Danguole Spakevicius
FemPartners

Marty Stango
Heritage Southwest

John Sulivan
Tucker Anthony

Jon Thomas
NovaMed Eyecare Management

Mark Toney
PricewaterhouseCoopers

Doug Townsend
Townsend Frew & Co.

Daniel Untch
MedPartners

Mark Wagar
American Physician Partners

Barton R. Wald, M.D.
UniMed

Stanley Weintraub
HCFA

Audrey Went
PricewaterhouseCoopers

Grant Wicklund
Heidrick & Struggles

Patricia Vogel
*Management Directions of North
 Carolina*

Robert Yeager
OrthoLink

CONTENTS

CHAPTER 1

The Push to Consolidate and Manage Physicians and Dentists

Sandy Lutz

Gary Garbrecht

During the past couple of years, the business of managing and investing in physician and dental practices has been a high-risk bet with no guarantee. Of the 40-plus publicly traded practice management companies, few have escaped without a major write-off, restructuring charge, or turmoil in the executive suite. Hospitals, health plans, and private investors have also been troubled by the complex problems of managing these practices.

For years, healthcare executives have smugly noted, "You know physicians, they're not very good at business. These guys need business managers to show them how to run these practices efficiently." Yet, as restructuring charges and write-offs mounted to more than $1 billion at the publicly held management companies in 1998, it became clear that doctors weren't the only ones with questionable business judgment. This business of practice management was testing the mettle of some of the industry's most savvy financial executives and investors.

In 1996, the market capitalization of the physician practice management industry towered at $14 billion. However, by April 1998, it had slipped to $10 billion and then sunk to half of that by year's end. Ironically, more physician practice management companies were publicly traded in late 1998 than in 1996, making the market less appealing for investors. At one point in the fall of 1998, only one physician practice management firm's stock was trading above $10. Several companies had shares trading in the penny-stock range, and the bankruptcy filings of FPA Medical Management, BMJ Medical Management, and PHP Healthcare Corp. led observers to question whether this was a viable business after all.

The publicly held practice management firm's woes were only the most visible because of their daily beating on the stock market. However, they weren't the only ones struggling. Many hospital systems and private physician groups were struggling to operate the physician practices they had rushed to buy. They found the practices were losing money and grappled for a way to stem the tide of red ink.

The failure of practice management to deliver value is alarming, touching nearly every segment of the nation's $1 trillion industry (Figure 1–1). Physicians control as much as 80 cents of the healthcare dollar. The way they practice, the treatments they prescribe, and the way they effect change in the health system will be influenced by whoever or whatever is managing them.

No accurate count exists of the number of practice management organizations in operation because there are so many different types of these groups and they're constantly merging and breaking off. According to the American Medical Association (AMA), however, there are 20,000 groups of three or more physicians. Most of those groups are likely to grow into their own practice management organizations or affiliate with a health system or management company in the future. Already, hundreds of hospitals systems maintain their own practice management arm.

Today's practice managers are asking many of the same questions: Is the business of practice management fundamentally flawed? Can anyone truly

FIGURE 1–1

U.S. Spending on Physician Services Projected to Rise Rapidly

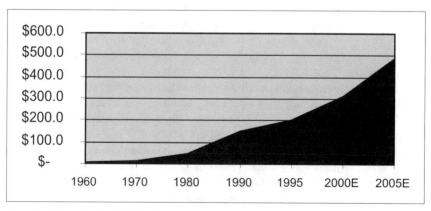

Source: Health Care Financing Administration.

manage physicians? Is the term *practice management financial controls* an oxy-moron? Is there an effective practice management development model?

The flaws are obvious. "The vast majority of PPMs have just bought assets and not added value," said Jonathan Coslet of Texas Pacific Group, a private equity investor in four healthcare companies, one of them a practice management organization. He also noted that although practice management companies are taking on more risk contracts, most are unprepared to underwrite medical costs. One observer noted that some of the practice management companies were merely "drive-by acquirers," moving from one deal to another, tossing their purchases in the back seat and driving right on.

In spite of practice management's problems, the momentum toward aggregating physician and dental groups continues to build. They continue to move toward organizations with a variety of schematics, practice management corporations being one of them. However, practice management companies are constantly trying to balance the autonomous nature of physicians with the more rigid framework of a fiscally responsible corporation.

"This is a huge and inevitable business," said Joseph Hutts, chairman, president and CEO of PhyCor, in October 1998. Speaking at a Nashville, Tenn., conference on the future of practice management, Hutts knew the financial woes of his own 56-clinic company would affect how capital sources view the physician practice management industry. "Physicians need capital, physicians need management, physicians need organization. They will find a way to come together with business to do that. The question is: Can we get it right? The opportunity to add value to physician organizations is increasing geometrically."

What is the future of physician organizations? Through the tumbling tiles of Wall Street's kaleidoscope, today's practice management companies are seen as an unworkable business model. If practice management companies can't work, what can? Where is the success story? Sadly, the pratfalls of other physician organizational efforts are evident as well. Hospital-owned practices are notorious loss leaders, costing hospitals from $25,000 to $150,000 per practice per year. Staff-model managed care plans are on the wane. The solo practice is a dinosaur. Foundation-model physician groups are experiencing a revival, but lack access to capital.

A crisis is at hand for physicians as they enter a period of acute business disruption. In the next few years, the industry is likely to witness a sizable disgorging or restructuring of physician practices owned by hospital systems. Until a couple of years ago, hospitals were on a buying binge of physician practices, which drove up acquisition prices and salaries. The most recent AMA figures show that as many as 45,000 physicians are employed by hospitals. However, that trend is now reversing itself. As their five-year contracts with physicians expire, many hospitals will either divest these money-losing practices or make the terms of staying so draconian that the physicians will ask to leave. It's impossible to predict how many physicians will be free agents in the next few years; however, one can assume the number is in the tens of thousands. Where will those physicians go?

Already accustomed to the organizational confines of hospital ownership, many are apt to look to similar organizations or health systems that have access to capital and can build infrastructure to handle the details of administration and managed care contracting. The practice management companies that survive the current shake-out will be one haven for them. However, so will integrated healthcare delivery systems and well-financed private practice management companies, financed either by retained earnings, bank debt, or healthcare-savvy investors.

It's a big job for practice managers of the future. They must be able to add value to physician groups through billings and collections, coding, contract negotiations, physician-hospital relations, compliance programs, Medicare and Medicaid arrangements, partnerships, practice assessment, revenue enhancement, and strategic business planning. There's not much room for error.

While many are ready to sound the death knell for practice management companies, some questions arise: Who or what is going to perform all of those functions? Can physicians really revert to their former organizational status? Or, will they seek out practice management organizations that can bring them value?

"The fact that some PPMs have stumbled or failed doesn't mean that the concept of PPMs is wrong, but rather that specific execution in some cases has been off the mark," said Steve Cooley, MD, president and CEO of a start-up physician organization, USCardioVascular. "The macro trends of declining physicians' reimbursement, population management, and risk contracting continue. The opportunity for the PPM industry is still there. What has become clear is that significant investment in infrastructure and practice development are the real challenges. Practice acquisition is only a platform, a first step."

Cooley compares practice management organizations to the early personal computer companies. The early 1980s was a time of chaos—companies forming, failing, growing, consolidating. Remember Osborne, Kaypro, Columbia, WordStar, and Ashton-Tate? All were early leaders who ultimately failed or were acquired; however, the industry as a whole grew at an amazing pace and, after 15 to 20 years, became a major part of the U.S. economy. Which management organizations will become the Compaq, Dell, and Microsoft of the 21st century? "I don't know, but it's going to be exciting to find out," Cooley said.

Filled with dreams of empowering a fragmented industry, physicians were dazzled by P/E multiples, stock options, and the prospect of fewer administrative hassles. What became painfully clear in 1997 and 1998 was that some practice management companies neglected the details of good management and infrastructure necessary to realize the dream.

"The inherent problem in these models is that what you have to do to build the business is the exact opposite of what you have to do to run the business," said Ira Korman, Ph.D., a Dallas area surgery center CEO who has worked with several medical groups. Too often practice management companies have been physician recruitment vehicles rather than management firms, he noted.

In this book, we attempt to step back and examine this nascent industry in mid-cycle. We've talked to dozens of physician organization executives, from companies that have succeeded and companies that have failed. We've heard stories from disillusioned physicians. And, we've delved into the logic of Wall Street bankers and venture capitalists who stoked the practice management fire, providing billions of dollars of capital to the growing legions of management organizations that are forming. We also examine the dental practice management business, which has shadowed the physician business in some ways but benefits from several distinctions.

It's hard to be objective when you're running through a hailstorm, but physicians, dentists, and the people who purport to manage them must realize that the turns and dips of the still-evolving practice management industry are just part of a cycle. There is no single workable model because the model is evolving, and the directions on how to put these businesses together and keep them running are changing. Not only is the model changing, but so are external factors. For example, government regulators, caught off guard by this booming business, are constantly tinkering with the accounting and anti-fraud guidelines that play fundamental roles in how physician organizations are operated.

As an industry, practice management companies have been viewed through the Wall Street success paradigm. If the stock goes up, it's a success. If the stock goes down, it's a failure. That's a one-dimensional view based on short-term returns. Instead, practice management companies must have a long-term strategy of how to build value within the changing, chaotic healthcare system.

Physician organizations have an opportunity to affect the nation's trillion-dollar healthcare system. Because physicians order the tests and treatments, they have the power to lower costs and improve care. Do physicians really want to miss that opportunity? If they do, they will cede more market share to larger health systems and payors. Figures indicate they're losing market share to other healthcare services. U.S. health spending increased 4.4% in 1996, according to the Health Care Financing Administration (HCFA). However, spending on physician services increased just 2.9%, the smallest increase for any category of professional services reported by HCFA.[1]

WHY CONSOLIDATE?

The provider side of the healthcare industry remains fragmented. While hospitals and health plans have made significant progress toward consolidating into larger

---

[1] American Medical Association: Highlights from the Socioeconomic Monitory System Surveys, *Aspen's Physician Management Bulletin,* March 23, 1998.

FIGURE 1–2

The Opportunity to Consolidate

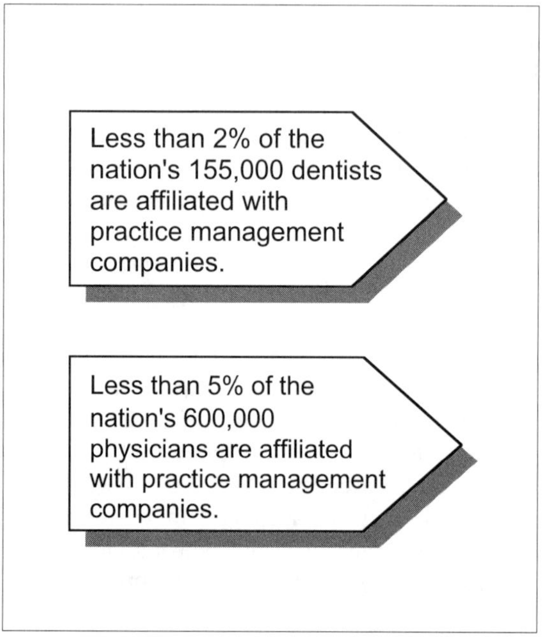

Less than 2% of the nation's 155,000 dentists are affiliated with practice management companies.

Less than 5% of the nation's 600,000 physicians are affiliated with practice management companies.

systems, physicians and dentists continue to work as small businesses. According to current estimates, only 2% of dentists and 5% of physicians are affiliated with publicly traded practice management companies. The supply of practitioners is robust, making it a consolidator's dream (Figure 1–2).

Physicians

About 600,000 physicians are active in patient care, according to the American Medical Association. The number of physicians practicing in group settings doubled between 1975 and 1995. About 200,000 are in groups today, although 70% of all group practices still have 10 or fewer physicians, according to the Medical Group Practice Digest.[2]

Some experts argue that the nation is on the cusp of an oversupply of physicians, particularly specialists. In fact, the Pew Health Professions Commission in 1995 recommended the closing of 25% of the nation's medical schools to prevent a glut of physicians. To further constrict the throughput of new practitioners,

---

[2] Part of the Hoechst Marion Roussel Managed Care Digest Series, 1997.

Medicare in 1997 began paying teaching hospitals to train fewer residents. That may sound screwy, but it's somewhat similar to how the government used to regulate farm prices by paying farmers not to farm. The incentive is to hold down supply.

Some areas of the United States have too many doctors, others too few. The conventional wisdom is that managed care influences will drive down the need for physicians, particularly specialists. One recent study contended that in tightly managed care areas only 125 physicians are needed for every 100,000 enrollees—that's less than half the current ratio nationally. Many managed care organizations are using physician extenders, such as nurse practitioners, nurse anesthetists, and physician assistants to stretch their healthcare dollars and better leverage their doctors' time.

What does this mean for practice management companies and other physician organizations? Physicians face a possible oversupply. When faced with this oversupply, the market will dictate who survives and who doesn't. By forming or affiliating with an efficient physician organization, an individual physician's likelihood of survival shoots up.

Large physician organizations also may be more attractive to young physicians who are burdened by $200,000 in medical school loans and interested in more family time. "I have visited every medical school and residency program in the state of California and am not aware of a single student who would go solo," said Jack Lewin, MD, president of the California Medical Association. "Even if they had help from independent practice associations and other resources, these young people don't want to be on call all the time, and they don't want the trouble of running office operations. They also enjoy the collegiality of consulting with each other."[3]

Dentists

For dentists, the situation is different. Rather than an oversupply, some experts predict a future shortage of dentists. The number of new dentists graduating each year has dropped from about 6,000 students in 1975 to 4,200 in 1995. One reason is that during the past decade, six private dental schools have closed. Most recently, trustees at Northwestern University in Chicago voted to close the dental school there when the freshmen who entered in 1998 graduate in 2001. Whether this downward supply trend will continue is debatable. Dental schools began closing because of an oversupply of dentists in the 1980s. When nurses were in oversupply, nursing schools closed as well. Then, when a shortage hit, they reopened.

---

[3] Gallagher, A. (1997). On Their Own: Bucking the Trend to Join Groups, Some Doctors are Staying Solo. *Modern Physician,* November.

The dental industry in the United States generates about $50 billion in revenues, representing just under 5% of all health spending. Dentistry remains even more fragmented than the physician side of the industry. Of more than 155,000 dentists practicing in the United States, only 12% of dentists work in groups of two or more, according to the American Dental Association.

The formation of dental practice management companies has been a catalyst for these practitioners to aggregate. On the medical side, physicians were already forming larger groups when practice management companies came along. However, dental care consolidation didn't really take off until a dozen dental practice management companies went public during 1997 and 1998. The emergence of dental practice management companies made dentists and orthodontists think for the first time about joining a larger group. Aggregation of dentists is "at the beginning of the beginning," says Bruce Broussard, CEO of Harbor Dental, a start-up practice management company based in Atlanta.

One reason dentistry has been slower to consolidate is that managed care is a smaller threat to these practitioners. Although managed dental plans have been growing, only about 19% of Americans with dental benefits are enrolled in a dental health maintenance organization (HMO).

FINANCIAL, GOVERNMENT, AND TECHNOLOGICAL MOTIVATORS

What factors made the physicians start to consolidate? The momentum comes from several factors. We see financial, governmental, and technological change as chief among these.

Financial Motivators

"This industry has great intuitive appeal," said Larry Marsh, who has staked his research franchise in practice management companies at the giant investment bank of Salomon Smith Barney. It is "in the throes of change, and that creates some real winners and losers," said Marsh.

Wall Street viewed physicians as a fragmented industry, lush with cash flow, but in need of capital to invest in infrastructure, information systems, and marketing. Health expenditures directly attributable to physician care are estimated at $246 billion annually. What's more, physicians control more than 80% of the overall healthcare industry expenditures of $1 trillion annually. In a report on the practice management industry, Marsh declared that "physician groups, if properly motivated, can meaningfully reduce costs in the U.S. healthcare delivery system." The potential is awesome.

Although the earliest publicly traded management organizations were geared to primary care and multispecialty practices, a host of single specialty firms came to market in the mid-1990s. Management organizations now operate in behavioral care, cardiology, emergency medicine, oncology, ophthalmology, orthopedics, pediatrics, pathology, neonatology, nephrology, neurosurgery, obstetrics and gynecology, urology, plastic surgery, and radiology. At least three start-ups seek to aggregate one of the newest physician specialties, hospitalists.

The financial push was that these specialty physician organizations have greater cash flow than primary care and also have the potential to bring in more revenues from ancillary services, such as outpatient centers. In fact, specialty management organizations could be the foundation to deliver a whole array of services that comprise an integrated delivery system. An example of this is MedCath, a company that specializes in inpatient and outpatient cardiology services. Management of cardiology practices is a building block for establishing and maintaining fully integrated cardiac care networks. MedCath lays the groundwork for the network by entering long-term management services agreements with local cardiologists and cardiovascular and vascular surgeons. Then, it constructs a heart hospital and other outpatient centers to support the practice.

The trade-off is fairly straightforward. MedCath agrees to perform the principal financial and administrative functions for physician groups, including billing, recruiting, record keeping, and negotiating with HMOs and other managed care plans for the services of the physicians. In return, MedCath takes a percentage of practice operating income (or, in one instance, a percentage of net revenue). In addition, MedCath also may provide working capital advances to the physician practices.

Yet, the financial push can swing both ways.

"We were in discussions with one PPM when another one came to us and doubled the offer for our practice," said a Texas physician who is part of a five-physician group. "My partners believed that the long-term future was going to be rough if they didn't sign up with somebody. In two weeks, the paperwork was signed." This physician was very impressed with the efficiency and speed of the acquisition process. However, once his group was part of the management organization, disillusion set in.

"I was shocked at what they did. They increased our prices more than 50%. The insurance companies said our rates were from outer space, so collections dropped to about 45%," he noted. The management company "doubled the number of office employees in our practice doing billing and collections. The only thing the PPM thinks about is its relationship with Wall Street."

Sound familiar? The doctor's dialogue seems to validate what many critics have contended are the chief reasons for physicians joining publicly traded management companies: "fear and greed." The doctors were afraid of what the future held, so they sold their practices for a huge price without thinking about what changes this might impose on their practice of medicine. Yet, the practice management firm isn't blameless either. Why weren't the physicians informed about what the acquisition would mean to them? Did the management company rush through the deal because they were afraid the specialists would get bought up by a hospital or another physician organization first?

Another financial motivator was dealing with managed care—both the discounts demanded from physicians and the expensive administrative cost of dealing with managed care plans. Certainly, the tendency of many HMOs to "deselect" physicians from their provider panels also motivates doctors to look for organizations that would provide them collectively with the clout they lacked individually. Undoubtedly, physicians are often out-maneuvered by managed care organizations with which they contract because they lack the information to negotiate contracts to their advantage.

Physician practices are unique economic models. Traditionally, most physicians have run their businesses as if they go out of business every year. A physician group paid all of its bills, then they split up what's left over, effectively zeroing out the books. They didn't want to hold onto the profits because they would have to pay taxes on it. However, holding some back is a common business practice outside the realm of physician practices. Some large groups did have the discipline to hold back, say, 10% of what was left and build cash reserves. These were the groups that attracted numerous venture capital principals and Wall Street bankers. Remember the old saw about how you can't borrow money unless you can prove you don't need it? The same axiom was true with physician groups attracting private capital. Groups that had retained a sizable war chest of cash reserves were more attractive investment vehicles than those that were functionally bankrupt because they paid everything out each year, or each month. As investor enthusiasm mounted, private capital began to widen its circle of physician enterprises worth investing in. Groups that had no concept of how to reserve cash received capital anyway, and some groups that weren't even groups yet received capital so that they could get together.

Finally, shrinking physician incomes (or at least that perception) pushed physicians to consider practice management collectives.

Actually, since 1984, physician incomes have declined only one year—1994. Even so, physician incomes haven't kept pace with inflation, the AMA argues. From 1993 to 1996, median net income increased an average of 2.1% annually, compared with an average 2.8% increase in the Consumer Price Index. That translates to an annual decline of 0.7% in real dollars, the AMA reported.

There's also a feeling that physicians may be losing ground as health spending expands. The AMA said that physician services spending rose 2.9% in 1996, the smallest increase for any category of healthcare services. Meanwhile, spending increased 3.4% for hospital care, 6.2% for home health, 4.3% for nursing homes, 9.2% for prescription drugs, and 6.4% for dental services, according to HCFA.

From a social standpoint, physicians want to realize value from their lifelong career and they want to have a nest egg for when they retire. Although this is a financial issue, it plays into physicians' needs for security. Interestingly, practice management companies were willing to pay physicians to join them. That was completely opposite what usually happened in medical practice. Usually, a physician had to pay to join a medical group, buying in to be a shareholder. So, here comes Best Physicians Corp. to a group of radiologists. No, no, we don't want your money. In fact, we're gonna pay you!

In another interesting twist in the practice management area, dentists are gaining ground on physicians in terms of compensation. In some parts of the United States, dentists are earning almost as much as physicians, according to a survey by the National Association of Healthcare Consultants.[4] The average U.S. dentist earned $181,586 in 1996, only about 10% less than the average physician.

On the west coast, where managed care has hammered reimbursement, the average dentist makes $202,166, compared with $173,383 for the average non-surgeon physicians. Surgeons earn appreciably more—$279,671.

According to Bruce Broussard, CEO of Harbor Dental, Atlanta, one factor driving dentists to management organizations is the fact that 40% of new graduates are females, "Because of family goals and objectives, they don't want to be tied down with a large debt," he said, noting that it costs at least $100,000 to establish a dental practice. "They would rather go into an employee-based model." The Harbor practices offer dentists flex time to work from 7 AM to 1 PM, or from 1 PM to 7 PM, he added.

In addition, Harbor puts about $50,000 in technology into its practices—equipment like intraoral video, voice activated charting systems, and lasers. It's hard for new dentists to come up with the capital to equip such state-of-the-art practices.

Government Motivators

The government push is two-pronged. One prong is the federal government's desire to make healthcare more productive, more businesslike, more efficient. Practice management companies are a business model that can achieve that for physicians.

The other prong is from a legal standpoint, Specifically, the government has created "safe harbors" from fraud regulations, which encourage the formation of medical groups. For example, the Stark legislation prevents independent physician practices from referring to their own ancillary services. However, group practices can be exempt from this rule, enabling them to capture the ancillary revenue that may have gone to others.

The group practice still cannot reward physicians based on the number of referrals made to those ancillaries. However, the potential for larger revenues and

---

[4] Average Dentist Income Nears or Tops Physician's, *Managed Dental Care,* October 1997.

profits exists, especially for certain single-specialty physician organizations, such as oncology and orthopedics.

However, the irony is that some of the legal regulations also set up road-blocks for physician groups becoming more of a business. While healthcare has been attacked as bureaucratic and expensive, the mechanisms to improve performance through financial incentives are being increasingly discouraged by government regulators. For example, most businesses have designed performance compensation arrangements for employees, and vendors often receive preferred status and discounts for sending business their way. However, those types of relationships run afoul of Medicare's fraud and abuse rules.

What's difficult for management organizations is that the fraud and abuse rules continue to evolve. That means healthcare organizations must be flexible in their contracts with physicians to allow for fall-back positions. The government's anti-kickback laws are a mainstay of the "risk factors" section in publicly held physician management company disclosure documents. We'll explore those problems in more detail in a later chapter.

In terms of fraud, physicians are faced with what many regard as a criminalization of misdeeds in medicine. According to the Health Insurance Portability and Accountability Act (HIPAA), passed by Congress in 1997, a physician who fails to fully implement the new documentation requirements could be convicted of a felony, punishable by a $10,000 fine and/or five-year prison sentence per occurrence. The government also warned that errors on forms, whether deliberate or due to carelessness or sloppiness, can be prosecuted as a felony.

The increasingly complex Medicare regulations pose more and more hassles for practitioners who look to their hospitals or physician organizations for legal expertise. For example, new Medicare regulations will require doctors to fill out forms with new mandatory guidelines for patient examinations. A musculoskeletal examination, for instance, will require the doctor's documentation that four out of six body parts were examined or that four out of six areas were palpated.

The second government push is the prospect of physicians forming organizations known as provider sponsored networks, which directly contract with Medicare. PSOs are basically are captive insurance companies, formed to serve specific needs of corporations. In 1997, 5 million seniors, or about 13% of the Medicare population, were enrolled in risk plans. Of those, 88% are enrolled with HMOs, compared with other at-risk plans. However, the growth of seniors in risk plans has been brisk, a 108% increase since 1993. It also differs significantly by geographic region.

PSOs could have several advantages over traditional managed care plans. In certain cases, the providers owning them will be known to the Medicare beneficiaries and have a local brand name or at least a local presence. Physician organizations may be in the best position of all providers to contract for Medicare on a risk basis because they will have the historical data to manage the patient's care.

However, Medicare risk contracting is a huge gamble and many HMOs have been pulling out of the business, saying it's financially untenable. It's unlikely small physician organizations can make it work either.

Technological Motivators

Information technology is seen as a necessary evil by today's physicians. They need sophisticated financial and clinical systems to make decisions on patient care and managed care contracting and to keep pace with payor systems.

It's not enough to understand how well one's own practice is doing. Physicians must compare outcomes—again, both financial and clinical—with one's peers. Also, many physician practices want to negotiate competitive capitated contracts, but they cannot do that with any accuracy without cost and utilization information

Yet, even large physician groups lack the capital to purchase the advanced information systems that provide such data. This is a major problem for physicians. Many a physician group has failed because it installed the wrong information system.

A few years ago, a start-up practice management company in Texas struck an agreement for a custom-built information system with a vendor whose background was primarily in hospital systems. "We contracted with them to do billing and collections and develop a practice management system," explained the group's former president. "We agreed to pay the vendor 4% of (total) billed charges."

The problem was the computer system development stalled and the vendor was collecting only 6% of total charges. When the vendor collected its 4%, the doctors were left with just 2%. The vendor had no incentive to collect additional billings and the physicians were left with an extreme cash flow problem.

Well, that's idiotic, an observer may say. Yes, but it shows the naïveté that physicians sometimes bring to the table when contracting for complex information systems.

Instead of solving problems, new computer systems can cripple basic bookkeeping tasks, delaying payments to doctors and hospitals and the billing of clients for months. Physicians want to join management organizations because they want to leave the business minutiae to someone else. Information systems that collect that minutiae with minimal work by the physician help accomplish that goal. However, many information systems don't do the job, creating havoc for all.

SO WHAT'S THE PROBLEM?

With so many moving parts, it's easy to understand why the practice management model has failed on so many fronts. The general business purpose for consolidating an industry is the creation of economies of scale, lower costs, and a more efficient, synergistic organization that is stronger than simply the sum of its parts.

What investors, physicians, and health system executives have learned is that practice management isn't just another consolidation play. These aren't the kinds of businesses that are going to roll up into neat little packages. Aggregating physicians isn't enough. The details of integrating and operating these complicated medical service businesses takes more time and effort than aggregating a retail industry such as fast-food restaurants or car dealers.

In other business models, start-up companies often begin with little infrastructure. They run lean and mean, shunning overhead so they can build up profits. However, experience has shown that practice management organizations cannot be similarly run on a shoestring. They must have a certain amount of infrastructure for billing, collections, compliance, and other administrative services.

The provision of healthcare through a physician organization has numerous constituencies—hospitals, physicians, payors, investors, and patients. Not all of these constituencies will be supportive of organized physician groups.

Expectations ran well ahead of reality, which is common in a nascent industry. Wall Street analysts relied on information provided by the executives of these pioneering companies to project growth. No wonder optimism reigned. Who would be the biggest promoters of practice management companies? The men and women being paid to run them.

However, this is not an easy business to grow or make money in. It looked deceptively easy when PhyCor was hitting on all cylinders. But, publicly traded companies found that they vastly underestimated the financial and personnel challenges of the business.

So, what's the problem?

- Physicians feel most accountable when they're responsible for their own production and compensation. When they join groups, accountability is diluted. **Result: Management organizations and health systems that acquire practices may dilute the accountability and subsequently the profitability of those practices.**

- Many physician practices do not have a high cost structure that can be better managed by large company. Doctors are notorious for being penny-pinchers on salaries, information systems, and office space. **Result: A practice management organization may actually add costs to practices.**

- To recruit physicians, many management organizations made the prospect of affiliation too appealing on the front end. Corporate resources were directed toward acquisitions, not operations. **Result: Physicians found themselves paying a 15% to 25% management fee, which amounted to a pay cut, on the promise that the** management organization would expand overall revenues and profits. When the clinic's revenues and profits stagnated, the physicians were left with a 15% to 20% pay cut.

- Management organizations aspired to grow to please investors. **Result: Physicians believed that the company's first allegiance was to shareholders, not physicians or the patients they treated. They were less faithful stewards of the practice's resources if the beneficiaries were faceless shareholders, rather than themselves or their patients.**

- Publicly held and privately funded physician practice management companies compete against organizations that do not have the same profitability requirements as they do. Some hospital systems bought physician practices and used them as loss leaders to make money on inpatient programs. Hospitals can sustain these losses because their physicians are bringing in admissions, a higher-margin business than running physician practices. The majority of these hospital systems are not-for-profit, which also puts them at a tax advantage to for-profit practice management companies. **Result: Management companies are at a competitive disadvantage because they must turn a profit. They're competing for acquisitions with organizations that can afford to pay higher prices and guarantee higher salaries because they don't have to make money on their physician practices. It's difficult to get physicians in a management organization to control their own costs and salaries when their colleagues across town work for organizations that don't hold their feet to the same fire of business discipline. Hospitals are effectively subsidizing their physician practices, although many are beginning to reassess this strategy.**

PRACTICE MANAGEMENT MODELS

Physicians practice in numerous types of organizations, some of which have done better than others. In some cases, the model itself was flawed. In others, poor leadership, lack of capital, or other forces contributed to failure. It's the nature of humans and money that conflicts will arise, egos will clash, and financial issues will divide loyalties. As we discuss numerous physician and dental organizations in the course of this book, we probably won't find the "perfect" model.

An array of different models has proliferated. Here's a listing, but keep in mind that many practice organizations fall into more than one category.

- Salaried physician model—Management company owns all the assets of the physician practices and employs the physicians. All of the revenue of the practice, except for physician compensation, is retained by the physician organization.

- Independent practice association (IPA) model—No assets are purchased. This type of organization has access to a large pool of physicians, but has limited control over them. It is not unusual for a physician to be in four or five IPAs as they strive to maximize their patient volume. Usually, arrangements with other payors, such as Medicare and Medicaid, are outside the realm of the IPA's operations.

  IPAs typically take a percent of revenue, although they often promise to pay physicians a bonus at the end of the year, depending on utilization and profits. The fee can also be described as a withhold, meaning that the IPA is holding back some of the physicians' compensation as an incentive to provide care efficiently.

  Some hospital systems and management companies manage IPAs, and at times that effort is a precursor to acquiring selected practices within the association.

- Medical services organization—A company owns the tangible and intangible assets of the physician practices and signs a long-term agreement with the physicians' professional corporation.

- Facilities-based model—A company manages physician practices, but the company's primary assets are its facilities, such as surgery centers, imaging centers, or radiation therapy centers.

- Fixed percent of revenue model—Some management organizations are gravitating toward this model, which is somewhat like a franchise in that the parent company takes a small percent of revenue in exchange for certain administrative and marketing services.

- Fixed percent of practice income model—Many practice management organizations are structured this way. The management company takes 10% to 35% of practice income after expenses are paid. In exchange, the company provides a suite of management services that may include billing, collections, information systems, medical transcription, managed care negotiations, human resources, payroll, legal services, and information systems management.

- Hospital-owned group practices—In a study of 460 physician practice acquisitions from 1994 to 1996, 83% were made by hospitals, according to the Center for Healthcare Industry Performance Studies, Columbus, Ohio. The trend of hospitals buying practices soared in the 1990s. In 1996, hospital systems owned 2,786 group practices, up 67% from 1995. The Medical Group Management Association found that hospital-owned practices are 50 times less profitable than those owned by medical groups or physician practice management firms. The group determined that the losses stemmed primarily from salary guarantees made to doctors, the purchase of marginal performers, and high overhead costs.

- Single specialty—By focusing on just one specialty, some physician organizations hope to attract specialists of like mind and eventually provide carve-out services to payors. Examples are American Oncology Resources (oncology), Pediatrix (neonatal pediatrics), and Specialty Care Network (musculoskeletal care). On Wall Street, these companies may be referred to as "category killers," in a reference to retail counterparts such as Just for Feet or Barnes and Noble. These types of companies are likely to have operations throughout the country, although they may get their start in a handful of regional markets.

- Regional management organizations—As management companies discover the expense and difficulty of duplicating their models over several time zones, more practice management companies may choose to take a more regional focus.

- Hospital outsourcing—In addition to managing physician practices, these management organizations also contract to manage hospital departments. The best examples are in the hospital-based specialties of radiology, emergency medicine, anesthesia and pathology. The economics of these physician organizations are different than those that manage doctors in private practice. Hospital-based physicians have less overhead; their offices are typically in the hospital setting.

- Multispecialty—These organizations seek to bring many specialties and primary care physicians under the same management umbrella. Examples are Scripps Clinic in California, Fargo Clinic in North Dakota, and PhyCor, a Nashville-based company.

- Private-pay players—These models are distinguished by the fact that they generate revenues from nongovernmental sources. Examples are Orthodontic Centers of America and Aesthetic Medical Management. Consumers pay for these out of pocket.

- Retailers—Primarily dental practice management companies that rely on marketing and high-traffic locations to draw in customers. An example is Denver-based Birner Dental, which brands under the name "Perfect Teeth." Nearly all of its units are in supermarket-anchored shopping centers.

- Physician hospital organizations (PHOs)—More than 150,000 physicians and 1,100 hospitals/medical centers participate in PHOs, according to the National Directory of Physician Organizations, published by the Managed Care Information Center. PHOs typically don't acquire physician practices, but they do provide contract negotiation and utilization management. The American Medical

Association reports that about one-third of physicians participate in PHOs. Usually, the organizations are 50-50 ventures in which the physician group and the hospital share equal ownership. The first reported formation of PHOs began in 1983, increasing steadily until 1994 when, in just one year, the number of PHOs doubled.

Most practice management firms have been an admixture of different models. Yet, successful practice management firms must focus on what makes their business different than other firms, not what makes them the same. These companies have stalled when they diluted their franchises rather than accentuated them.

AN EXPERT'S PERSPECTIVE: R. DALE ROSS, CEO OF AMERICAN ONCOLOGY RESOURCES

Among the 40-plus publicly traded practice management firms, American Oncology Resources (AOR) has been a consistent performer and its CEO one of a handful of top management organization executives to survive the industry's dips and spins (Figure 1–3).

R. Dale Ross' experience in healthcare is extensive, and his credentials (including building a healthcare company, then merging it with a larger firm) demonstrate the business acumen that Wall Street admires. Before joining AOR in 1992, Ross was founder of HMSS, a home infusion therapy company based in Houston, Texas. HMSS was bought by Secomerica in 1989. Among physician management organizations, AOR's stock is among the most closely watched on Wall Street. Sixteen healthcare analysts follow it.

At AOR, Ross has been careful to build a management company that isn't just an aggregator of practices. It is one that strives to bring value to oncologists who battle one of the nation's biggest killers.

FIGURE 1–3

American Oncology Resources, Houston, Texas

STATS:

- 111% annual growth rate from 1992 to 1997
- 1997 net income of $22.9 million, or $.48 per share, on revenues of $322 million.
- More than 300 physicians under management

Company statistics would nearly double under pending merger with Physician Reliance Network, Dallas, which was announced in December 1998.

The company's 1997 annual report notes that an American dies from cancer every minute. One in every two men will eventually be diagnosed with cancer. One in every three women will have cancer in her lifetime.

The survival rate for people with cancer has risen dramatically in recent years, and that has increased demand for cancer treatment. AOR has the largest and most profitable network of cancer specialists in the country, with more than 300 affiliated doctors. It targets only markets where it can quickly become a significant player: four-fifths of the company's revenue comes from areas where it has a better than 40% market share.

The company's first network was in Colorado, where AOR started with six physicians in December 1992. That has grown to about 30 physicians reaching from Boulder to Colorado Springs. The company also is building three new comprehensive cancer centers in the state, part of a $50-million program to build 10 cancer centers in 1998.

By building oncology networks, AOR brings value to both physicians and patients. To a cancer patient, the medical oncologist typically takes the role of a patient's primary care physician, coordinating all necessary treatment. AOR goes into a market where it can acquire the practice of a leading medical oncologist, ideally an opinion leader that other oncologists respect. Then, AOR brings on other practices such as radiation oncology. The network often branches out to include stem-cell transplant specialists and obstetric/gynecological oncology practices. Ross has seen the forces pushing physicians toward practice management companies and has watched the industry change and grow.

In AOR's early years, managed care prompted physicians to talk to AOR. "The fear was driven by the managed care side of the business. Five years ago, there was this dark, ominous cloud hanging over the provider side and physicians feared a loss of control. More than anything else, managed care was pushing physicians to consider affiliating with large management organizations.

Now, managed care hasn't gone away, but it hasn't turned out to be this terrible, horrendous thing.

Physicians also feared that in terms of clinical decision making, someone was going to tell them how to practice medicine. Back then, a physician practice management company was a new phenomenon. Nobody understood it—it was new and untried." Ross said there were other forces at work as well, "Hospitals were reaching out, trying to create networks and buy physician practices. However, physicians were clearly very suspicious of hospitals. Also, payers were reaching out to physicians, but they had problems getting compliance and controlling costs.

"Now, physicians are looking for more value providers in PPMs. They want to know how do you drive market share, how do you do a better job in drug purchasing, how do you integrate things like clinical research. The fear of the AORs of the world is not as great because the whole concept of PPMs is more acceptable and viable."

In terms of management organizations for oncologists, AOR has plenty of company and competition for acquisitions. Three other publicly traded companies focus on oncology: Physician Reliance Network, Dallas, Texas; Response Oncology, Memphis, Tenn.; and EquiMed, State College, Pa. (A merger with Physician Reliance was pending.) In addition, at least two private companies target this niche. "In the early days, you would differentiate yourself by affiliating with the quality practices," Ross said. That's still true today, but there's more to it, he said. "You have to differentiate yourself with your information systems, managed care expertise, and access to capital for construction projects to get physicians to come on board."

In terms of information systems, Ross is quick to say, "People have a tendency to think systems are going to solve their problems. All too often, we think systems can overcome poor structure and inadequately defined operational processes."

However, AOR recognizes the need to improve on administrative and clinical functions. AOR supports four different operating platforms in the physicians' offices. Those platform systems are used to standardize office functions such as billing, scheduling, and collections. The company is moving to a standardized system, but has focused on other needs first. While other management organizations have been plagued with billing problems, AOR has stayed on top of its collections. "This is an area that requires constant monitoring and you can expect to see continued improvement in this area," Ross said.

By the end of 1998, all physicians will be on the same general ledger. Also, in 1998, the physicians' offices began moving to a central clinical information system.

AOR has profiled the top 20 oncology diseases to determine best treatment patterns. When more data is available through the clinical information system, Ross says the results will be extremely valuable to clinicians, payors, and manufacturers.

However, he added: "There aren't going to be any secrets in treating cancer. There's not going to be proprietary data that you're going to keep to yourself." Any clinical breakthroughs that AOR physicians discover will be shared with other physicians inside and outside of AOR because of the dreaded nature of the disease. "That's what makes oncology different from other PPMs. It's probably possible for an orthopedic surgeon to have the best outcome on a knee surgery because of some proprietary technique he used. In oncology, there aren't going to be any secrets. "Our advantage is that we can document the best outcomes faster within the AOR network. These outcome improvements will translate into better patient care as well as more cost effective care for the payers," he said.

As an oncology company, AOR deals with the exploding costs of new drugs for cancer treatment, a factor that affects this specialty more than others. New drugs are often among the most expensive to purchase, presenting a challenge to payors and providers. About 45% of AOR's revenues are eaten up by drug costs, which obviously is an area of concern to management. "There has been a tremendous genetic revolution in the last three or four years. There have been more new chemical compounds in the last year alone than in the last 10 years, and that will be true again this year.

"A number of these are single-source drugs that are available from only one manufacturer. Getting favorable economic terms can be a challenge," he noted.

The whole premise behind affiliating with a management company is that scale brings certain advantages. At AOR, one of those advantages is the ability to participate in clinical trials. AOR-affiliated oncologists treat 80,000 new cancer patients annually. In comparison, most major metropolitan cancer centers treat between 5,000 and 10,000 new cancer patients yearly.

That puts AOR in a perfect position to do clinical trials, claiming a piece of an industry generating $3.4 billion in revenues annually.

PricewaterhouseCoopers Tips for Practice Management Companies

- Realize that healthcare is a local business and the practices must remain market focused.
- Find physician partners who will remain committed for the long haul. Don't sell them on the potential of equity ownership.
- Design an infrastructure that focuses on operations.
- Put together a management team that has experience working with physicians.
- Establish incentives that are linked to accountability.

2
CHAPTER

Operations: Practice Managers' Achilles Heel

Sandy Lutz

Jane Sarra

A tale of two practice management organizations.

Organization A is buying physicians' practices at a furious pace. Initially it struggles with losses, but executives pacify health system administrators and investors by telling them that the company is trying to attain "critical mass." Although profits are elusive, investors are pleased because Organization A is ramping up revenues, driving momentum, and creating a buzz in the marketplace. Surely profits will follow. Once the organization gets to the "critical mass," executives promise that it will begin building outpatient centers and buying state-of-the-art information systems. "Critical mass" occurs, but profits are ephemeral and little capital is left to build or buy the promised infrastructure. Investors balk at financing a new round of capital. Meanwhile, physicians are reviewing their five-year, non-compete clauses to see when they can bolt.

Organization B also is buying physician practices. However, this organization stays focused on its hometown market. Instead of blowing all of its capital on buying more practices, executives spend time and money on information systems, manuals, and ensuring that its physicians have the appropriate referral systems in place. Rather than sending development people hither and yon to get "dots on a map," Organization B works at internal growth and integrating the practices it already owns with standardized procedures and physician-driven clinical systems. It begins working with local providers to capitalize on the already-growing trend toward outpatient procedures.

Which organization will survive long term? Which organization will see a surge in momentum, followed by capital constraints and unhappy physicians? Which organization characterizes most of the practice management companies that have gone public in the past few years?

Following the stellar implosions of several practice management firms and the losses suffered by hospitals in their physician practices, investors, physicians, and payors are asking: Is practice management a viable business model? Can anyone operate these organizations successfully?

The answer is yes, but success must be grounded in the following four precepts.

1. Incentives must be clearly communicated and consistently implemented and that rewards productivity.

2. Management fees must be fairly structured and reward the business and clinical partnership process.

3. Reductions in overall costs must be achieved.

4. Growth must be generated from within—through ancillary development, financially sound managed care contracts, and/or clinical research pacts rather than from multiple acquisitions.

These precepts need to be implemented at the clinic level. It's not enough to have a corporate organization that follows these guidelines. Each practice must have a hands-on administrator who guides the clinic to operational excellence (Figure 2–1).

FUNDAMENTAL FINANCIAL DRIVERS IN PHYSICIAN MANAGEMENT

Why do so many organizations fail at operations? Part of the answer is that a complex set of interlocking factors helps determine success. Health systems and practice management companies that operate a practice need to look at the practice's operations, its contracts with physicians and payors, and the market to determine whether this business will succeed or not. Suppose the physician contracts are fair and reasonable and operations are running smoothly and efficiently, but the payor contracts are so inadequate that there's no way to turn a profit. That's why operations must be considered within the context of key variables. While some variables are specific to operations, two impact the overall area: physician compensation and management fees.

Physician Compensation

Practice management organizations can drive value to physicians, patients, and payors, but they must be motivated to focus on efficiency and productivity. Under

FIGURE 2-1

Duties of Hands-On Clinic Administrators

- Administrative, financial, personnel, and purchasing functions
- Fine-tuning procedures and standards
- Developing training for new employees
- Ensuring that collections are current
- Reviewing all invoices
- Implementing clinical policies agreed upon by physicians

the old fee-for-service model, many doctors were productivity machines. They knew how to maximize their revenues—the more procedures they performed or patients they saw, the more compensation they earned.

However, productivity fell when these once-entrepreneurial physicians' practices were bought by hospitals or practice management organizations. The incentives and feeling of ownership were no longer there.

From those early failures, physician organizations are learning that compensation, if structured correctly, will stimulate productivity (and thus produce revenues) and efficiency (and thus hold the line on costs) without sacrificing quality.

Practice management organizations often stand at a crossroads. They know that the industry is moving toward capitation, which operates under different financial incentives than does fee-for-service medicine. Yet, many medical groups are still living off discounted fee-for-service; for them, capitation is not yet a reality.

To succeed, physician organizations must structure financial incentives—compensation, vacation, bonuses—around the productivity and efficiency goals set by the group. We'll talk more about that in Chapter 5, which deals with compensation models.

Management Fees

Someone must pay for operational talent and systems. In some practice management organizations, that is handled through the management fee.

Generally, practice management firms charge fees ranging from 7% to 35% of a practice's revenues or profits. In addition, the practice manager also may charge fees of up to 50% or 100% on ancillary revenues. These fees pay for corporate and local administrators of the practices. Physicians also may receive marketing, legal, and accounting expertise from the practice manager in exchange for the fee.

During 1998, the industry started reassessing its traditional management fee structures, particularly after PhyCor, the nation's oldest publicly traded physician company, announced that it was going to start offering a different model to new groups—less cash paid up front for practices acquired in exchange for a lower management fee. This new structure allows Nashville-based PhyCor to incur lower capital costs in growing its physician base. In exchange, physicians— who were beginning to question what they were getting for their management fees anyway—might find a lower fee more palatable, especially early on while the practice management firm is proving its worth. Following PhyCor's lead, other practice managers began reassessing their fee structures, and the fees themselves became a more important negotiating point in the acquisition process.

Management fees should be an incentive for both the physicians and the management organization. Physicians need to ensure they're getting their money's worth, and practice management organizations need to make sure they're earning their fees. Fees are an investment by both parties. In fact, many practice management organizations apply half of the management fee received toward capital purchases for the practices. In that light, it's an enforced savings plan for future capital needs.

There are several types of management fees: percent of revenues, percent of profits (otherwise known as predistribution earnings), flat fee, and percent of collections. The percent of revenues model tends to reward growth, because it doesn't focus as much on profits. However, since it's easier to grow revenues than cut costs, this has been a preferable model for some practice management organizations that aren't as focused on forcing changes on their practices. The percent of profits model is more cost-conscious and encourages physicians and the practice management organization to watch their costs more. However, physician groups need to be aware of fraud and abuse concerns over management fees. More on that is included in Chapter 7.

OPERATIONAL LEVERS OF CHANGE

There are a number of levers of change with which a management organization can drive changes to cost structure, enhance quality, or increase revenues.

In manipulating these levers, practice managers must realize that they are shooting at an evolving and evasive target. Like Ben Hur astride two chariots, practice management organizations must manipulate these levers with one foot in capitation and one foot in fee-for-services.

Here's another way to look at it. Historically, physician practices operated under a manufacturing model. They focused on churning out a product—an office visit, an MRI scan, or a hip implant. Fee-for-service payment encouraged physicians to produce more of that product. As the industry has shifted to capitation, a retail model was adopted with more emphasis placed on customer satisfaction issues.

When examining operational issues, physician organizations must look at both the manufacturing and retail aspects of their practices. For many, the customer service issues have long been ignored. In some cases, the practices didn't have the time or money to devote to market analysis and customer service. However, paying attention to those issues will benefit the physician organization in the long run. In addition, under the fee-for-service model, the physician is focused on one patient at a time. Under managed care, physicians must look at groups of patients. This requires them to put more emphasis on prevention and outcomes research.

Physician organizations must drive value to stay in business. As we said earlier, because investors are now frowning on acquisition-dependent strategies, physician organizations that need capital must focus on growth generated by improving operations—growing revenues, negotiating favorable risk contracts, enhancing quality, and controlling costs. In the absence of demonstrated success in those areas, physician organizations won't be able to attract the capital they need to grow.

Controlling Costs

One reason physicians began to consider affiliating with practice management organizations was to combat the rising tide of overhead expenses. The amount of money spent on overhead nearly doubled between 1985 and 1995, according to the American Medical Association. The average total expenses for a self-employed physician was $201,600 in 1995, compared with $102,700 in 1985, the group reported.[1]

In the early years of managing a practice, a management entity gains savings from consolidation of certain administrative functions—what investment bankers term "low-hanging fruit." Thereafter, there may be some additional savings that the practice management organization can bring through consolidation, but it's not likely to be in the double-digit range year after year.

The Medical Group Management Association publishes averages that are used as benchmarks for operating expenses in different types of multispecialty and single specialty practices. Those figures give practices a starting point to talk to physicians and staff about what percent of the practice's income is going toward the following.

- Salaries and benefits
- Rent
- Malpractice insurance
- Laboratory and radiology fees
- Marketing
- Professional services
- Other general and administrative services
- Supplies

Even small practices can do some rudimentary analysis of revenues and expenses (Table 2–1).

---

[1] AMA Socioeconomic Monitoring System, 1997 report.

TABLE 2–1

Sample Patient Cost Analysis

Patients	$8,000
Expenses	$250,000
Revenues	$450,000
Profit	$200,000
Revenue/patient	56.25
Cost/patient	31.25
Profit/patient	25.00
Fixed expenses	$165,000
Variable expenses	$85,000
Fixed expenses/patient	20.625
Variable expenses/patient	10.625

Purchasing

Hospitals have long subscribed to group purchasing organizations that trade volume for discounts on hundreds of different medical supplies. Physician groups are starting to do the same, combining their buying clout to get lower prices. For example, OrthoLink formed a resource development department that manages all vendor partnerships, supplier contracting, and inventory control. The organization's preferred vendor contracts include diagnostic imaging, hotels, business forms, pharmaceuticals, and orthotics.

Entering into such relationships can produce significant cost savings. However, physician managers may encounter problems with compliance with national contracts. When a group practice signs a national purchasing contract with a vendor, physicians must comply with that contract to receive the promised discounts. Typically, vendors will offer different levels of discounts, depending on the group's loyalty to the contract. Physicians may feel this encroaches on their preferences, and preference level can vary greatly from product to product. For example, physicians may not feel as strongly about sutures as they do about hip implants.

It's amazing how healthcare providers can be controlled by the vendors from whom they purchase supplies. It's not uncommon for physicians to allow pharmaceutical and other supply salesmen access to their supply rooms to see what they're low on. By doing so, the vendor not only takes stock of its own on products, but learns what and how much the doctor is purchasing from other suppliers. How much should vendors know? In addition, by allowing the vendor to conduct inventory, there's a strong chance of oversupplying certain products. Reorder systems should be set up on only need level so the physician organization doesn't get stockpiled with excess items.

Physician groups can profitably put vendors to work in another way, however—by requesting historical data about ordering habits. Analysis of this data may yield information about practice efficiencies. If that data can be linked to specific physicians and/or diagnoses, other efficiencies are bound to be discovered. Taking that analysis one further step, physicians can be profiled according to equipment usage. For example, some practice management organizations own lasers, mammography scanners, and other scanners. By analyzing per-physician use of that equipment, the practice can determine whether the equipment is paying for itself and whether physicians are overutilizing or underutilizing this equipment.

When a practice management firm contracts with a physician practice, it often acquires many of the practice's employees. As a result, opportunities abound for savings in the employee benefits area. When the employees of a doctor's office (a small business) become employees of a large practice management organization, health insurance premiums may fall. However, hospitals have often found that this cost goes up because their benefit structure is more generous. Also, an evaluation should be made whether "successor employer" rules apply with respect to the Federal Insurance Contributions Act (FICA) and state unemployment taxes. For example, the practice management organization may be able to get credit for the FICA taxes already paid by the physician group that year on certain highly compensated employees, which could reduce its outlay for FICA taxes in the first year. If the physician practice had enjoyed low employee turnover, the practice management firm also may be able to "succeed to" the practice's state unemployment tax rates, which may be more favorable. These rules are discussed more in Chapter 9.

Practice managers should consider outsourcing certain departments or functional areas, such as billing, collections, information systems, marketing, lab, transcription, accounting, and diagnostic services. Outsourcing considerations for billing and collections are discussed in Chapter 3.

A final note: groups should always be careful about perceived conflicts of interest with respect to purchasing. Some management organizations have found themselves in trouble because they bought computers or consulting services from officers, board members, or other friends of the firm. It's a good idea to give board members a statement of policy on conflicts of interest and have them sign a disclosure statement. Even though board members may believe they're getting the practice management organization a good deal, it may be seen otherwise if things go south. For example, one practice management organization was sued when it bought a computer system from an organization in which top executives had an ownership interest. When the system failed, it led to cash flow problems and accusations of kickbacks.

Malpractice Premiums

One area in which physician management organizations can generate tremendous savings is malpractice insurance. MediSphere reported malpractice premiums dropped an average of 20% for its OB/GYNs, and some saw drops of as much as 50%. OrthoLink gained a 90% decrease in premiums for one of its groups. "The kind of physicians that we are going after have very good malpractice records," said CEO Robert Yeager. "Yet, they often are lumped in actuarially with other surgeons (which causes them to have to pay higher premiums.)"

Pharmacy Utilization

If the physician groups are in capitation contracts with pharmacy caps or global capitation contracts, they are having to bear risk with respect to pharmacy costs. These costs escalate rapidly and are often difficult to manage.

There's a widespread presumption that because physicians are the ones who issue prescriptions, they can exert significant controls over pharmacy costs. For example, many managed care contracts financially penalize physicians who exceed a set budget on prescriptions, requiring them to bear the additional costs themselves. To keep within budget, the practice may want to consider making generic pharmaceuticals mandatory or at least encourage the use of generic drugs. Another option is to create a formulary of only the 50 most commonly used drugs.

The recent onslaught of direct-to-consumer advertising by pharmaceutical companies is making it harder for physicians to control those costs today. Pharmaceutical companies have ratcheted up spending on consumer advertising to get patients to ask their physicians to prescribe certain name-brand drugs. As a result, drug spending continues to rise with no abatement in sight. In fact, U.S. spending on drugs is expected to double from $62 billion in 1996 to $171 billion in 2007, according to the latest estimates from HCFA.

Another way to reduce prescription drug costs is to use drug samples wherever possible. These can reduce pharmacy utilization by as much as 10%. Ordering those samples may become even easier. In July 1998, IMS Health announced plans to build an online pharmaceutical sample fulfillment system in which physicians can request samples through their desktop computers. The service is coordinated through its Clark-O'Neill unit in partnership with Physicians' Online.[2]

Real Estate and Equipment

Take stock of the real estate used by the practices. Can physicians be housed in common office space with shared services?

If physicians aren't using all of the office space, the practice management organization may be able to sublet excess space. Or, they may be able to put the excess space to other uses. Under old standards, practices allowed between three and four exam rooms for each primary care physician. Today, the standard should be more like five to six exam rooms. Why? Practices need to focus on patient

---

[2] Physicians' Online is the largest Internet physician community and Clark-O'Neill is the largest U.S. pharmaceutical sample fulfillment company. IMS HEALTH provides information solutions to the pharmaceutical and healthcare industries.

flow—getting patients out of the waiting room and into exam rooms with physician extenders and physicians.

If equipment is being underutilized, consider mobilizing it. Equipment that can be moved from room to room is likely to used more often.

Sharing Resources

Look around for partners who can share overhead costs. For example, managed care organizations may be willing to help with reports or other analysis in physician profiling. These organizations also may be willing to provide computer systems or upgrades. After all, it's in the best interests of these organizations to have their providers be as efficient as possible.

The managed care organization may also be willing to give practices a hand with marketing expenses (e.g., to share the expense of brochures on a disease management program). Or, they may be willing to underwrite the cost of other educational efforts, such as seminars and brown-bag lunches at work sites. If a practice wants to establish a lending library of educational materials—both print and video—for patients, a managed care organization may be interested in contributing to this effort.

Other resources that a managed care organization may be willing to share include after-hours call centers or utilization management nurses. Obviously, the physician group will want to weigh resource sharing with becoming too dependent on a particular managed care organization.

Taxes

Practice managers' eyes may glaze over at the mere mention of tax planning. Their interest is quickly piqued, however, when they see how much can be gained in cash flow and cost savings when a few savvy tax-planning strategies are implemented. Tax planning isn't just about the opportunity to find dollars left on the table, however. Practice management organizations sometimes encounter unexpected tax liabilities when they find that state or local taxing authorities assess taxes on services, activities, or transactions they would never have dreamed were taxable. Under the tax laws of some states and municipalities, for example, a medical practice would have to pay sales tax on management services provided by a physician management organization. With proper planning on the front end, such taxes can often be reduced or eliminated altogether. Tax-planning considerations are discussed more in Chapter 9.

Productivity, Efficiency, Quality, and Patient Satisfaction

Practitioners

Just as a hospital must stay efficient by making best use of its bed capacity, a medical practice must make the best use of its physicians' time. If a physician can see 32 patients a day, but he's only seeing 28, then he's not working to capacity. That might not be the physician's fault; it may be a scheduling problem (see Figure 2–4 later in this chapter).

Orthodontic Centers of America (OCA), a dental practice management firm based in Ponte Vedra Beach, Fla., believes that that its orthodontists are nearly twice as efficient as their colleagues. Its centers treat an average of 77 patients per nine-hour patient treatment day compared to the industry average of 45.[3]

The organization's proprietary patient scheduling system groups appointments by the type of procedure. Certain types of cases are seen on specific days and new patients are only seen on certain days as well. Longer appointments are scheduled for new patients to allow for the initial consultation and preliminary procedures such as teeth impressions and x-rays. Patients are scheduled to come in monthly. On each visit, the patient must make payment before proceeding. Then, the orthodontist reviews the status of the treatment and prescribes adjustments to the braces, which are made by an orthodontic assistant. The orthodontist then sees the patient for a final examination and adjustments that must be made by an orthodontist. Before leaving, the patient makes next month's appointment. This type of patient flow, which is notably preceded by payment, enhances the company's cash flow. Since 1991, only 1.3% of net revenues have been uncollectible, the company reports.

Orthodontic Centers, which operates 260 dental centers in 39 states, believes center efficiency not only increases profits to the company, but allows it to charge less. Patients sign a contract to make monthly payments of $98 per month during treatment, with no down payment. At the end, patients make a final payment of $398. A standard case (which lasts between 26 and 32 months) amounted to $3,100 in 1997. The company reported that this was below the 1996 national average of $3,650 to $3,950 for other companies for the same period of treatment.[4]

OCA's fast throughput of patients is due, in part, to its use of orthodontic assistants to better leverage the orthodontists' time. Each of the company's centers has an average of five orthodontic assistants. The use of assistants is widely accepted in dentistry. General dentists have long made use of the services of dental hygienists and dental assistants to perform certain routine tasks, thereby, freeing them up to concentrate on seeing more patients. In states where it is legal to do so, physician practices might be wise to analyze work flow to determine if the practice could benefit from physician extenders. A good rule of thumb is two physician extenders for every primary care physician; the ratio will differ depending on the specialty. In specialties such as orthopedics and radiology, the use of technicians and physician assistants can add greatly to the efficiency of the practice.

Physicians also may benefit from some assistance in utilization management. Physicians often spend many hours on the phone handling matters such as weekend hospital discharges that could be worked out on their behalf by a nurse. Practice managers may look at hiring a utilization management nurse who can handle these concerns, freeing up more of the doctor's time to spend with patients.

---

[3] Orthodontic Centers of America 10-K for 1997.
[4] Ibid.

What about efficiency after hours? Practice managers should take a hard look at that area. Does the management organization use an answering service that has established protocols for calling physicians? An effective call center system that does triage on calls will ensure that physicians aren't unnecessarily fatigued when they come into the office during the day. Larger practice management organizations may want to consider outsourcing this service to a "demand-management" firm that specializes in handling after-hours calls through a central call center.

Another area is how physicians handle hospital rounds and discharges. These duties take physicians away from the office, which can lower productivity. In some practices, it may be appropriate to consider hiring a hospitalist—a physician who spends all of his or her time working with hospitalized patients (see Box 2–1).

No discussion of physician efficiency would be complete without mentioning phone calls. Some doctors try to catch snatches of time each day to return their calls. However, it may be more efficient to establish a block of time each day to perform telephone tasks rather than have periodic interruptions. This also can improve relations with patients.

Other Medical Office Personnel

Opportunities for efficiency lurk at every turn in a medical office. Here are some to consider.

Analyze staff workloads to ensure that the right staff are performing appropriate tasks. Cross-training is a popular strategy, but don't take it so far that capabilities are stretched beyond the breaking point. It is a good idea to cross-train staff to work with different doctors or to cover one another during vacations or illnesses.

Make sure employees are in an environment that helps them be efficient. For example, telephone operators should be in a quiet location. Away from a bustling office, these workers make fewer errors and have a shorter average call rate.

Consider separate phone lines. Practice administrators may want to consider getting separate phone lines for patient services, referring physicians, laboratory, and the business office. Once the practice has installed these separate lines, the next step is to measure productivity on them. The telephone company can provide reports, such as how long phones are ringing before they're answered and how many callers hang up before the phone is answered.

If the practice is cyclical, use part-time workers to handle peak times. Look at flex-time schedules. For example, many hospitals, particularly in the South, institute flexible schedules that give workers more time off in the summer when kids are out of school and units are less full. Then, full schedules resume during the winter flu season. If workers know what to anticipate with such flexible schedules, they'll plan vacations around them as well.

Review compensation strategy. Many physician offices pay office workers by the hour, but converting them to salary has two benefits. First, it will reduce

BOX 2-1

THE ROLE OF A HOSPITALIST

One way a physician organization might handle hospital duties is to hire a new type of specialist—a hospitalist. A hospitalist is a physician who spends all of his or her time working with hospitalized patients. A hospitalist can help expedite tests, rehabilitation, and discharges, as well as reduce length of stay.

More than 2,500 hospitalists are now working in hospitals, up from 500 three years ago, according to the National Association of Inpatient Physicians.[1] The number is growing rapidly as some managed care companies are beginning to mandate their use because they help control inpatient utilization.

A practice management organization can either hire its own hospitalist or contract with a hospitalist physician organization for this service. There are five firms devoted to hospitalists.

1. InPatient Consultants, North Hollywood, Calif.

2. Hospitalists Inc., Laguna Hills, Calif.

3. Cove HealthCare, San Diego

4. Hospital Inpatient Management System, San Antonio

5. IntensiCare Corp., San Diego

To shift their duties to a hospitalist, physicians must be able to trust the decisions made by this person, which may be no small task. Physicians who are used to controlling their patients' courses of treatment may have a hard time letting go.

The use of hospitalists allows physicians to spend more time on office visits. In fact, a 1998 report to the American Medical Association's Council on Medicare Service showed that in one pilot program, office patients reported easier access to appointments, decreased waiting times, and better preventive advice because physicians were spending more time in the office.[2]

Although hospitalists can make physicians' offices flow more efficiently, the greatest dollar savings will likely be enjoyed by the hospital itself through more timely patient discharges. For that reason, physician practices may want to enter a cost-sharing program with the hospital, which may not be aware of the potential savings.

---

[1] Jaklevic, M.C. (1998). Hospitalists Gain Ground: The Next Issue Is Whether Using Them Should Be Mandated. *Modern Healthcare*, June 15.

[2] Ibid.

overtime payments. Second, workers will feel like they're part of a team. Hourly workers punch a clock; salaried workers participate in the long-term success of an organization.

Patient Satisfaction

Rewarding employees for outstanding service is common in retail industries such as lodging, restaurants, and fashion stores. It's far less common in healthcare. Yet, that's changing: today's medical consumers are better informed and are more likely to make changes in providers and carriers if they are dissatisfied. Five ways to increase satisfaction are shown in Figure 2–2. Among retail employees, customer service standards are a way of life. That expectation is becoming the same for physician practices.

Adequate appointment time. Surveys show that patient satisfaction correlates directly with the amount of time spent with a patient. One physician group found that the quality of that time also is important. In this physician group, the physician who spent the longest amount of time with each patient had one of the lowest satisfaction rates. Why? Because when he was in the room, he spent most of the time with his hand on the doorknob, giving the impression that he was ready to rush out.

Wait times. A major determinant of patient satisfaction is how long patients must sit in the waiting room (or "reception area," as some practices prefer to call it). This is a "hot button" issue with consumers of all stripes. Besides calling it something different, physician groups need to look hard at how long they keep patients waiting. (For average times, see Figure 2–3.)

What is a reasonable waiting time? Physicians should not make patients wait more than 30 minutes. Beyond that, patients should be offered an explanation, and/or the option of rescheduling the appointment.

Practices can decrease waiting times by doing the following.

- Making sure physicians have a patient's chart, including lab or diagnostic results, so they don't spend time searching for them.

FIGURE 2–2

Five Ways to Increase Patient Satisfaction

1. Offer evening and weekend hours.
2. Call patients a few days after a visit or treatment to see how they're doing.
3. Call promptly with lab results.
4. Mail forms and instructions to new patients to decrease waiting room time.
5. Provide videos and big-print books in reception areas.

FIGURE 2–3

Average Waiting Times (in Minutes)

- Solo practice: 18.3
- Two-physician groups: 21.2
- Three-physician groups: 20.3
- Four- to eight-physician groups: 19
- Physician groups of nine or more: 23.5

Source: AMA Physician Marketplace Statistics, 1995.

Organize charts so that progress notes, test results, and hospital reports are easy to find.

- Scheduling extra time for new patients or special procedures.
- Avoiding overbooking patients.
- Informing patients of delays in their appointments and offering options.
- Calling patients at home or work to advise them of unexpected delays.
- Blocking time each day for walk-ins and emergencies.

Friendliness of office staff. Just as patients sometimes judge hospitals by the palatability of their food, patients often weigh the quality of a physician practice by the friendliness of its office staff. In many cases, nonphysician employees talk to patients as much as doctors do, and they can be responsible for how satisfied patients are with the practice.

If the practice is measuring patient satisfaction, results can be linked to bonuses for office workers who go above and beyond the call of duty in providing positive customer service. This can be implemented in the form of an employee-of-the-month award or a periodic award given as the occasion arises.

Clinical Benchmarking

Measuring physician performance by using scorecards—issued either monthly or quarterly—is one way of communicating expectations to physicians and other clinicians. Suggested categories include the following.

- Volume of work and service
- Quality of care
- Patient satisfaction
- Utilization of resources
- Teamwork
- Citizenship

- Patients per hour
- Average revenue per patient
- Hours of operation per physician

These scorecard items may have to be constantly reviewed and fine-tuned. Depending on the specialty, there may be specific reference points that are far and above the most salient information. For example, an important scorecard item for cardiovascular surgeons is the morbidity rate. For obstetricians, it's the C-section rate. OrthoLink, a Nashville-based orthopedic practice management company, provides its orthopedic physicians with customized monthly reports on the following items.

- Number of visits
- Waiting time
- Supplies per physician
- Revenue per procedure
- Revenue per visit
- Lab tests per physician
- Radiology procedures per physician

Through clinical benchmarking, physician practices can determine the strengths and weaknesses of each physician, and then operate off those strengths. For example, suppose a cardiology practice includes a surgeon who is particularly good at heart valve surgery. Then, the practice would want to direct more patients to that surgeon because his or her outcomes are likely to be better than a surgeon who doesn't do as many of those procedures.

Practice management organizations also would be wise to consider the scorecard items used by the managed care companies with which they do business. Health plans are measuring enrollees' satisfaction because employers are demanding that data. Enrollees' satisfaction with their health plan often stems from how well they like their physicians. Health plans and employers are beginning to invest in timely patient satisfaction reports to provide more information to consumers. Probably the

F I G U R E   2–4

How Productive Are Physicians?

On average, they:
- Spend a median of 56 hours a week on professional activities
- Work 48 weeks a year

Source: American Medical Association.

most comprehensive example of this is provided by the California-based Pacific Business Group on Health, which uses its Web site to publish report cards on patient satisfaction, chronic care, preventive care, and accreditation report cards on physician groups. On its Web site (www.healthscope.org), the business coalition rates physician groups on a 0 to 100 scale on the following attributes.

- Overall satisfaction
- Overall rating of care
- Ease of getting care
- Promptness of care
- Quality of care
- Doctors' communication skills
- Courtesy of office staff

Physician group scores that are below average are highlighted in red. Above-average scores are in blue. In terms of clinical quality, the business group also rates physician groups on how they treat chronic care by looking at cholesterol and blood pressure checks. In terms of accreditation, the group publishes how physician groups fared on accreditation with the Medical Quality Commission. That commission evaluates medical groups on 155 standards and IPAs on 149 standards within the following areas.

- Anesthesia services
- Facilities and environment
- Governance
- Management and administrative services
- Medical laboratory/pathology services
- Medical records
- Nursing services
- Office surgery services
- Patient rights and responsibilities
- Prepaid health services
- Quality management
- Radiology services
- Urgent care services
- Utilization management

Policies and Procedures Documentation

Practice management organizations and hospital systems should make sure their clinics know what corporate and network resources are available to them. For example, OrthoLink distributes an administrator resource manual that provides an overview of the organization and its practices and contains answers to frequently asked operational questions. The manual is divided into the following sections.

- Corporate overview
- Regulatory compliance
- Human resources
- Technology
- Risk management
- New programs
- Personnel
- Finance
- Marketing
- Managed care
- Materiel management
- Model contracts
- Web site access
- Glossary

The manual also provides a detailed outline to the organization's protocols in each of those areas, plus the following.

- Personnel policies and procedures
- Employment procedures
- Benefits information
- Federal statutes and regulations
- Accreditation standards and guidelines
- State statutes and regulations
- Corporate compliance program
- OSHA requirements
- Information technology documentation

Communicate, Communicate, Communicate

Many practice management organizations and health systems recognize that their biggest challenge is communication. Lack of it can cause massive operational difficulties, particularly if physicians believe they're being left out of the loop or are constantly reinventing the wheel. It's good business to keep up the flow of communication with physicians, staff members, and board members. Have meetings; publish newsletters; use e-mail, fax, and phone—whatever it takes.

Most physician management organizations have regular meetings of physicians, administrators and others to monitor the organization's progress. Depending on the size of the organization, annual or quarterly meetings of regional directors, medical directors, and physicians may be appropriate. Some organizations have practice advisory boards that meet annually or biennially to discuss clinical issues. Others have subcommittees dealing with finance, new services, managed care, best practices, or other operational issues that meet regularly. Those types of committees help physicians feel involved in the organization's direction.

Physicians want to know what's going on in the organization even if they don't ask about it on a regular basis. This is particularly true with financial matters. "What doctors respect is someone who will tell them the news just as it is—not sugar coat it. Give them the good and bad news," said MediSphere's chief financial officer Cynthia Dotson. One Texas-based practice management organization that went bankrupt did not provide regular financial statements to physicians. When the organization became insolvent, the physicians weren't aware of it because the organization was borrowing from vendors and creditors without their knowledge. A well-communicated financial plan wouldn't have kept physicians in the dark. However, because there was no requirement to communicate with physicians on a monthly or even yearly basis, the corporation didn't do so.

As the practice management organization grows, it becomes harder to stay in touch and understand the capabilities of everyone involved. Monthly newsletters can do more than just market a practice. They can share best practices and hail accomplishments of the organization or individuals. They also can help the practice run more efficiently. For example, a newsletter can include prescription refill policies, which will decrease office phone calls and increase physician productivity.

Growing the Revenue Line

"We don't make our groups change anything," says one practice management organization executive. Indeed, many practice management organizations appeal to physicians' desire for autonomy. Rather than trying to get physicians to be more efficient in their practices, they choose instead to focus on new revenues.

Traditionally, many practice management organizations believed in a strategy of buying lots of practices first, then focusing on growing revenues through ancillary services.

Ancillary Development

In terms of growing revenue, getting physicians to see more and more patients a day isn't a sustainable formula. Eventually, the hours in the day run out. The opportunity for practice management organizations is to leverage capital to create wealth by accessing the ancillaries that are part of the physician's business.

Thanks to the well-publicized financial disasters at some practice management organizations and questions about the amortization life of intangible assets like a practice's goodwill, practice management organizations in 1997 and 1998 began looking toward developing facilities. The move back to bricks and mortar as an asset base represents a new cycle on an old theme. Physicians have long talked about developing their own treatment facilities. However, they've often lacked the capital to develop them and have been wary of the vague legal guidance available on self-referrals.

Developing ancillary services such as outpatient and inpatient centers can give a practice management organization more predictability in revenues and earnings. Properly structured, these sectors may derive only a small portion of their profits and revenues from the practice management business itself.

The bulk—as much as 80%—could come from the outpatient surgery, imaging and diagnostic centers, or even the inpatient centers that they operate. In that sense, successful practice management organizations in the future may be more akin to the outpatient surgery centers of the 1980s than the practice management organizations of the mid-1990s.

One model that many practice management organizations are studying is MedCath, a Charlotte, NC–based cardiology physicians company that expanded into building heart hospitals (Figure 2–5). MedCath is difficult to categorize. It's a practice management organization, hospital, and outpatient provider all rolled into one. It founder and CEO, Steve Puckett, is a former hospital administrator who had overseen the construction and operation of an 80,000-square-foot heart institute at Carolinas Medical Center.

MedCath was started in 1988 as a mobile cardiac catheterization lab. It went public in 1994, and opened its first heart hospital in McAllen, Texas, in 1996. By mid-1998, MedCath operated four specialty heart hospitals and had four additional heart hospitals under development. In addition, it was managing over 100 physicians and was operating 33 mobile or fixed-site cardiac catheterization laboratories and diagnostic centers.

Puckett has strong feelings about the role of ancillaries in the future of physician practice management organizations: "I don't think a stand-alone PPM is sustainable strategy," he said.

At MedCath, three-fourths of its 1995 revenues were from its diagnostic centers, primarily mobile cath labs, and one-fourth were from practice management. By 1997, when it had opened three heart hospitals, 50% of revenues stemmed from the hospitals, 33% was from the outpatient centers, and just 17% was from practice management. What about profits? It's hard to judge profits out of the hospital division since the company is opening so many new hospitals, and new hospitals lose money during the first six to nine months. However, operating margins in the practice management division were 12% —35% in the diagnostic centers.

Because MedCath doesn't depend on the physician practices to drive the company's revenues or earnings, it has been unscathed by the accounting changes

FIGURE 2–5

MedCath's Heart Hospital Strategy

60-bed McAllen (Texas) Heart Hospital, includes 3 surgery suites and
3 cardiac cath labs. Total cost: $28 million. Opened 1/96.

84-bed Arkansas Heart Hospital, Little Rock, includes 3 surgery suites
and 6 cardiac cath labs. Total cost: $45 million. Opened 2/97.

66-bed Tucson (AZ) Heart Hospital, includes 3 surgery suites and
4 cardiac cath labs. Total cost: $35 million. Opened 10/97.

58-bed Arizona Heart Hospital, Phoenix, includes 3 surgery suites and
3 cardiac cath labs. Total cost: $52 million. Opened 2/98.

In Development

58-bed Heart Hospital of Austin, Texas, includes 3 surgery suites and
4 cardiac cath labs. Total cost: $49 million. Scheduled to open 1999.

54-bed Albuquerque (NM) Heart Hospital, includes 3 surgery suites and
4 cardiac cath labs. Total cost: $43 million. Scheduled to open 1999.

54-bed Bakersfield (CA) Heart Hospital, includes 3 surgery suites and
4 cardiac cath labs. Total cost: $43 million. Scheduled to open 1999.

48-bed Dayton (OH) Heart Hospital, includes 3 surgery suites and
4 cardiac cath labs. Total cost: $38 million. Scheduled to open 1999.

---

pertaining to amortization of intangibles that recently rocked the practice management industry. In fact, when MedCath filed documents with the Securities and Exchange Commission to go private in 1998, the topic of amortization schedules never even came up, Puckett said.

Operating small heart hospitals brings certain economies of scale. For example, Puckett estimates that his heart hospitals shave 50% off the costs of labor. In a $40,000 bypass surgery, nearly half of the cost is tied up in labor expense. Reduce that, pass the savings along to payors, demonstrate good outcomes and you've got a marketable service. What's more, heart surgery is one of those risky procedures where the more you do, the better you get at it. High-volume heart centers whose physicians and personnel concentrate only on cardiac procedures have better outcomes than hospitals where heart surgery is done less frequently.

Each MedCath hospital is a joint venture with physicians. MedCath serves as manager and owns a majority interest (generally 51%) in these ventures, into each of which it has invested between $730,000 and $2 million. Because hospital ventures are exempted from the Stark II anti-kickback legislation (discussed in Chapter 7), MedCath doesn't have to worry about fraud problems arising from physician ownership. In some cases, MedCath owns the practices of its physician partners in the heart hospitals; in other cases, it does not. "We would ultimately like to work with all of them," Puckett said. However, affiliation with MedCath's practice management division isn't a requirement for physicians who want to invest in the hospitals.

As a former hospital administrator, Puckett enjoys working at a company where the financial incentives are aligned rather than at loggerheads. "We recently had a meeting in Dallas in which two to four of our senior physicians from each market came together to brainstorm. They have a keen interest in the quality of medicine being practiced, and in riding the cost curve down," Puckett said. "Things are so much easier to manage when the right incentives are in place."

The MedCath facility-based model is being viewed as a preferable one by some practice management organizations that want to have tangible assets and leverage their physician networks. Clearly, facilities-based organizations, such as HealthSouth Rehabilitation Corp. and Health Management Associates, have been able to weather changes in reimbursement and physician preferences. However, this is a capital-intensive strategy and the start-up costs of such facilities can put a damper on earnings. This lack of strong earnings growth prompted the publicly traded MedCath to revert to a private company in August 1998 through a buy-out financed by two New York investment firms, Kohlberg Kravis Roberts & Co. and Welsh, Carson, Anderson & Stowe.

Although many specialty organizations are intent on studying the MedCath model, Puckett cautions that each niche has its own unique opportunities. "Every clinical segment has a unique cost structure," he noted. He gave this rule of thumb: For every $1 of physician revenues, a practice management company can generate $5 of inpatient revenues.

MediSphere, a Nashville-based organization, is pursuing a similar strategy in women's health. It hopes to develop women's hospitals. "For us and our affiliated physicians, the gain doesn't come from saving on operations and overhead," said Cynthia Dotson, chief financial officer of MediSphere. Practices won't necessarily become more efficient or economical through consolidation, she pointed out. Instead, the organization is focusing on developing inpatient and outpatient women's health centers. "What we see as the end game is creating value," she added. "We listen to our physicians as customers and develop those services they're interested in."

In smaller markets, a more outpatient-oriented facility can provide the needed services. Such a combined outpatient surgery, diagnostic, and birthing facility was being developed in Northern California with an affiliated group.

In other markets, the organization also is pursuing development of comprehensive women's hospitals in Phoenix and Fayetteville, Ark., as of early 1999. Building a women's hospital for physicians can bring operational efficiencies, particularly for doctors who were splitting admissions among two or more hospitals.

Convenience becomes an economic issue for those physicians. On the other hand, these types of moves must be carefully weighed. What if the location for the new hospital is far from where the OB/GYNs are now practicing? The efficiencies of moving physicians into a central location where they can attend to both inpatient and outpatient care may be overwhelmingly positive. However, actually getting the physicians to physically move is likely to be a long and arduous process.

Obviously, when planning inpatient facilities, practice management organizations are more likely to look to states without certificate of need (CON) laws. Those laws, designed to staunch overbuilding of healthcare facilities, require state agency approval for large capital expenditures that would add patient beds or provide new services. In states with CON laws, it may be best to look for hospital partners. Sometimes established health systems will have a better chance at navigating through the CON process to gain approval.

Building hospitals is in vogue now, but the risks are high as a practice management organization takes on debt for a large capital-intensive venture. Consider the experiences of a Denver-based physician group, Precedent Health Partners. When its hospital, Precedent Health Center, began losing money, the Precedent doctors voted to forego salaries until the organization's financial fortunes turned around.[5]

Physician specialties that may be well suited to capture ancillary revenues and corresponding practice management organizations in that business include the following.

- Cardiology (Cardiology Partners of America, MedCath, Corda, Care Select)
- Oncology (American Oncology Resources, Physician Reliance Network)
- Ophthalmology (NovaMed)
- Orthopedics (OrthoLink, Integrated Orthopedics, U.S. Orthopedics)
- Women's health (MediSphere, FemPartners, Women's Health Partners)
- Radiology (American Physician Partners)
- Pathology (AmeriPath)

Referrals from Other Physicians

Clinics also can increase revenues by increasing referrals from other physicians. Referral trend patterns should be analyzed on a clinic-by-clinic (and even physician-by-physician) basis. It's important to know what those patterns are and why are they the way they are. In fact, referral patterns should be analyzed both coming and going—i.e., referrals into the practice and referrals out to other specialists.

---

[5] "Doctors on brink of failing; Bankruptcy possible for Paramount group," by Martha Austin, Denver Business Journal, Oct. 26, 1998.

Ways to increase referrals from other physicians include the following.

- Convenient scheduling
- Physician-to-physician personal visits. How competent are the physicians that are receiving the practice's referrals? What types of physicians are making referrals into the practice?
- Patient referral forms
- Brochures on specialty areas

Clinical Trials

Clinical research organizations (CROs) are outsourcing companies that have cropped up to take overflow work from pharmaceutical companies in conducting clinical trials to test new drugs. CROs and SMOs (site management organizations) contract with physicians to serve as investigators in conducting clinical trials on human volunteers. During the past five years, the CRO industry has ballooned to more than 500 firms as drug companies realized the savings in outsourcing research, manufacturing, and sales of new drugs.

The more time that pharmaceutical companies can shave off the development process, the more they save. Suppose a new drug is estimated to generate $500 million a year. Shaving one day off the development process can generate more than $1 million in sales. One of the key delays in clinical trials is getting the right volunteer population. Say a company wants to test a new blood-pressure drug for the elderly who are overweight and diabetic. Advertising for and recruiting volunteers with those particular characteristics is expensive and time-consuming. Yet, a quick search of a physician's files—assuming they're in a patient database—can make this a simple matter.

That's one reason that CROs are interested in affiliating with physician organizations. Physicians organizations are equally interested because clinical trials can be a real revenue generator. Additionally, involvement in such activities may attract other physicians to join the group because they want to be on the cutting edge of drug development.

In some cases, practice management firms have bought or formed CROs and SMOs. ILEX Oncology, a CRO that focuses on cancer drugs, gave Physician Reliance Network, an oncology practice management firm, $5.6 million in stock in exchange for access to PRN's patient network. In 1997 PhyMatrix, a West Palm Beach, Fla.–based practice management company, bought Clinical Studies Ltd., a site management organization, for about $85 million in stock and about $9 million in debt. PhyMatrix likes this business so much it decided in 1998 to focus exclusively on it by divesting its practice management operations.

Managed Care Contracting

Risk contracting is an activity that, properly structured and managed, can bring great financial rewards to physician organizations. Chapter 6 is devoted to a discussion of risk contracting issues, so we won't dwell on them here. Suffice it to say that managed care contracting has a profound impact on medical practices' cost structures. On the one hand, managed care is designed to reduce consumption, which requires vigilant monitoring of fixed costs and cost reduction efforts by the practice and its physicians. On the other hand, entering into managed care contracts requires a practice to take on additional staff—thus, incurring additional cost—to deal with the administrative requirements. In a 1998 survey, two-thirds of Newark, NJ–area doctors said the overwhelming paperwork demands of managed care had forced them to increase the hours their administrative staff works, and more than half said they added staff.[6]

Adding Physicians and Physician Groups

How many physicians should a practice management organization add in a given period of time? There are no hard and fast rules on this because it depends on markets, infrastructure, and specialty. Growth for growth's sake, however, clearly has not worked for management organizations that spiraled out of control in the past year.

Some management organizations were encouraged to grow at the exclusion of other priorities. For example, one organization received succeeding rounds of capital from its venture source as a reward for reaching selected milestones in physician numbers. That prompted the organization to add physicians rather than slow down and work on operating the integrated practices. Early practice management firms had a somewhat similar experience with Wall Street. Just like today's Internet-related stocks that have soared despite the lack of earnings, investors bought them on the basis of rising revenues and future promise. Early practice management stocks received the same vote of confidence from shareholders, who believed they were buying a warrant toward future earnings. Fueled by that vote of confidence, management firms signed up as many physicians as they could to show growth.

If a firm wants to show a bunch of dots on a map to investment bankers, they can sign up groups throughout the country. However, it's going to be harder to support those groups on a continuing basis. Adding 10 physicians to an already thriving group in Atlanta will be much less costly than adding a new 10-person group in Seattle.

Marketing

Although many physicians abhor blatant advertising, some may be agreeable to "soft" marketing techniques that can help to increase their business. Following are some examples.

- **Referrals.** Marketing programs should focus on increasing revenues to the practice's physicians through referrals from other physicians,

---

[6] "A World Turned Upside Down: HMOs Put Medical Professional to the Test," by Lindy Washburn, The Record, Northern New Jersey, July 12, 1998.

managed care plans, and hospitals. Ideas will depend on the specialties within the group. Physicians should get to know their referral sources through luncheons, breakfasts, and other personal communications. Referral source phone calls should be returned promptly.

Often-overlooked referral sources are operators at managed care organizations. They field hundreds of calls from members wanting to select a physician, yet may be unfamiliar with the physicians on their referral lists. These operators are more likely to make referrals to the practices that they know, so physicians who want to increase referrals need to ensure that these operators understand their practices. That's also true for physician groups associated with hospitals, many of which list "Find-a-Doctor" telephone numbers and ads in the Yellow Pages.

Don't overlook alternative-medicine providers. Clearly, many physicians will have problems with the types of treatments offered by these sources. However, one out of four Americans who see their medical doctors for a serious health problem may be using unconventional therapy in addition to conventional medicine for that problem; seven out of 10 such encounters take place without patients telling their medical doctors that they use unconventional therapy.[7] Physicians should realize that it may be their patients' best interests to coordinate care with these providers in certain circumstances. Organized alternative medicine companies often are seeking physicians who have an understanding of both traditional medical techniques and the alternative disciplines.

- **Printed materials.** Dentists, orthodontists, and ophthalmologists are excellent at sending reminder cards to patients. Yet, other medical providers seem to falter in this regard. There's nothing wrong with sending a card reminding patients about annual check-ups, needed inoculations, or other health screenings. It's estimated to cost five times more to attract a new patient than keep an existing one.

  Many management organizations and large practices use newsletters—either monthly or quarterly—to communicate with patients and referral sources. To improve patient volume, it's important to "mine" one's own patient files regularly. A newsletter that goes out to the physician's patients keeps the physician's name in front when they need medical treatment or choose some type of elective treatments.

- **Print advertising.** Only a few specialties—for example, plastic surgery, orthodontics, and ophthalmology—generally benefit from print advertising.

---

[7] www.americanwholehealth.com.

Orthodontic Centers of America (OCA) believes that marketing brings patients in the door, especially since its services are elective and its practitioners have traditionally relied on referrals from dentists. During 1997, the company spent an average of $65,230 per orthodontist on direct marketing costs and advertising. That's particularly remarkable considering the average orthodontists spends $4,400 per year.[8] To kick off its marketing effort, the company hired Brett Favre, quarterback of the 1997 Super Bowl champion Green Bay Packers, as a spokesperson for its commercials.

The results were impressive. The marketing efforts generated an average of 505 new case starts during 1997 for each OCA orthodontist who had been affiliated with the company for at least one year. That's three times as many as the 1996 national average of about 180 new case starts per orthodontist.[9]

- **Web sites.** Web sites can be designed and launched in nearly any price range, and many physician organizations now have them. Both PhyCor and MedPartners have extensive Web sites. From a marketing standpoint, a Web site can enhance a practice's viability and allow it to stay in touch with a growing population that increasingly gets the majority of its information from the World Wide Web. A physician management organization may want to establish a corporate Web site that provides links to individual home pages for each practice or clinic. Examples of some provider Web sites are listed in the Resources section at the end of this chapter.

For many, Web sites will merely be electronic marketing brochures. However, some firms may want to consider more advanced applications that allow patients to make appointments or check the status of lab results. This is discussed in Chapter 4.

- Items to include in a Web site include the following.
- Physician/dentist biographies
- "How to Find Us" page, including address, map, and phone number
- Frequently asked questions (FAQ) page
- Prevention information
- Health education information
- Prescription refills information

Marketing efforts are wasted unless the physician group approaches them with a strategy based on strong research. It's a good idea to sketch out the

---

[8] Orthodontic Centers of America 1997 10-K.
[9] Ibid.

strengths and weaknesses, threats and opportunities of the practice before moving into a marketing strategy discussion. Healthcare is a local business and physicians should know how they're getting their patients, payor contracts, and referrals. If a local physician group is large enough, it may be cost effective to have a marketing director or director of patient relations to handle these tasks. If not, the marketing duties likely will fall to the local administrator or office manager.

We should say a word here about branding. There aren't many "name brands" in healthcare. Each market may have a handful of healthcare "brands," but they're usually associated with a particular medical center. Physician branding is almost unheard of. It's extremely costly to launch a brand name from scratch, and it's expensive just to maintain one. In San Diego, Scripps is a recognizable brand name. The problem is the name is associated with both a hospital system and a physician clinic. That was great when these groups were part of the same organization. However, when they parted ways in 1996, both groups wanted to keep using it. After months of negotiation, the groups reached an agreement that each could continue using the Scripps name, but Scripps Clinic would forego that privilege if it ever decided to become a publicly traded company. (Scripps Hospital System was worried that the appearance of a for-profit company being publicly traded under the name of Scripps would compromise its own philanthropic efforts.)

Meanwhile, Scripps Hospital started its own physician organization, also called Scripps, adding to confusion in the marketplace. Ironically, both Scripps the hospital and Scripps the clinic are spending a combined $12 million annually on marketing their own organizations in the community. In other words, even when a medical group has an easily identifiable name, the brand may be confused with a hospital or health system of the same name.

AN EXPERT'S PERSPECTIVE: JACK CASTLE, JR., CHAIRMAN AND CEO, CASTLE DENTAL CENTERS

Practice management organizations should take "breathing lessons." That term, coined by fiction author Anne Tyler, could easily apply to fast-growing practice management organizations. Operational excellence means taking time to breathe, digest, and assess.

Put those institutional salesmen from Wall Street on hold for a while. Look inward. If you staff your practice management company with too many glass-half-full types who don't recognize the downside of growth, your company will be courting disaster.

Near the end of 1998 several practice management companies tried to put a good face on the lack of continued cash in the equity markets. "We can hone in on our market and not be distracted by outside markets," one practice management executive commented.

Translation: They're taking breathing lessons because the market has knocked the wind out of them. They're being forced to focus on operations, because they've been cut off from the capital sources they need to fund acquisitions. That's good for the industry.

"The companies in the healthcare business that are going to emerge as the break-away leaders in their sectors are the companies that are best in operations," said Jack Castle Jr., chairman and CEO of Castle Dental Centers. "If you're not good operators, you can't add value." Castle led his Houston-based company through a rapid growth streak from 1981 to 1985. Then, they took a break. "We stopped building for three years," Castle said. Castle realized that the centers they were building were too big and wasteful. "Back then, we thought bigger was better," he explained. They found out it wasn't. They trimmed them back from about 5,000 square feet to 2,800 square feet and cut back on reserving specialized suites for certain professionals, such as periodontists. They refined the model. Castle selects metropolitan markets where it has adequate access to dentists and where the company can have a minimum 5% market share. They want to have one dentist for every 75,000 to 100,000 residents.

Using standardized operating models allows Castle to practice "management by exception." Corporate headquarters handles marketing and administrative functions, including billing and collections. The same profit and patient satisfaction standards are used judge each of the dental centers. "Having a standardized operational model and management process enables you to get your hands around the business," Castle said. "And you can create a lot of incentives and opportunities for people."

Castle went public in late 1997 and as a public company is expected to achieve certain financial targets. To achieve those targets, the centers themselves have profit targets they must meet. They're responsible for making sure patients are happy and employees are productive. If business is slow one day, the clinic administrator can send employees home. Each office is its own profit center and must meet or beat its profit target to pay out bonuses to employees and the dentists themselves.

As a public company, Castle has a goal of 15% operating margins and 30% same-market annual growth (Figure 2–6). How does Castle achieve such growth? Through branding and having a customer-friendly business system with a retail business orientation. "We can drive demand through advertising," Castle said.

Castle believes that it's a failed strategy to roll up practices, go public, and hope to save money through consolidation. "The costs of running a public company will eat up any back-office savings," he noted.

PricewaterhouseCoopers Tips for Operational Excellence

- Set realistic expectations for physician productivity that are backed up with financial and nonfinancial incentives.

FIGURE 2-6

Castle Dental Centers, Houston, Texas

1997 Revenues—$46.2 million
1997 Operating income—$3.3 million
Number of dental centers >55
Affiliated dentists, orthodontists, and other dental specialists—165
States—Texas, Florida, Tennessee, California
Payor mix—53% fee-for-services, 36% traditional indemnity, 7% managed care, 4% Medicaid

The Castle Strategy: Five Operating Goals

1. 90% patient satisfaction
2. Grow each region's revenues by at least 30%
3. Double-digit revenue growth in each region
4. 15% operating margins in each region
5. Grow profits faster than revenues in each region

- Ensure that officers and physicians receive timely reports on the financial condition and clinical guidelines of the practice and the corporation.
- Direct utilization to the most cost-effective providers and services.
- Don't overspend on practice acquisition. It doesn't leave enough capital to add ancillaries and infrastructure.
- Set reasonable management fees that are justified through shared services and efficient operations.

Resources

Examples of provider/payor Web sites.
- **www.chw.edu**—Catholic Healthcare West.
- **www.choiceplus.com**—Minnesota-based Buyers Health Care Action Group, which does direct contracting with providers
- **www.phycor.com**—Nashville-based PhyCor
- **www.healthscope.org**—Pacific Business Group of Health
- **www.mdpso.com**—Lifespan/Physicians PSO in Providence, R.I.

3

CHAPTER

Billing and Reimbursement: Blocking and Tackling for Practice Managers

Sandy Lutz

Cynthia Fry

Physician organizations that were lax about billing and collections have paid the price in recent years. They wrote off millions of dollars in past-due receivables. Publicly held ones were forced to make embarrassing apologies to shareholders. Some blamed information systems failures; others admitted that they just weren't getting bills out on time or making sure the collections came in.

Physician practices send out bills based on CPT (Current Procedural Terminology) and the ICD-9-CM (International Classification of Diseases, 9th Edition, Clinical Modification) codes contained in voluminous reference books. Each year, billing seemingly becomes more complicated; in 1998 alone, billing systems had to be updated for 81 new ICD-9 codes and 15 codes that are no longer considered valid.

BILLING ISSUES

Gathering Information

The first chore of billing correctly means gathering the right information on the front end. All new patients should fill out registrations that gather demographic, clinical, and insurance information.

Sure, most practices already do this. However, practice management organizations will want to look at how the registration forms are designed. Here are some questions for physicians and practice administrators to ask.

- Are the forms too complicated for the average person?
- Do the forms use jargon that a patient won't understand?
- Does the patient have sufficient time to fill out the form?
- Is the form so long that the patient simply tires of filling it out?

Consider taking a few minutes with a new patient to talk about the form. This should be done in a treatment room or some other private area—not amid other patients in the waiting room. Ensure that a new patient understands the questions and is answering them fully. Some patients may consider the questions an invasion of their privacy, so this would be a good time to respond to their concerns.

Subsequently, the front desk person should verify that the information in the system is correct each time the patient returns. This is vital because some patients change carriers frequently. Patients may become irritated at being asked the same questions every visit, but they'd be more upset if it turned out their visit or procedure was no longer covered by insurance.

Consolidating Billing Operations

Physician billing systems are driven by specialties, each of which bills in different ways. For example, anesthesiologists bill by time, primary care physicians bill by office visit, and surgeons bill by procedure.

Although today's physicians are more astute than ever about business issues, their primary interest lies in the clinical arena. That's why so many have turned to physician management organizations to relieve them of their billing and reimbursement hassles (Figure 3–1).

Unfortunately, some physicians have found that joining a practice management company can actually worsen reimbursement problems.

Take the case of an anesthesiology practice management organization that was purchasing physician groups at a rapid clip. Part of the physician organization's strategy was to cut costs by centralizing the practices' billing functions.

This was welcome news to the smaller practices, because they had struggled for years with billing and collection issues. Yet, most of the larger practices

FIGURE 3–1

Advantages of Local Billing Operations

- Stay on top of billing and collection problems with local payors
- Proficiency of working the local Medicare carriers

had already woven together well-oiled billing and collections operations. For them, joining the physician organization actually bogged down payments. In addition, centralizing the billing didn't result in lower labor costs, because the management organization wasn't willing to cut employees.

This is not to say, however, that no benefits were derived from this effort. A major benefit was consistency in billing—practice management executives found that the physicians were billing in many different ways, some of which weren't consistent with government regulations. Centralizing the billing function allowed review mechanisms to be put in place, ensuring that physicians were in coding compliance. The anesthesiologists also found that the practice management organization offered advantages related to third-party payment issues, such as clout in contracting, more sophisticated information systems, a top-notch management team, risk management, and analysis of practice costs.

IPA Billing Systems

Billing systems can be a real concern for independent practice associations (IPAs). Traditionally, IPAs start out as a group of physicians who band together in order to contract with health plans. Many IPAs were merely organized panels of physicians for one or more payors.

In recent years, IPAs began taking on additional duties for those physicians, such as billing and utilization review. The physicians are usually assessed for such services based on a percentage of their reimbursement. For start-up IPAs, the fees may be high because the IPA must invest in systems to provide those services. For mature IPAs, those fees should range between 5% to 11%, according to Albert Holloway, president and CEO of The IPA Association of America. His group counts nearly 900 IPA members representing 335,000 physicians.

Most physicians belong to more than one IPA because they want to be included in a wide array of managed care plans. As a result, they have an opportunity to compare and contrast billing systems and possibly shift more business to the more efficient IPAs.

Holloway said one of the most frequent pitfalls for IPAs has been buying systems that are more sophisticated—and expensive—than what they really need.

Electronic Billing

For a long time, commercial payors did not subscribe to electronic claims processing. However, that's changing. In the summer of 1998, Aetna U.S. Healthcare pledged to pay doctors who filed claims electronically within 15 business days. The program, called E-pay, was set to start on the East Coast and be nationwide by the end of 1999.[1]

---

[1] "A different tack: Aetna to pay docs faster, in contrast to other HMOs" by Scott Hensley, Modern Healthcare, June 15, 1998, p. 24.

As this practice gains acceptance, physician companies may find that it's worthwhile to contract with a clearinghouse that electronically processes claims for several commercial payors. The cost-effectiveness of such a move will depend on the volume of claims that can be run through the clearinghouse. Typically, there's an up-front set-up charge for hardware and software as well as a licensing agreement that must be maintained. In addition, some volume payments may be required.

Some computer vendors also are marketing systems that do real-time claims resolution. These interactive computer systems are designed to assist with a provider's billing and collections simultaneously. The systems allow physicians to do on-line account inquiries about the status of a patient's insurance. They also capture, store, and retrieve patient charge information as well as produce bills, accept receipts, and generate refunds. However, these systems are solutions for the future, not necessarily considerations for today's practice management organizations.

Coding Compliance

Fraud investigations almost always revolve around billing and reimbursement issues. Practice management companies will be wise to review their compliance programs, as discussed in Chapter 7, to ensure that they have a coding compliance program that includes an internal audit process. At a minimum, the audit process should review a representative sample of each physician's patient records and compare billing practices among physicians. An internal audit process should itself be consistent and the results of these audits should be communicated with physicians in a timely manner to correct any problems detected.

Following are examples of billing fraud red flags.

- Upcoding—using a code that provides a higher reimbursement rate than is called for by the treatment.
- Duplicate billing—sending more than one bill for the same service.
- Unbundling—submitting separate bills for tests or procedures that are required to be billed together.
- Medically unnecessary services—submitting a claim for payment that does not have adequate documentation showing that the service was warranted.

Many software vendors are now offering billing compliance products that alert physicians to possible Medicare and Medicaid program violations by flagging bills that appear to be out of compliance. They also will monitor payment of claims that need to be refunded.

Assignment of Claims

Because some physicians are employees of practice management organizations or maintain other arrangements within physician organizations, they need to heed Medicare's regulations with respect to assignment of payments. Payments for services provided to Medicare beneficiaries, for example, must be made directly to the physician provider. There are the exceptions, however. Payments also may be paid to the following.

- *Physician employers,* if it is a condition of employment for the physician to turn over fees for his or her services. According to Medicare regulations, the employer must have a signed and dated statement on file acknowledging that the employer has the right to receive the payment for physicians services. Medicare's recommended language is, "I acknowledge that, under the terms of my employment, only (Name of Employer) is entitled to claim or receive any fees or charges for my services."
- *Facilities,* if there is a contractual agreement between the physicians and the facility, such as an outpatient center.
- *Organized healthcare delivery systems,* where there is a contractual arrangement (for example, a group practice prepayment plan).

COLLECTIONS ISSUES

It used to be that when physicians sent out bills, they collected their charges in full. In recent years, however, they've seen less and less coming back. In 1992, physician practices collected 90 cents on each dollar of gross charges. By 1995, that had dropped to 73 cents thanks to bad debts, managed care, and discounted payment arrangements, according to the Medical Group Management Association. That trend makes it critical for physician organizations to tightly manage collections, in order to maximize cash flows.

Collecting from Patients

Through an effective information system, practices can link the patient appointment scheduling system with the accounts receivable system to look for uncollected balances. That prompts the receptionist to ask patients to pay outstanding balances at the point of service. If a patient cannot pay at the time of service, the billing office should make arrangements for payment before the patient leaves.

It's also important to collect any co-pays that may apply to a patient's insurance coverage. Obviously, front office clerks need to know what the required co-pays are. Failure to try to collect co-pays from Medicare or Medicaid beneficiaries may be interpreted as fraud, so don't let this slide with patients.

If the practice has a high volume of patients that want to pay with a credit card, it may be worth the expense to accommodate that process. Practices will need to evaluate the financial cost of that against the benefits derived from the acceleration of cash flows. Some patients won't want to use a credit card because if they carry a balance with the physician practice, they're unlikely to be charged interest; with the credit card, they'll be hit with double-digit interest rates.

Unless the practice is very small, it's best to have segregation of duties with respect to billing and collections—i.e., some clerks handling nothing but collections, others handling nothing but billing. Obviously, collections clerks will want to focus on the largest outstanding bills to ensure that their time is well spent.

Practices will want to institute certain basic front-office policies with respect to collections. For example, if a patient's account is delinquent, their patient record should be flagged so that it can be discussed with them on their next visit. Other policies involve when to turn over delinquent accounts to an outside collection agency. Collections agencies typically take between 30% and 40% of what they collect. If the collection agency hasn't collected the account within 120 days, the account should probably be written off as uncollectible.

Collecting from Insurers

The biggest collection problems usually don't stem from patients who don't pay. The vast majority are third-party payor problems that aren't resolved.

It's important to maintain some benchmarks that can be followed at the practice level and in the billing office. Once collected, the following information can be shared among practices to determine how efficient they are performing in collections.

- Collection ratio—Billings divided by collections.
- Cost to collection ratio—Collections divided by expenses. Hospitals spend about 3 cents to collect each dollar, but the rate for physicians is going to be higher because outstanding bills will be lower.
- Days revenue outstanding—Accounts receivable divided by annualized billings (360 days).

Collecting from managed care payors can sometimes be more frustrating than collecting from patients who are unwilling to pay. Before signing contracts with insurers, it's wise to ask about their claims payment record. Most should be able to document what percent of claims are paid within 30, 45, and 60 days. A physician group will want to see nearly 100% paid within 60 days.

Experience has taught physicians that contracting with the wrong managed care insurer can mean big collection headaches. One notorious example in 1997 and 1998 was Oxford Health Plans, whose failure to make timely payments for services provided to Oxford enrollees enraged doctors. After intervention from the New York attorney general, Oxford agreed to pay physicians interest on claims that weren't paid within 30 days.

That being said, it's important for practice management organizations to monitor monthly payments from payors to ensure that they don't become delinquent. If a delinquent payor isn't contacted at least once a month, they often won't pay. They'll assume that the provider's system isn't organized enough to know that the bill is overdue, so they'll pay those providers who seemingly are more on top of their claims status. If a physician practice continues to run into a brick wall with an HMO or insurer, it's wise to get the patient involved. The patient is paying premiums to the insurer and, therefore, should be notified if the insurer isn't honoring its agreement to pay for services provided on their behalf.

Tax Considerations

In certain states, the provision of billing and collection services by a management company to a physician can have significant sales and use tax consequences that are many times overlooked. Several states impose sales and use tax on the performance of these types of services. In some cases, physician organizations are able to minimize debt collection services taxes by keeping the billing and collection functions at the medical group level. In other situations, taxes can be avoided if the management company purchases the professional corporation's receivables, thereby causing the billing and collection function to relate to the management company's own assets, which, of course, are not taxable. Management organizations should consult with experienced tax advisors in evaluating their (or their groups') exposure to sales and use taxes.

Outsourcing

Start-up physician organizations may want to consider outsourcing billing and collections functions until they've acquired enough practices to make it cost-efficient to bring them in-house. Generally, groups tend to bring those functions in-house as they start billing for 50 or more physicians.

A 1997 survey by the National CPA Health Care Advisors Association found that 25% of groups with more than 50 physicians outsource some of their billing and collections functions; however, none were outsourcing all of those functions (Figure 3–2).

Another motive for bringing billing and collections inside is so that the organization can own and analyze the data. "I want to be able to get to my data when I want it," said one practice management executive. In some cases, outside billing companies can provide data to do benchmarking in terms of procedure,

FIGURE 3-2

Percent of Physician Groups Using Outsourcing for Billing and Collections

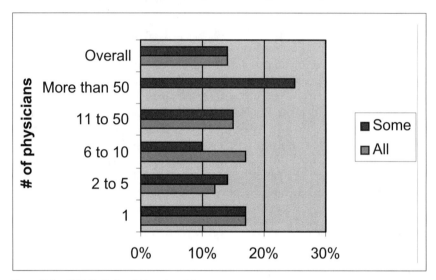

Source: National CPA Health Care Advisors Association.

coding, payor mix, and cash flow at the various practices. Yet, this is the exception rather than the rule.

Groups considering outsourcing should consider the following points.

- Ask for competitive bids.
- Make sure that the contract specifies goals, service levels and scope of work.
- Understand what types of services will be charged at an extra rate.
- Evaluate the vendor's work regularly.
- Negotiate a termination rate that's reasonable and won't make it too expensive to get out of the contract in case the vendor does not perform as expected.
- Contract length should be one year as opposed to multi-year to limit their commitment.
- Have an attorney review the contract.

Special considerations apply when Medicare, Medicaid, and other federal claims are outsourced. In that situation, keep these Medicare requirements in mind.

- Payments generally must be in the name of the physician or physician group (other than the exceptions we mentioned previously).
- Physicians must have a specified agreement with the agency.
- The billing agency's fees cannot be related to amounts collected or billed; the preferred method is based on claims volume (i.e., a per-claim charge).
- Likewise, the billing agency's employees may not be compensated based on collections.
- The billing agent acts under instructions from the provider.

Most important, deal with an outsourcing company whose reputation is beyond reproach. In particular, make sure the outsourcing company is aware of all of the federal regulatory requirements related to billing and submission of false claims. If they violate them, the physician is held responsible and could be charged with fraud.

REIMBURSEMENT ISSUES

Physician groups must stay on top of reimbursement trends to properly forecast how their billing and collections functions will operate going forward. Although it's difficult to gauge what commercial payors will do, Medicare's moves are telegraphed early on.

As physicians know, Medicare's resource based relative value scale (RBRVS) was implemented in 1992 as a way to pay physicians based on costs and the value of their labor. There are three components to RBRVS: labor, practice expense, and malpractice. The first component of RBRVS—the labor component—focused on valuing the physician's time. The second component, which was implemented on Jan. 1, 1999, determines the level of reimbursement for physicians' practice expenses—things such as rent, office labor, equipment, supplies, and technology. This "practice expense" component accounts for about $4 billion annually and represents as much as 45% of total physician reimbursement.

The U.S. Department of Health and Human Services (HHS) said the new formula, which is required by a 1994 law, is designed to correct some of the inequities in the system, which tended to overpay surgeons and underpay primary care physicians. HHS said that under the old system, surgeons performing coronary bypasses received practice expense payments that were in excess of 100 times that paid for a routine office visit. Yet, the actual practice expense costs for bypass surgery are only about 18 times higher than for a routine office visit, according to the agency.[2]

---

[2] "HFCA Proposes New RVU-Based Payment for Physician Practice Expenses," by Stratton Shartel, Aspen's Physician Management Bulletin, June 15, 1998.

Physician organizations need to review how their physicians will fare under the new formulas. The readjustment could be draconian for some specialists. For example, the formula initially cut cardiologists' income by 17% while boosting reimbursement to primary care physicians by 12%. However, the Health Care Finance Administration (HCFA) went back and reworked the formula after Congress required the agency to rewrite the rule and delay its enforcement. The revised schedule, announced in June 1998, drops cardiologists' Medicare payments by only 13% and raises primary care incomes by only 6%.[3] The American College of Emergency Physicians estimated that emergency department (ED) physicians would experience a 13% drop in Medicare-allowed charges over the four-year transition to the resource-based practice expense system.[4] Other specialty reductions were: cardiology (-13%), gastroenterology (-14%), neurosurgery (-10%), pathology (-10%), plastic surgery (-10%), radiology (-13%), and thoracic surgery (-13%). Among the specialties with expected increases in reimbursements are dermatology (27%), family practice (6%), internal medicine (1%), and ophthalmology (11%).[5]

HCFA based its estimations of practice expenses on data from the American Medical Association's Socioeconomic Monitoring System. The average practice expense per hour was then multiplied by the total number of physician hours worked by that specialty according to Medicare claims data. Working with "clinical practice expert panels" and the relative value units already calculated for physician reimbursement, the total pool of practice expense payments for each specialty was determined. However, HCFA also proposed applying what it calls a "behavioral offset" to account for an expected increase in volume and intensity of services. HCFA has determined that for every dollar that fees are reduced, physicians will increase the volume and intensity of services to make up 50% of that reduction. For practice expense declines, however, HCFA proposed only a 30% behavioral response. Some specialties object to the behavioral response, saying that their patient services are based on need and that physicians can't alter that.

The final component of physician payment will be the calculation of malpractice costs. HCFA is expected to tackle that issue in the year 2000.

On a different front, the Evaluation and Management (E&M) guidelines proposed by HCFA may drastically affect reimbursement for primary care physicians. Those guidelines describe what a physician must do to receive reimbursement for different levels of office visits. The requirements are so complicated that physicians will likely be unable to memorize them. In those cases, the easiest thing may be to embed them in the software for the practice's electronic patient record system. HCFA is set to field test the guidelines and implement them in 2000.

---

[3] "Doc-Fee Rules Revisited: New Regs Shift Less Money to Primary-Care Physicians," by Jonathan Gardner, *Modern Healthcare,* June 8, 1998, p. 10.
[4] Technical Summary of HCFA's June 5th Practice Expense Proposed Rule, www.acep.org
[5] Ibid.

Many primary care physicians, however, will find a benefit in tying in an electronic version of the E&M guidelines to a billing system that records the appropriate reimbursement amount. Even a system that provides an electronic version of the guidelines for physicians to check will be a useful tool.

These types of systems will help physicians who may have been coding their office visits too low, as well as keep in check any possible problems with upcoding.

AN EXPERT'S PERSPECTIVE: STANLEY WEINTRAUB, SENIOR POLICY ANALYST FOR PHYSICIAN PAYMENT, HCFA

Physician reimbursement policy has gone through a slow, but steady transformation during the past two decades. After revolutionizing hospital payment with the advent of diagnosis-related groups in the mid-1980s, HCFA and Congress set their sights on reconstructing the way physicians are paid.

Stanley Weintraub, a CPA and MBA, has witnessed the cycles of change, having joined HCFA in the mid-1970s when the agency was created to oversee Medicare and Medicaid reimbursement. Weintraub is a seasoned Washington insider who knows the context of the current reimbursement matrix. He also has ideas about where the future lies for physician payment.

Looking at physician payment through his eyes, it's clear that the agency—which is guided by congressional mandates—has been making physicians more accountable for their payments, and the level of accountability will increase in the years to come.

For physicians, this emphasis on increased accountability has translated into more work in terms of documentation and justifying their work to the federal agency and its carriers that approve Medicare payments. "You're asking the government to pay you, yet you don't want to tell us what you're doing? Unless there's something in the record, we don't know what type of office visit you did that day," Weintraub argued. "What about your patients? Don't your patients deserve a medical record that's appropriately noted about what you did that day?"

"The fear with documentation is that Medicare auditors are going to come in, look at a few records, and haul you off to Leavenworth," Weintraub said. He noted that regulators aren't nearly that ruthless about ensuring physicians receive the proper reimbursement.

He acknowledged, however, that his employer will remain vigilant about pursuing fraud. "The news is full of stories about how people are cheating the Medicare program," Weintraub said. "Unfortunately, 90% of the rules are for 10% of the people."

He hears some physicians say they want more guidance from HCFA, others want less. "Documentation is risk aversion," he said, noting that the more clear the guidelines, the easier it is for physicians to know if they are in compliance or not.

Weintraub also talked about HCFA's work on reimbursing physician practice expenses. Although drawing up the new RBRVS practice expense reimbursement methodology has been excruciating, he said, determining how to keep it up to date may be even more so. "There are many unanswered questions about how this is going to be refined," Weintraub said. In particular, questions will be raised as new technologies are approved that are not yet included in the reimbursement methodology. Weintraub mentions PET (positron-emission tomography) scans as an example. The work of reading a PET scan is much the same as reading a single photon emission computer tomography (SPECT) scan, Weintraub said. However, the cost of the technology is much higher and the "practice expense" component of reimbursement needs to reflect that cost.

Another unknown is how practice expenses will increase or decrease in the future. Clearly, this is an issue for physician management organizations. One of the prime notions is that consolidation of practices will lead to lower expenses. "We know that practice patterns are changing," Weintraub said. "The treatment models are changing, the way HMOs use these models is shifting things. In some cases they make physicians more efficient; in others, less efficient. How do we reflect these things in the payment methodology?"

HCFA relied on information from the American Medical Association to develop its practice expense figures. If HCFA similarly bases future refinements on the AMA data, Weintraub wonders whether it will affect the way physicians respond to those surveys—specifically, will they report inflated expenses? Doctors are "not sworn to give us accurate data," he noted.

Another issue focuses on the objectives of a massive reimbursement system like Medicare. Should reimbursement be designed to reflect or guide the marketplace? "That's a pretty important question," Weintraub said. For example, as physicians perform more procedures in their offices, HCFA must grapple with how to reimburse for that. "Should we establish a higher fee when services are done in an office or should we let the marketplace take its course?" Weintraub noted. "Would we force the shift by encouraging it through higher payments?"

Weintraub acknowledged that research-oriented professionals rather than business professionals do much of the analysis. "Some researchers have concluded that the fewer people working in a practice, the better. I could not see how they came to that conclusion," he added. "For example, is it more efficient for a practice of a certain size to have three office workers or another with two? Can you simply look at that and make a conclusion about which is the most efficient practice? I don't think so. The three-person office may have one person dedicated solely to collecting co-insurance payments. That practice has a 98% collection rate and brings in $40,000 or $50,000. The two-person office doesn't have that extra person and only collects 10%. In that case, can you say that the two-person office is better?"

The dissection of costs within the physician payment system could be moot if Medicare moves toward more risk-based contracting. Currently, about 5 million American seniors are enrolled in managed care risk plans. Some predict that number will triple to 15 million in three years, thanks to financial incentives offered by risk plans such as free pharmaceuticals and vision care. At that level, Medicare risk plans would represent almost half of the nation's 33 million seniors.

The final component of physician payment will be the calculation of malpractice costs. However, that component makes up only 5% of physician reimbursement, so Weintraub doesn't expect it to raise as much controversy. HCFA will tackle that issue in the year 2000.

Weintraub said he's not sure which direction Congress will lead HCFA. Congress hasn't yet proposed requiring Medicare beneficiaries to enroll in HMOs, and disposing of indemnity coverage entirely. However, that could change in the coming decade as pressures grow to cut costs. Between 1980 and 1995, Medicare spending increased at an average annual rate of 11.3%, and its share of the federal budget increased from 5.4% to 10.6%.

What can physicians do to benefit themselves in this area? "Get friendly with your Part B carrier's medical director," Weintraub recommended. "Stay on top of developments in payment. When you hear about something going on affecting someone else, don't assume it doesn't affect you—the complexity of the healthcare delivery system means that it may."

Also, Weintraub encouraged physicians to talk to HCFA officials when they believe the agency is making a mistake. "We rely on input from people who do this for a living and we do listen to their concerns," he added.

PricewaterhouseCoopers Tips for Billing and Reimbursement

- Consider redesigning the new patient intake process to ensure that information is gathered correctly on the front end.
- Standardize business office policies for collections.
- Ensure that one or more persons is assigned to stay on top of regulatory changes.
- Consult your tax advisor about potential minimization of sales and use taxes on credit and collection services provided, if applicable.
- Make use of benchmark information for collections, fee schedules, and other important indicators of performance.

RESOURCES

Organizations

Healthcare Financial Management Association, Chicago

American Collectors Association, Minneapolis, Minn.

Association of Healthcare Internal Auditors

American Academy of Procedural Coders, Sylacauga, La.

National Association of Claims Assistance Professionals, Downers Grove, Ill.

Medical Group Management Association, Englewood, Colo.

American Medical Association, Chicago

Internet

www.hcfa.gov—Health Care Financing Administration

www.aspenpublishers.com—healthcare business newsletters such as Health Care Biller, Health Care Collector and Receivables Report

4

C H A P T E R

Information Systems Chapter: Moving Practices into the 21st Century

Sandy Lutz

Frank Cavanaugh

When Eric Thrailkill joined PhyCor six years ago, the practice management company's corporate staff could meet over a single pizza at lunchtime. Now, the chief information officer muses, they'd need to order 25 or more pizzas.

It's not just a catering problem. CIO Thrailkill must ensure that the rapidly expanding practice management company serves the technology needs of its 28,000 affiliated physicians. Directing an information technology (IT) staff that includes six corporate employees and an information systems (IS) director in each of 56 clinics, Thrailkill converts, installs, and supports practice management systems that must be ready for the 21st century.

"Eventually, the cost equation is going to settle out and physicians are going to compete on the basis of quality," Thrailkill said about PhyCor's strategy. As PhyCor launches Internet-based solutions to share information among its clinics, it moves toward the kinds of systems that will help its physicians compete for business on the basis of quality.

Like any techie, Thrailkill knows all about the cutting-edge technologies of voice recognition and personal digital assistants. Yet, he must weigh the desire to deploy those high-tech toys against the benefits offered by them and the desires of PhyCor's physicians.

It's a tug-of-war that all physician companies and health systems that work with physicians face. Some physicians simply don't want the high-tech gadgets.

They like their paper-choked offices just the way they are, thank you. At the other end of the spectrum are doctors who want the most powerful systems on the planet, but don't really need them in their offices.

Practice management CIOs like Thrailkill must keep one foot in reality while reaching for a cost-effective technology that will improve operations and patient care in the years ahead.

Healthcare has been behind the curve in adapting technology to its business operations. Information technology's penetration in the healthcare industry is one-third to one-fourth of that in industries such as insurance or manufacturing. However, that means physician groups may be in an ideal position to embrace tomorrow's technology without the baggage of past loyalties to outdated systems (Figure 4–1).

The goal isn't merely to automate current records. Instead, it's to create new systems that support improved patient care and reduce time and costs spent in managing information.

FIGURE 4–1

IS Buzzwords

ANSI—American National Standards Institute's Healthcare Informatics Standards Board provides an open, public forum for the voluntary coordination of healthcare informatics standards among all United States' standard developing organizations. The U.S. Department of Health and Human Services has proposed using ANSI's ASC X12 transaction sets for electronically submitted claims and related transactions.

CDR—Clinical data repository—clinical information maintained for operations and outcomes analysis

CPR—Computerized patient record, often used interchangeably with EMR (electronic medical record); also called virtual patient record

EDI—Electronic Data Interface

Health Level 7—A data transfer protocol designed to simplify the flow of clinical data among disparate information systems.

Graphical-User Interface (GUI)—Systems that use icons and graphics to guide users through a task rather than just words and text.

MPI—Master Patient Index. Enterprise-wide software systems that use matching algorithms to retrieve data on patients from numerous locations. Such systems can load millions of patient records and match them at speeds of more than 1,000 matches per minute.

Unix, DOS and Windows—The way a computer communicates with its user. Both Unix and DOS use character screens. Windows is a graphical-user interface, which office workers and physicians may like because they use one, such as Microsoft Windows, on their home personal computers.

Physician groups and health systems need to plan for fundamental changes in healthcare computing, particularly clinical computing. In the next few years, healthcare computing will move from proprietary, monolithic application suites to modular software components and universal standards. Modular components will be able to share data across networks, managing information according to universal standards (Box 4–1).

The complexity of billing and reimbursement makes information systems a necessity. Without information, physicians and dental groups wage a losing battle in today's cost-conscious environment.

Practice management companies' philosophies on information systems vary widely. "At Monarch [Dental], the only non-negotiable issue (in an acquisition) is that they have to convert to our common information system," said Gary Cage, the company's chief executive officer. "Without a common information system, the Dallas-based practice management company couldn't operate as efficiently as it does," Cage said. The system selected by Monarch is used widely in the dental industry, and includes several modules for administrative, financial, and clinical reporting and analysis. Many of the acquired practices are already

B O X   4–1

STARTING FROM SCRATCH: NOVAMED EYECARE MANAGEMENT, CHICAGO

When Jon Thomas joined NovaMed Eyecare Management, a practice management organization based in Chicago, as vice president of information technology, company founder Steve Winjum was already sold on the importance of information systems.

In fact, Winjum had already spent $1 million on information technology when he hired Thomas to make it all work. Although he had no experience in healthcare, Thomas had spend 12 years in information integration development work where he specialized in integrating islands of information. He saw physician practices' use of information "severely lacking in their ability to reporting and analyze their operations."

What Thomas found was that NovaMed's practices were using several different information systems, most of which were developed 10 to 15 years ago using proprietary operating systems and databases. This made it difficult to retrieve information to support decision making. "In a market where reimbursements continue to decline, a practice must be able to capture and report on areas that affect their operational efficiency. The inability of these older systems to provide flexible reporting puts the practice at a distinct disadvantage," said Thomas.

Starting from Scratch: NovaMed Eyecare Management, Chicago, Continued

Thomas wanted to move the company toward a system that could integrate operational, financial, marketing, and clinical information. The centerpiece would be a new practice management system that could provide extended reporting and better focus on patient marketing capabilities. Each practice management company needs to find the system that works best for its specialty, which in NovaMed's case is ophthalmology. Most patients see their ophthalmologist without a referral from a primary care physician, meaning that customer service is probably more important for these patients than for those who visit other specialists.

"The selection of a software system must be heavily dependent on the business problem you are trying to solve," Thomas noted. "Too many people view computers as a black box, rather than as a tool. The real value is created when the tool is used by someone who knows how to use it." Practice management company executives, physicians, and staff need to understand and learn how to use their information system to its greatest potential.

Thomas, whose staff includes 14 employees, said NovaMed considered numerous practice management vendors before narrowing it down to 10 to 12 companies. The finalists consisted of both large and small companies that were past their first and second versions of the software NovaMed needed and that had an installed base of at least a dozen practices.

In July 1997, NovaMed selected its system; in September 1997, it was approved by the board; and in December 1997, the first practice went live on the system.

The system selected is built around a client/server relational database management system to provide flexible reporting and a graphical user interface to minimize training and improve productivity; it was implemented using Microsoft NT to provide scalability. In addition, the IT team chose to implement a centralized topology, in which all the information is stored at a central database, versus a decentralized approach, in which there's a separate database at each practice.

"We wanted to enhance the consolidation efforts and provide better customer service," Thomas said. "By choosing a centralized model, we could provide cross-scheduling of patients and resources, provide practice and regional reporting, and at the same time significantly reduce our operating costs." In Kansas City, for example, NovaMed needed to combine 14 satellite offices that included 17 physicians and two ambulatory surgical centers. NovaMed's system includes a master patient index that allows all of the

Starting from Scratch: NovaMed Eyecare Management, Chicago, Concluded

locations to share patients' clinical and financial information as well as schedule appointments within the network. This type of index also gives the practices a record of no-shows and recurring appointments.

For the Kansas City network (the practice management company's largest) only 10 personal computers were installed for 120 users. Everyone who doesn't have a PC has a dumb terminal with a Windows interface that connects to four servers. The terminals, which have a fixed number of icons on the screen, can be upgraded through the servers. By keeping the functionality of the terminals low, Thomas and his staff save themselves work in supporting the network. For example, users can't install their own software on these systems (e.g., software such as screen savers that might have viruses).

In all, NovaMed plans to spend about $1.5 million on building and maintaining the new information system. By using a combination of PCs and dumb terminals, Thomas figures the cost is about $3,000 per user, or about half the industry average.

John Hunkeler, MD, a NovaMed board member, gives this advice to physicians going through conversions: "Get out of the way and let it happen."

Hunkeler heads the Hunkeler Eye Centers in Kansas City, which includes 11 ophthalmologists and four optometrists. Prior to affiliating with NovaMed, the practitioners were on three different systems, two of which were compatible with each other. All were at least seven years old. Although the physicians knew how to use their own systems, they "didn't have a clue" how to use those at the other offices, Hunkeler said.

Now, an administrative clerk at one clinic can schedule a patient at any one of the four clinics. The centralized scheduling also helps with arranging vacations among physicians and staff members. Workers can fill in at the other clinics because they know how to use the system; prior to the conversion, that was difficult because staff members at one clinic didn't know how to use the system at the other clinics.

In addition, physicians are using e-mail, accessing the Internet, and own a Web site.

"Obviously, the next step is the electronic medical record," he added.

Thomas agreed, although he said he's still waiting for the standards necessary to take that next step. However, the company wants to begin to develop outcomes data on cataract and refractive surgery and may start a beta site for electronic medical records within the next year.

using the system. If not, the cost of converting is usually reimbursed through future earn-out payments to the dentists.

PhyCor's practices, on the other hand, often run on legacy systems. "It doesn't make sense for us to convert just for conversion's sake," said Thrailkill. Since PhyCor is a decentralized company, decisions about upgrading information systems are made at the practice level through a joint decision between the physicians and PhyCor. From a financial standpoint, it makes sense to leverage the existing assets—including the information systems—Thrailkill said. If the local practice decides to convert, it must use one of PhyCor's two preferred software vendors.

BUDGETING FOR IS

Expense is a prime concern to physicians. The cost of a new information system often comes out of their own budget, rather than a health system or corporate budget. Getting up to speed may cost more than physicians ever dreamed of spending.

Physician organizations, including independent practice associations, will spend between $20 billion and $40 billion over the next five years on information technology, according to estimates from the GartnerGroup, a Wakefield, Mass.–based information technology research firm.

That level of spending signals a major break with the past. Most medical groups have been frugal in buying computers. In fact, they spend less than 3% of their total operating expenses on information technology, according to a survey by PricewaterhouseCoopers (PwC) and *Modern Physician* magazine. The 1998 survey found that 18% of respondents spent less than 1%; 26.9% spent 1% to 2%, 21.1% spent 2% to 3%; and 13.5% spent 3% to 4%. Only 12.7% spent more than 4%.

Although information technology will dictate how much a physician organization is paid, how much it's spending, and how it will fare economically, few groups make strategic decisions about this part of their practice. Only 21% had a written strategic information technology plan, the PwC survey showed.

Ironically, the Year 2000 problem may be just the kick in the pants these companies need to boost their IT investments. For the nascent practice management industry, upgrading to Year 2000–compliant systems often brings additional benefits.

Vendors that have heretofore focused on other industries are beginning to use their talents in software development for healthcare providers. The healthcare application software market recorded 20%-plus growth in 1997 compared to 1996—making it the fastest growing software market—according to International Data Corp., Framingham, Mass.[1]

---

[1] "New IDC Survey Results," Healthcare Informatics, June 1998, p. 48.

Information technology offers challenges along with opportunities. Let's address the challenges, which can be organized into four areas.

1. Hiring and retaining IT staff
2. Running on legacy systems
3. New systems integration
4. Other IT priorities

HIRING AND RETAINING IT STAFF

As group practices attempt to link their administrative, financial, and clinical resources, they soon realize they need help from an information specialist.

Information technology staffing is a problem for all industries, and healthcare is no exception. The classified pages of healthcare IT trade journals are filled with advertisements for IT managers, programmers, and technicians. Hiring and retaining high-quality staff was listed as the top IT priority of healthcare organizations in 1998, according to the latest HIMSS Annual Leadership Survey, sponsored by the Healthcare Information and Management Systems Society (HIMSS) and IBM Global Healthcare Industry (Figure 4–2). IT staff adept at the singular business of operating large-scale practice management company systems are especially rare.

One of the initial IT decisions facing organizations that manage physicians is whether to hire a CIO. Most do, because even in their formative stages, physician organizations want a technology-savvy management leader to help direct the company's business strategy.

F I G U R E 4–2

IT Priorities for Heathcare Organizations in 1998

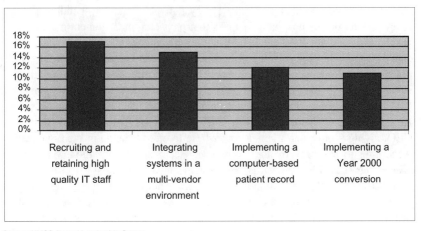

Source: HMSS Annual Leadership Survey.

However, before hiring a CIO, a physician organization must establish its priorities. For example, an organization facing a major systems conversion would be wise to hire a CIO who has been through that process. If the organization is rapidly consolidating multiple group practices, it should look for someone with those credentials.

It's a given that CIOs need to know technology issues, but for a practice management firm, it's essential that they understand the business issues as well. Walk into the office of a CIO at a practice management company, and the bookshelves are likely to be stacked with issues of Business Week, Healthcare Informatics, and PC magazine.

That's certainly the case with John Lacy, CIO of USCardioVascular, who was the third executive hired when the Dallas-based cardiology practice management company was formed in late 1997. "We want to use our information systems as a strategic advantage," Lacy said about the reasons behind his hiring so early in the company's founding days. "We believe that through rolling up practices and analyzing outcomes data, we can gain a competitive edge. With that type of strategy, the CIO is one of the most important positions," he said, noting that his job includes everything from technical support for an e-mail problem to compiling spreadsheets for long-range planning. Lacy believes that physician services groups will need to proactively use outcomes data to gain strategic positions in their markets. If they don't, giant payor organizations such as HMOs will gather their own outcomes and physician profiling data to select—or exclude—physicians. Lacy's early months were spent looking at systems that could be used by the practices to produce outcomes analyses. As the company adds practices, Lacy will evaluate their needs carefully, then decide on an enterprise-wide information system.

Because information technology professionals are in demand throughout the country, finding the right CIO can be very difficult for an independent physician practice management company, especially a small one that can't compete with the salaries offered by large hospital systems. However, hospital systems managing physicians may have other problems. The system's CIO may be spending so much time working on the hospital's IT tasks that physician management matters never get the time and attention needed. Hiring an information executive just for physician management may be difficult because the system is competing with smaller practice management companies that may be able to offer stock options or other advantages, such as the power to influence the organization. In a health system, the CIO typically reports through a chief financial officer, who holds the purse strings. At a practice management company, a CIO is more likely to report directly to the CEO, giving him or her a larger power base to effect change in the organization. According to a survey by the College of Healthcare Information Management Executives (CHIME), power is a heady incentive (Figure 4–3). The top way to increase CIO job satisfaction is to give him or her more authority in the organization, the survey reported. In other words, money isn't as important as authority to healthcare CIOs. This is important for small physician companies in the start-up stages of stepping up their information technology strategies to bear in mind as they recruit.

FIGURE 4–3

How Can Healthcare Employer Increase CIO's Job Satisfaction?

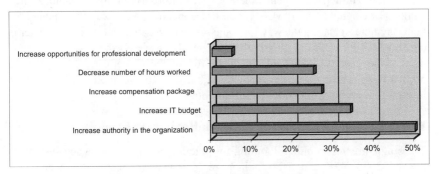

Source: ADVANCE for Health Information Executives and College of Healthcare Information.

The survey also found that, overall, healthcare industry CIOs were a pretty happy lot: 78% were satisfied with some or all aspects of their job. That contentment level can make recruitment difficult. (The survey did not provide a separate break-out of physician group CIOs' responses.)

RUNNING ON LEGACY SYSTEMS

Practice management organizations in growth mode often will run for awhile on their acquired practices' legacy systems Rather than jumping immediately into a conversion, the IT manager will analyze both the market and the practices' specific needs. PhyCor's practices, for example, often run on incumbent (i.e., legacy) systems. Since PhyCor is a decentralized company, decisions about upgrading information systems are made at the practice level. This is a challenge, however. Typically, a practice that affiliates with PhyCor takes a year and a half evaluating whether or not to sell. During that period, the practice usually will postpone making large capital expenditures, such as buying new computers. Then, it might be another year until the transaction is completed. That means that even the newest information system will be at least $2\frac{1}{2}$ years old when PhyCor acquires it.

Another issue associated with acquired practices' legacy systems is making sure that they are legally licensed. Some healthcare organizations have bought practices only to find a dozen or more personal computers (PCs) using the same copy of Windows 95, for example. A Texas hospital recently paid a $1 million-plus fine for operating a spreadsheet program without a license. A whistleblower at the hospital apparently called the Business Software Alliance, an antipiracy watchdog group based in Washington, DC, to report the hospital's use of unlicensed programs.[2] Although it's unlikely that individual physicians

---

[2] Morrissey, J. (1998). Pirates of Pasadena: Texas Hospital Pays Fine for Using Unlicensed Software. *Modern Healthcare*, June 15.

would be hunted down for such practices, larger physician groups could eventually be targeted.

Even with legacy systems, there are ways to transition toward uniform networks. For example, one PhyCor group has standardized the way they dictate patient care notes, clearing the way for some standardized elements to be used later in outcomes analysis. Others have built templates that use embedded data elements.

"One day, you'll be able to query for all the diabetic patients over age 50 that have used a particular medication because you've already collected this information on the front end," Thrailkill noted.

Year 2000 Bug—A Kick in the Pants for Healthcare Companies

The single greatest problem looming for practice management legacy systems is the Year 2000 (Y2K) glitch. Physicians aren't alone here. Most of healthcare is behind the eight ball in ensuring their computers will still run on Jan. 1, 2000. Why is healthcare so backward? An article in Healthcare Informatics explained it in the following way.

> Sometime around 1970, banks that sold 30-year mortgages became the first to say "Oops." Computers spit back mortgage applications that terminated in 2000 because the little cyber neurons assumed '00' was ancient history. From there, the succession of industries, ranging from insurers with multi-year policies, to brokerages selling long-term bonds, replaced or updated their computer systems to bring them into the 21st century. Healthcare's reach didn't stretch so far into the future, so rewriting business and clinical applications wasn't a priority until recently.[3]

According to many healthcare CIOs, the average physician is using a system that's about five years old and is not Y2K compliant. As practices are acquired, the CIO must determine whether their information systems will be able to do business in the Year 2000.

Unfortunately, some practices may encounter problems even before the calendar turns to January 1, 2000. In some older software programs, for example, "99" was used to indicate the end of a file. Even more important, physicians schedule office visits months ahead, which means they'll start encountering problems in 1999 as they attempt to schedule into the year 2000.

The GartnerGroup estimated that many healthcare firms would spend at least one-third of their 1998 IT budgets on Y2K testing and remediation. Industrywide, the GartnerGroup estimates the Y2K problem could cost healthcare companies between $10 billion and $50 billion.

How much will it cost to fix physician organizations? For a mid-sized company—which defines most practice management companies—the GartnerGroup estimated the cost at about $4 million to find and make the changes needed line by line in computer code. Publicly held physician companies are required to dis-

---

[3] Joch, A. (1998). Late Testing Your Systems for Y2K Problems? So's Everyone Else. Here's What to Do About It. Healthcare Informatics, October.

close this information in filings with the Securities and Exchange Commission (Figure 4–4). For example, in its 10-Q filed for the third quarter of 1998, PhyCor reported:

> To date, the Company has spent approximately $250,000 on the development and implementation of its Year 2000 compliance plan. The Company estimates that it will spend a total of approximately $28 million to complete all phases of its plan, which amounts will be funded from cash flows from operations and, if necessary, with borrowings under the Company's primary credit facility. Of those costs, an estimated $24 million is expected to be incurred to acquire replacement systems and equipment, including certain amounts spent in connection with standardizing certain of the Company's systems (Figure 4–5).

Other practice management companies have not put dollar figures on the problem, but have explained what they're doing. For example, Occupational Health and Rehabilitation Systems, Hingham, Mass., reported the following.

> The company is utilizing both internal and external resources to identify, correct or reprogram, and test its systems for Year 2000 compliance. It is currently anticipated that all reprogramming efforts will be completed by December 31, 1998, allowing adequate time for testing. A preliminary assessment has indicated that some of the Company's older personal computers and ancillary software programs may not be Year 2000 compatible. The Company intends to either replace or modify these computers and programs. The cost of this replacement is not expected to be material as the shelf life of the Company's personal computers is 3 to 5 years, and as a result historically each year approximately 25% of all personal computers are replaced or upgraded. All personal computers purchased in 1997 and through March 31, 1998 are Year 2000 compatible.

FIGURE 4–4

What the SEC Requires in Year 2000

A public company must provide Year 2000 disclosure if:

- Its assessment of its Year 2000 issues is not complete, or
- Management determines that the consequences of its Year 2000 issues would have a material effect on the company's business, results of operations, or financial condition.

If the issue is material, the company must disclose:

- State of readiness
- Costs to address Year 2000
- Risks to the company
- Contingency plans

FIGURE 4–5

Year 2000 Accounting Issues

Costs That Should Be Included in Financial Statements

- Modifying software
- Operating losses from failure to be Year 2000 Compliant
- Payments related to becoming Year 2000 Compliant
- Revenue and loss recognition due to Year 2000 issues
- Impairment of assets

"Going Concern" Issues

The SEC requires that auditors of publicly traded companies evaluate whether there could be substantial doubt about the entity's ability to continue as a going concern. "Year 2000 issues, either alone or when considered in relation to other conditions and events, may indicate going concern issues about an entity. The going concern issues may affect the disclosures in the financial statements and result in a modification of the auditor's report," the SEC reported.

Source: Disclosure of Year 2000 Issues and Consequences by Public Companies, Investment Advisers, Investment Companies, and Municipal Securities Issuers (http://www.sec.gov/rules/concept/33-7558.htm)

Orthodontic Centers of America, Ponte Vedra Beach, Fla., gave the following details in filing.

> The Year 2000 issue may affect the systems of various entities with which the Company interacts, including the Company's suppliers, and the Company is coordinating its efforts to address the Year 2000 issue with those entities. There can be no assurance, however, that the systems of other companies on which the Company's systems rely will be timely converted, or that a failure to convert by another company, or a conversion that is incompatible with the Company's systems, would not have material adverse effect on the Company.

The Y2K bug is a legal issue as well as an operational nuisance. Unless practice management companies take what attorneys view as "reasonable and prudent" measures to avoid problems potentially caused by Y2K bugs, they could be liable for harm or damage caused to their practices' patients. Therefore, practice management companies must implement a Y2K strategy that envelops both business and clinical operations. On the business side, practices need to ensure that their managed care and fee-for-service payors have worked out the bugs in their systems that might prevent claims from being received, processed, or paid. On the clinical side, they must ensure that their equipment and devices are Y2K compliant.

Elements of a Y2K strategy for physician groups include the following.

- Inventory all systems to determine whether they're Y2K compliant.
- Be sure that the inventory includes medical equipment, monitoring systems, and other devices containing computer chips that may be outdated. Don't forget to include low-tech equipment such as air conditioning systems, elevators, cash registers, and telephones.
- Contact the vendors of all equipment to find out what they've done to make their equipment and devices YK2 compliant.
- Take an especially close look at accounting and billing systems. These will affect the cash flow and patient satisfaction of the practice. It may be necessary to find the programmers who developed the practices' legacy systems.
- Have a written Y2K compliance statement ready to give to potential acquisitions. Savvy physicians will ask the practice management company to give them documentation of how the company is complying with Y2K issues.
- Prioritize. If you're starting in mid-1999, you won't get everything done.
- Document what you've done in case legal problems arise later.
- Set aside reserves to offset potential cash-flow problems.

Physician groups must also consider the effect that Y2K may have on third-party payors with which they do significant business. For example, if the government does not complete fixes to the Medicare program's computer systems on time, HCFA and its contractors may be unable to pay claims to providers or make eligibility determinations for the nation's 70 million-plus Medicare and Medicaid beneficiaries. Although the programming changes required for reimbursement updates are relatively simple, HCFA officials were concerned that making such programming changes while simultaneously attempting to modify the systems' Y2K programming could, among other things, obscure whether breakdowns were caused by the computer changes or by underlying faulty code.

NEW SYSTEMS INTEGRATION

When selecting a new system, a practice management organization is primarily making a software decision. Hardware has become a commodity and a secondary consideration. It's getting cheaper and cheaper to upgrade hardware, but software remains an expensive decision.

When buying either a whole new system or a single application, physician organizations should first organize a work group to follow the project from beginning to end. The work group should be multi-disciplinary and consist of eight to 12 persons, including physicians and nonclinicians. Including staff members and physicians in the selection and implementation process is likely to increase acceptance of a new system because the work group members can help sell the idea to their colleagues. The work group takes ownership of the solution and is more likely to work toward its successful implementation.

Here's one approach to this time-consuming process.

- Choose a selection team that includes operations managers, physicians and office workers. Recognize that physicians' time on the panel may be more limited because of patient care time constraints.
- Research the various systems by reading trade journals and talking to colleagues.
- Send out requests for proposals to about a dozen vendors.
- Narrow the selection to five vendors who will do demonstrations.
- Get two references from each of the five vendors and schedule site visits with as many of those references as possible. While on-site, make note of how many staff members it takes to run the system in the clinics and at the corporate office, and of how the practices are using the software.

Sorting out the Products and Vendors

The basic information system for a PhyCor practice, which averages 30 physicians, includes scheduling, billing, managed care information, and referrals management. Thrailkill and his staff install a local area network infrastructure to support the system that provides transcription services, lab results, and clinical information to the physicians' practices.

Some practice management companies, however, will want to add other features to their information system. For example, many clinics are incorporating patient education into their medical records system. Before a patient leaves the office, the appropriate health education information needed is printed out to take home. This may be wise to consider because physicians are being pushed to see more patients, meaning they spend less time with them. On the other hand, patients are demanding more information, and it's in the physicians' best interest to ensure that the patient is well informed about treatment and prescriptions.

More than 2,000 companies sell computer systems to physicians. With such an array of choices, it's difficult for a practice management company, let alone an individual physician, to sort out the differences. What's more, vendors are constantly merging or being acquired, making the landscape even more confusing.

Unless physicians have an individual or team of individuals dedicated to IT, it's difficult just to keep up with the players. National vendors are buying regional vendors, which are buying niche solutions companies. Most vendors are small. Fewer than 30 national vendors of physician practice management software had achieved national prominence with regionally deployed sales forces and support staff, according to the GartnerGroup.[4] However, numerous hospital

---

[4] Categorizing Physician Practice Management Vendors. *GartnerGroup*, January 8, 1998.

information system vendors also had developed products aimed at the physician market.

Most physician companies employ one of the following strategies.

1. Buy "best of breed." Separate systems for scheduling, practice management, and billing are purchased. If this approach is adopted, interfaces must be developed to integrate the systems. These interfaces can be seamless to the user, but they add programming and support expenses to the project's overall cost.

2. Buy single integrated solution. These systems run on their own proprietary databases. However, it's difficult to find vendors with solutions that perfectly address all of a physician company's needs. There is no perfect system. A physician company may find a system that solves 80% of the clinic's needs. If the other 20% is really important, it can become a negotiation point when it's time to close a deal.

Internet

Today, most physicians use the Internet for e-mail, new services, or educational research. However, a 1998 PricewaterhouseCoopers/*Modern Physician* survey found that 36.4% of the groups don't use the Internet at all. Those that don't said they simply didn't need it from a clinical standpoint. Others voiced concerns about security, cost, difficulty of use, or said that they simply didn't have the technology to surf.

Recent innovations in call center technology, among others, may start to change that mind-set. Call centers allow multilocation businesses to consolidate a number of vital functions through a centralized telephone system utilizing the Internet.

The use of centralized call centers is ingrained in service industries such as hotels and banking, where customer service representatives have information they need at their fingertips through computer access. Many managed care organizations also use call center technology to consolidate scheduling, patient information, and billing functions, which helps customer service representatives respond to patients in an effective, organized manner.

Physician groups, particularly those that manage capitated populations, may find that they, too, can make effective use of call center technology. Advantages include the following.

- Centralized scheduling for more than one clinic or practice
- Ease of use for staff
- Pop-up windows that can prompt office staff to remind patients about vaccinations, medications, or overdue bills
- Useful for waiting lists

What's more, the newest generation of medical call centers allows practices to create personalized Internet Web sites for each of their patients. Patients can access their Web sites to obtain information on lab results or treatment regimens; schedule appointments; enroll in special events, such as prenatal classes; or obtain health education information about their condition. For a generation of adults that increasingly are using the Internet for everything from news gathering to stock portfolio management, a personalized health Web site is ideal, and could win over a patient's loyalty to the physician group.

Computer-Based Patient Records

Vendors spout a great deal of information about computer-based, or electronic, patient records. These products range from text-based systems to sophisticated integrated suites.

Computer-based patient records (CPRs) can increase the efficiency of clinic operations and improve patient care. Ideally, they provide physicians and other caregivers with instant access to the information they need to make treatment decisions. For example, they would allow an on-call physician to retrieve patient records on his or her home PC.

A PricewaterhouseCoopers/*Modern Physician* survey found that medical groups want the following core elements in an electronic patient record.

Chief complaint	80.5%
Vital signs	67.4%
History	83.5%
Problem list	81.4%
Medication list	84.5%
Prescriptions	73.3%
Test orders	63.1%
Radiology reports	64.5%
Radiology images	23.1%
Telephone inquiries	50.9%
MD consultation	55.4%
Discharge information	49.8%
Outcome measures	66.5%
Cost information	45.7%
Preventive medical reminders	52.3%

Some CPR applications also offer disease management guidelines and clinical decision support, and can be integrated with practice management tools, such as billing, collections, and eligibility determination. However, most are application-centric: The patient record opens as an application, and patient information is entered and updated within that application. The downside of this is it cannot interface with software from other vendors or distribute information to other applications. It also lacks Internet capabilities.

The future, however, lies in patient-centric computing in which the application programs are embedded in the patient object. All the medical information collected on a patient would be contained in the computer-based patient object (CPO). The CPO is the healthcare version of the object-oriented technology moving into other industries. Unfortunately, healthcare lacks the EDI standardization that allows so many other industries to exchange information in a common standard methodology. However, development of those standards is underway by groups like the American National Standards Institute's (ANSI's) Healthcare Informatics Standards Board.

Once the industry agrees on standard properties and events for chart-note objects, then chart-note objects can be developed by a vendor to be part of a computer-based patient record.

The HIMSS survey referenced earlier reported that the top three roadblocks to fully implementing a CPR system industry wide are lack of a standardized vocabulary (23%), inadequate IT infrastructure (15%), and resistance of administrative staff (14%). Lack of adequate funding is a roadblock for 9%.

Within medical groups, initial cost was identified as the top roadblock to an electronic patient records system, according to a 1998 Pricewaterhouse Coopers/*Modern Physician* survey. Other challenges (in order of most mentioned) were ease of utilization, incomplete product development, time consuming for clinicians, security concerns, user training requirement, and vendor stability.

The issue of time consumption hinges primarily on data input. The data that previously has been stored on paper must be inputted into the electronic patient record. Getting physicians to input (rather than dictate) this data will require overcoming some sizable obstacles to time-honored processes of delivering and documenting care. In some cases, practice management companies are considering palm-sized devices that physicians can take into the treatment room and enter the data themselves at the point of care (Box 4–2).

Some physician practices have made the leap. For example, Mayo Clinic in Jacksonville, Fla., moved to paperless medical records in 1998, making measurable productivity gains[5] (Figure 4–6).

Sorting Out the Finances

When a healthcare organizations makes the decision to invest in an information system, the most difficult decision is justifying the cost. In the selection of a computerized patient records system, for example, once the work group has

---

[5] Systems: The Mayo Clinic's Experience in Implementing a Paperless Medical Record. Reginald Smith, chief information officer, Mayo Clinic, Jacksonville, Fla., presentation to the National Congress on the Future of Medical Practice and Practice Management.

B O X 4–2

PALMING IT

It's a common sight at a '90s business meeting. When the discussion turns to scheduling the next meeting, at least one participant pulls out one of those palm-size personal digital assistants (PDAs) to check his or her schedule. Business executives have turned to palm-sized tools to keep themselves organized and on schedule; similar tools may soon change the way in which physicians document and retrieve patient information.

Pen-based computing, used daily by rental car and Federal Express agents, could one day ingrain itself with physicians (into a physician's modus operandi). Point-of-care devices that slip nicely into the pockets of a lab coat are being developed that enable physicians to input data, check medical records, or review test results in hallways, the cafeteria—in short, anywhere they happen to be.

However, acquiring this freedom from paper charts requires challenging one of the most unshakable traditions in healthcare—dictating notes into a recorder. For physicians, dictation is a way of life. Will they abandon this age-old process to take on what they view as data entry?

"You have to transition the physicians away from concept of the paper chart and away from dictation and transcription," said John Lacy, CIO of USCardio Vascular. "Our challenge is to have this process (data entry) result in enough added value that the physicians accept the change in practice patterns. If ultimately, the value perceived by the physicians is significant, they will not only accept the change—they will demand it."

In some cases, getting physicians computer-friendly is a generational issue. Those who grew up playing Nintendo are likely to be much more technology friendly than those who grew up with black-and-white television. The technology-challenged physicians often contend that paper charts are easier to use, they don't want to do data entry, and the text-based software programs they've tried in the past were monotonous to pore through.

To encourage those doctors to start typing, practice management companies must convince them that it will improve patient outcomes and, even-

narrowed down the choices, the CIO or CFO should begin preparing a financial spreadsheet on each proposed system. Ideally, this spreadsheet will stretch out five years to give the physicians, executives and board members a full picture of the entire project's life cycle. Specific items should include the following.

- Cost of software and hardware
- Consulting costs

tually, make more efficient use of their time. "It's about improving their quality of life; but more than that, it's about improving the quality of care they can provide. Initially, they'll experience a decrease in productivity," Lacy said. "But once they get into it, there will be a significant increase in productivity."

Other aspects that may motivate physicians to use electronic rather than the transcription service include the following.

- Stress that the electronic records will be useful for research purposes. Physicians who want to have the research benefits of electronic records collection may be motivated by that desire.

- Involve them in designing the electronic templates used in the new system.

- For physicians whose compensation is based in part on collections, emphasize that the devices can help get bills out the door faster because the office manager isn't waiting for a physician to sign off on the charts.

- Test palm-sized technology and physician data entry in a clinic where physicians are willing to be on the leading edge. Then, if the trial is successful, it can be expanded.

Despite all of the advantages, PhyCor's CIO, Eric Thrailkill, doesn't believe physicians will turn away quickly from their dictation habit. "Physicians' clinical processes are very difficult to change. Some physicians are very efficient from a process standpoint at using a cassette recorder. I'm not sure there's a better way for them."

If palm-sized technology doesn't signal an end to transcription, voice recognition may. Although these products have been plagued with problems, the technology is moving at such a rate that experts predict they will be in the mainstream within five years. For physicians who have resisted the move to inputting data themselves, voice recognition could be a turning point toward an electronic patient record

- Costs of writing new interfaces
- Depreciation
- Training costs, including employee overtime during the conversion process
- Temporary help added to fill in while full-time employees go through training
- Travel costs to send employees to vendor's training sessions

FIGURE 4-6

Experiences of Mayo Clinic, Jacksonville, FL

Improvements from implementation of paperless medical record

- Patient waiting time
- Scheduling of appointments
- Timeliness of correspondence
- Telephone response
- Availability of chart on demand
- Better reimbursement

Results:
20% increase in physician productivity
Reduced the number of steps in processing patient records by one-third overall
Number of FTEs per physician dropped from 6.6 to 4.5
2.5 years break-even for IT investment

Nothing makes information technology vendors and gurus more nervous than talking about return on investment (ROI). It's difficult to compute, requiring financial data on revenues and expenses, in addition to the capital outlays required. In the medical environment, it's further complicated by the fact that quality improvements are so difficult to quantify for inclusion in the equation. Issues to consider in evaluating ROI include the following.

- *Lag time.* The goal of these systems goes beyond automating paper-based records to actually improving the quality of patient care. Yet, the financial return on that won't be measurable for three to five years. In the medical environment, it's complicated further by the fact that the system may be collecting data that won't be used for a year or more. As clinical and outcomes data are collected, they'll need to be analyzed before they're used for contracting purposes. In some ways, practice management companies and their physicians must make a blind leap of faith.

- *Other cost savings.* If physicians are inputting their own data, it will take time before their efforts become a seamless process. Initially, it may take longer for physicians to do that input and the practice may want to retain the services of its transcriptionists on a part-time basis (Figure 4-7). Obviously, transcription costs may eventually go to zero, but initially that may be offset by productivity losses by physicians.

- *Lower maintenance costs.* Quantifying savings starts with the information system the practice was using. Did it constantly need maintenance and expensive tech support from the vendor? Did the practice maintain its own staff of programmers to deal with coding problems?
- *Improved efficiency.* One item practices might measure after installing an electronic records system is chart pulls. With the records on the system, staff members should be spending less time looking for charts. That will give them more time to answer phones and other administrative functions.

Negotiating Tips

Most physician organizations end up selecting one or more preferred vendors. A company can have 25 of the best systems around, but supporting that many systems will be a nightmare for the IT staff. Selecting a few preferred vendors may mean savings through volume pricing. It also makes conversions and support easier for the IT staff (Table 4–1).

Before signing a deal with a vendor, a practice must decide what it wants to haggle over. Once a deal is signed, the physician organization's negotiating leverage will be gone. Points to consider include the following.

- Make a list of items that the system does not offer, but your clinics want or need. Make them negotiating points in the contract.
- Have a preliminary planning session with the vendor's installation crew. These are the people who will be installing the system and their opinions on how the installation will go may be markedly different than those of the marketing representatives.

FIGURE 4–7

Medical Groups That Have Reduced Their Staff Size by Use of Software

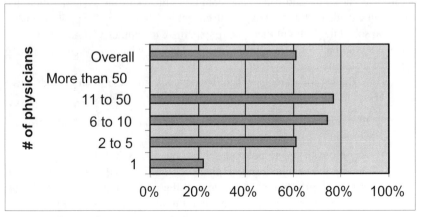

Source: National CPA Healthcare Advisors Association.

TABLE 4-1

How Medical Groups Obtain Their Technology

Through an MSO	9.9%
Directly purchased from IT vendor	70.6%
Through a group purchasing organization	9.4%
Through a hospital affiliate	13.8%
Through a time-share outsourcing agreement	3.2%
Other	5.1%

Source: PricewaterhouseCoopers/Modern Physician.

- Carefully talk about the resources needed for an implementation. Negotiate for as much training assistance as possible. Vendors tend to underestimate the amount of training needed.

Where decisions are made by the clinics themselves, rather than by the practice management organization, the practice management company's information technology staff can play a helpful role as advisors. Traditionally, most groups have made decisions based solely on information received from vendors themselves, according to a survey by PricewaterhouseCoopers and *Modern Physician* magazine.

Installation and Training

Practice management companies and their clinics tend to expect a speedy installation and implementation of a new information system. The most common mistake is underestimating the time and resources required.

Practice management companies may want to hire outside consultants to help with the installation process. Hire a consultant who has installed this system before and knows the intricacies and common glitches of the system. Often, the cost of an outside consultant pays for itself in time savings by keeping the installation on schedule. Without that type of expertise, the clinics will have to rely on managers who have other responsibilities to take on what can be overwhelming duties of installing a new system.

Time frames for training will differ depending on the practice and physicians' level of understanding of technology. Here are some tips.

- Offer training during the week, nights, and on weekends. Budget for overtime.
- Advise physicians to put themselves on a 50% schedule during the training, then again during implementation. That will give them time to learn and adjust to the new system. If there is a big difference in ability levels among physicians, individual training sessions may be best for some. If the physicians are on a production-based compensation

system, the management organization or health system administrator may have to compensate them for the time spent in training.

- Bring in temporary workers to cover for nonphysician employees in training.
- On the first day of implementation, have trainers in the offices to answer questions.
- Plan for a 9- to 12-month implementation schedule in each clinic. Any schedule longer than that runs the risk of causing people to lose interest.

OTHER IT PRIORITIES

Security Issues

Physicians operate in an interconnected world and security is of prime importance, especially in terms of patient records. Security problems are costly and can erode the confidence of payors and patients. In addition, for clinics seeking accreditation from the Joint Commission on Accreditation of Healthcare Organizations (JCAHO), data security is a basic requirement.

Sharing of information heightens concerns about security issues—yet information systems can actually increase security, experts argue. Vendors brag about the built-in security features of their systems, networks, databases, and applications. However, these features only provide a baseline of security that is inadequate for a medical business. Here's a security issues checklist for physician clinics to consider.

- Develop a comprehensive security evaluation program.
- Purchase a firewall product to protect against outside hackers.
- Set controls on patient records, such as using different levels of password security.
- Keep computers physically locked up.
- Institute passwords and require employees to change them every 30 to 60 days. Passwords should be a minimum of seven characters.
- Evaluate secure links across the Internet with payors, suppliers, and other providers. By securing these links, the practice management company and its physicians may find increased ways to collaborate and open new opportunities.
- Remember that employees (including temporary personnel) represent a practice's biggest security threat. A well-designed information technology architecture that gives employees access only to what they need is necessary to guard against these security risks.
- Establish a policy on confidentiality. Make sure employees know the importance of confidentiality and the penalties for violating the policy. Require employees to sign confidentiality agreements.

Some physician companies are looking into the leading-edge security technologies used in some highly-sensitive banking, government, and manufacturing environments. These biometric systems employ technology such as fingerprint imaging and eye scans. Fingerprint identification is one of the most secure methods available. In addition, users don't have to worry about changing or forgetting passwords.

Data Confidentiality

Practice management companies will want to roll up data for analysis—that's the whole push behind outcomes management. However, it's a problem if patients haven't given permission for their data to be shared. In such cases, the practice must ensure confidentiality by masking identities.

The issue of patient confidentiality and medical record privacy promises to be a lightning rod for politicians in the years ahead. For example, prior to making his unsuccessful 1996 presidential bid, Sen. Robert Dole (R-Kan.) co-sponsored legislation that would make the improper disclosure of confidential medical records a federal crime. This issue gains sympathy from politicians of all stripes: Dole's co-sponsor for the legislation was his ideological opposite, Sen. Edward Kennedy (D-Mass.).

Although that particular piece of legislation did not pass, the Health Insurance Portability and Accountability Act, passed in 1997, includes a provision that requires Congress to pass legislation ensuring medical records confidentiality by 1998. If that fails, the Secretary of Health and Human Services must implement regulations governing medical records confidentiality by February 1999.

In addition, Rep. Louise Slaughter (D-N.Y.) and Rep. Joseph Kennedy (D-Mass.) have each introduced bills focused on protecting genetic information contained in patient medical records.

Data Ownership

Although this may not seem important initially, questions eventually will arise about ownership of the data. Do the physicians own the data, or does the physician practice management company own the data? A PPM may decide that it is like a bank—it keeps the data and makes sure it is secure, but the data belongs to the physicians. At the practice level, ownership of data may ensure that physicians remain involved with system upgrades and maintenance.

If a physician organization craters, data? ownership questions could become critical. In the case of one ophthalmology group in North Carolina, more than 1,000 patient records were reported missing when the management company filed for bankruptcy. The North Carolina Medical Board said it had no jurisdiction over the management company since it was a nonmedical entity.[6]

---

[6] Stiff, C. (1988). Complications Arise in Simel Eye Bankruptcy Case. *Greater Triangle Area Business Journal,* November 16.

PricewaterhouseCoopers Tips for Information Systems

- Determine an information systems strategy, then develop a transition plan to get there.
- Don't automate processes that should be eliminated. Look at the overall work flow in the office and try to eliminate work rather than maintaining it through a new information system.
- Select an IT vendor that has resources and staying power.
- Communicate often with physicians and staff about a conversion or installation project. Ensure that all parties remain current on how the system will be used and benefit their practices.
- Invest in a change management effort. A system dependent on paper records will not easily adapt to a change in information technology. Despite all assurances that the system will be easier and cheaper to use, it will probably start out being more difficult and more expensive.

Checklist of IS Functions

- Scheduling of resources (physicians and office staff)
- Scheduling of patients
- Registration
- Master patient index
- Encounter tracking
- Encoding support
- Connectivity with hospital information systems
- Billing
- Workers' compensation
- Collections management
- Accounts receivables management
- Health plan eligibility
- Referrals and referral management
- Claims processing
- Capitation
- Risk pool management
- Electronic claims
- Remittance processing
- Electronic funds transfer

RESOURCES

www.fda.gov/cdrh/yr2000.html—Food and Drug Administration issues on Y2K

www.year2000.com—Y2K technical and legal information

www.healthcare-informatics.com—*Healthcare Informatics* magazine, a monthly source of information on healthcare information systems and regular articles on Y2K

www.hcfa.gov/y2k—Y2K information from Medicare

www.rx2000.org—Minneapolis-based institute to help healthcare organizations navigate Year 2000 problems

www.isaca.org—Information Systems Audit & Control Association (ISACA), a Rolling Meadows, Ill.–based association of information systems technical experts; publishes a journal, plus bulletins on Year 2000 and other information systems issues

www.healthprovider.com/library/hippa.chklist4.asp—A checklist for getting ready for the Health Insurance Portability and Accountability Act requirements

www.po.com—Physicians Online, a subscription service that has medical news, journals, on-line discussion areas, and searchable databases such as MEDLINE

www.amia.org—American Medical Informatics Association

www.himss.org—Healthcare Information and Management Systems Society

www.mdconsult.com—Web-based service that includes the full texts of medical textbooks, searchable drug interaction databases, and practice guidelines from more than 45 professional associations and organizations. Also includes patient education handouts that physicians can customize for their own use.

http://208.192.104.178/y2k/y2k_search.cfm—The U.S. government's online database of biomedical device compliance. The site includes a survey of vendors on Y2K compliance.

www.medrecinst.com—The Medical Records Institute, which sponsors an annual meeting, Toward an Electronic Patient Record.

www.uthscsa.edu/2000/test1.html—Tool kit for testing embedded devices for Y2K. Site is maintained by the University of Texas Health Science Center at San Antonio.

5

CHAPTER

Compensation: Physician Organizations Move Toward Incentives

Sandy Lutz

Charles Goldberg

Want to hear some real war stories? Compensation experts talk of no bigger battles with physician organizations than those involving compensation. A doctor's paycheck can be hallowed ground—tamper with it at your own risk. Even the most congenial physician group can turn into a vicious mob when the conversation turns to drastic changes in compensation and distribution of incentive pools. Just the process of formulating incentives can be expensive in time, money and human toil.

For these reasons, some practice management organizations do not dictate how much each physician is going to make. After taking their management fee and paying expenses, the practice management firm leaves it up to the physicians' professional corporations to determine how the remaining dollars will be divided up. "That's what the doctors liked most about joining our PPM," said one former development executive. "We didn't tell them how to pay each other."

However, that won't work for other physicians organizations and health systems that manage doctors. These physician organizations believe that money is a big motivator that, properly applied, can have a positive impact on the organization's overall profitability. They believe that operational success is grounded in incentives and that they must take a hand in guiding physicians toward compensation

FIGURE 5-1

More Healthcare Organizations Are Rewarding Performance

In a PricewaterhouseCoopers compensation survey, 46% of healthcare organizations participating said they used short-term executive bonuses or incentive plans. The most prevalent award criteria are performance-related: 64% for individual performance and 49% for unit or division performance.

According to the survey, 54% of clinical department heads and 22% of staff physicians were eligible for short-term incentive payments. In terms of long-term incentive programs, 17% of clinical department heads and 8.8% of staff physicians were eligible.

systems that provide those incentives[1] (Figure 5–1). This chapter deals with those types of organizations.

In designing compensation systems, physician organizations need to keep these guiding principles in mind.

- The perfect compensation system does not exist.
- To be successful, compensation systems must be structured so that physicians believe they are making more money with the organization they would without it.
- Most compensation models will beget winners and losers. Therefore, criticism from some quarter will be inevitable.

Physicians who have left (or are trying to leave) practice management companies or other organizations have an almost universal complaint: their compensation dropped once they signed up. The physician management organization's response to this complaint is that their compensation would have dropped regardless because of changes taking place in the marketplace. It may be impossible to quantify how the physician group would have fared apart from the physician organization. That being said, the onus is on the practice management firm, physician organization, or hospital system to make the doctors feel that they are better off with them than without them.

In the days of rising stock prices, the compensation debate wasn't nearly so important for physician management companies. As long as stock price increases

---

[1] For example, physician practices affiliated with American Oncology Resources receive about 23% of the medical practice's revenues and 50% of the cash flow if it rises above the negotiated EBITDA target. This gives physicians an incentive to work with AOR in controlling operating costs and growing the practice.

were offsetting declines in compensation, physicians didn't mind. But, once stock prices started to decline in 1998, physicians who had sold their practices for stock witnessed their net worth spiraling downward. If their compensation was declining as well, physicians understandably became disgruntled.

But the physicians aren't the only ones who have complaints. Practice management companies that have divested (or are trying to divest) themselves of physician practices also had an almost universal complaint: productivity dropped off after the physicians signed the affiliation agreement. In organizations in which physicians have no incentive to meet performance targets or build the practice, productivity and profitability fall—we've seen it happen time and again. Some physician organizations have structured compensation so that the physicians make the same as before they affiliated with the organization. However, in addition to guaranteeing this salary, the organization provided the physicians with better benefits—more vacation, an extra day off during the week, or shorter hours during the day. The result was that the physicians were working less to earn the same amount of money—and that didn't even take into account the amount the physician had received for selling his or her practice to the management company or health system in the first place.

A dose of incentive compensation may be the cure for this ailment. Physicians see the value in incentives, and often understand why they're necessary. Nearly every study shows that without incentives, physicians will not be as productive. Employing physicians almost ensures less productivity (Table 5–1).

"Economically and emotionally, you cannot have the physicians feeling like they're employees," said Danguole J. Spakevicius, president and CEO of FemPartners, a Houston-based OB/GYN practice management firm. "If you do, their drive to produce goes by the wayside."

T A B L E 5–1

Productivity for Self-Employed versus Employee Physicians

	Self-Employed	Employee	Percent Difference
Mean # of office hours per week	30.8	25	23%
Mean # of hours in surgery per week	7.3	4.8	52%
Mean # of total patient visits per week	115.3	98.4	17%
Mean # of office visits per week	88	63.1	39%
Mean # of visits on hospital rounds per week	16.3	15.2	7%
Mean # of surgical procedures per week	4.1	2.3	78%

Source: AMA Socioeconomic Characteristics of Medical Practice, 1997.

DEVELOPING THE COMPENSATION FORMULA

Most physician organizations are trying to move toward a blend of base and incentive (bonus) compensation, and away from a straight guaranteed salary (Figure 5–2). Moving physicians from a base salary without any incentive-based compensation to one in which part of their income is at risk can be difficult, but it is not impossible (Box 5–1). Change must evolve gradually or the practice management firm could have an uprising on its hands. For example, some physician groups are tightly controlled by a few older physicians. They started the practice and even though they allowed other physicians to buy in, they still reap the most compensation because of their standing in the group. When a physician management organization or hospital buys the group, it may want to instill incentives to retain the younger physicians—incentives that weren't there under the previous regime.

The ratios used (for example, 80% base/20% bonus) are all over the map, depending on how much compensation physicians are willing (or are required) to put at risk.

Base Compensation

The base salary component of the compensation equation provides financial stability for physicians because it is a guaranteed source of income (e.g., in an employment contract) and because it carries a low level of risk with respect to the total compensation package.

Part of ensuring a fair and equitable compensation system is determining whether base salaries are in line with those of the local market. For physician organizations that are moving into new markets, it is important to define the comparable market for base pay as part of the market assessment. Understanding that no one

F I G U R E   5–2

Evolution of Physician Compensation

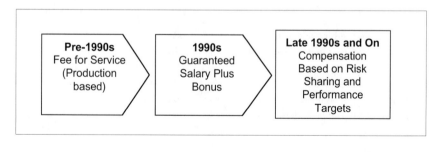

B O X   5-1

PHYSICIAN INCOME BENCHMARKS

A year after a physician has sold his practice, he'll look at his income and that of his peers. If it's less than what he was making prior to affiliating with the physician management organization, he'll be unhappy.

In fact, a typical squabble between physicians and their practice management firms revolves around past and future compensation. The physician's typical argument: "I'm making less than I did last year." The practice management company's typical answer: "You would have made even less without us because the market is changing."

Is that response valid?

Except for a dip in 1994, physician income has risen steadily during the past few years. In 1996, overall physician income climbed 3.8% to a median of $166,000, according to the American Medical Association.

The data also show that physicians employed by organizations were getting bigger raises even though their income level lagged. Employed doctors' median income rose 4.4% to $142,000, while the median income for self-employed physicians decreased a half percent to $198,000. Even so, employed physicians made about 40% less than those who were self-employed.

How accurate are the statistics, though, and how usable are they for organizations that manage physicians? For example, how many of those seemingly lower-compensated employed physicians also received non-cash compensation such as stock or notes from the sale of their practices?

Some physicians have complained about the accuracy of the data, which is based on a sample of 4,000 physicians—a relatively small slice of the nation's 600,000 practicing physicians. In fact, delegates to the AMA's annual meeting last year questioned whether the AMA income data accurately reflect the negative impact of managed care on reimbursement rates.[1]

Another question to consider is whether the physician incomes in 1996 and 1997 were inflated because acquisitive practice management firms and hospital systems were paying high salaries to attract physicians. In truth, it may be impossible to quantify how the physicians would have fared apart from the physician organization.

---

[1] Jacob, J. (1998). Delegated Voice Concerns with AMA's Collection and Release of Physician Income Data. *American Medical News*, July 13.

"ruler" should be used to determine appropriate base pay levels, the following factors must be considered in determining the structure of base salary for physicians.

- Type of specialty—primary, obstetrics/gynecology, cardiology, etc.
- Type of practice—hospital-based, solo practitioner, managed care environment, academic setting, partnership, group setting.
- Stage of practice—start-up, growing, established
- Geographic region

To assess base salary, benchmark positions are selected to compare the appropriate local, regional or national levels of base salary and salary range. Any number of published survey sources are available that provide timely data for benchmarking physician compensation sliced and diced in a variety of ways. (See Resources at the end of this chapter for a listing). For example, one widely-used survey, the *Physician Compensation and Production Survey,* is produced by the Medical Group Management Association (an industry group) and Cejka & Company. (Recent data are in Figure 5–3.) It provides the following data classifications.

- Specialty
- Years in specialty

FIGURE 5–3

MGMA's Report on Doctor Compensation in 1997

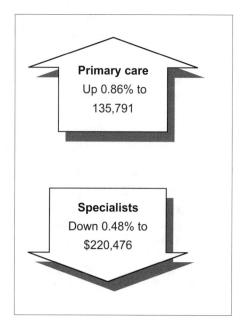

- Gender
- Geographic region
- Legal organization structure
- Hospital ownership
- Practice management company affiliation
- At-risk managed care percent of revenue
- Per-RBRVS units
- Hours worked

Most such surveys are published annually and report data from a variety of practice settings, including HMOs, hospitals, group practices, solo practitioners, and physicians in academic settings. Additionally, published surveys are available that provide information on other forms of physician compensation, including clinical income and stipends.

When benchmarking, bear in mind that a compensation model must reflect the pulse of its own market. It's great to analyze data from national surveys, but that data may be meaningless in Biloxi or Seattle. For example, primary-care physicians in the South make about $20,000 more a year than their colleagues in other parts of the country, according to MGMA data. Specialists, on average, make nearly $80,000 a year more in the South than do their cohorts do in the West. Why is this? Factors that affect base salaries in specific regions include cost of living; supply and demand for healthcare services and certain specialties; the desirability of a region as a place in which to live; and the region's overall market/economic conditions with respect to managed care.

Users of benchmarking data also must bear in mind that the most recent published data may be skewed by the bidding wars that developed for physician practices in certain markets. In many cases, physicians were offered salaries by hospitals and/or practice management companies that exceeded market rates. In retrospect, these providers regret the guaranteed salaries they gave physicians. Now, they are facing the arduous process of renegotiations to make their organizations profitable. Organizations in those markets should bear in mind that base compensation levels going forward will not be as high as they may have been in the past, and adjust their assessment accordingly.

Once established, base salary levels should be reviewed and updated annually to ensure that they remain in line with the market (i.e., with comparable organizations and the local, regional, or national market for pay).

Incentives and Bonus Pools

Different incentives work in different practice settings. For example, in a fee-for-service environment, it may be appropriate to create an incentive that focuses in part on net collections. Likewise, in a capitated managed care environment, it may be more appropriate to create incentives to increase physicians' accessibility to patients (patient encounters), which in turn can link to potential revenue growth and practice efficiency.

Some incentives may work better when applied to the group (i.e., when they work toward the single objective of satisfied patients), and some incentives may work better at the individual physician level.

Following are the most common components of incentive compensation.

- Production—How much business is the physician generating?
- Cost savings—How efficient is the physician's practice?
- Patient satisfaction—How happy are patients with the care they receive?
- Quality—What are the physician's clinical outcomes?
- Citizenship—How involved is the physician in governance, clinical pathways, and other business committees?

These components are described briefly below.

Practice Productivity/Production Bonuses

There are many ways to measure physician productivity, all of which work in different settings. Practice productivity measures include net collections, patient encounters/weighted average visits, active patient records, and covered lives/covered life equivalents, to name a few. Different methodologies of measuring productivity include paying out upon meeting productivity measures, exceeding them or establishing specific incentive compensation as a multiple of base salary. Methodologies differ in their complexity. Organizations that manage physicians must keep in mind that the more complex the methodology, the more difficult a compensation system may be to administer.

Many physicians groups are moving to systems in which all or part of a physician's income is based on relative value units (RVUs), which are a way of measuring work.[2] Physicians already understand RVUs because Medicare uses them as the basis of reimbursement for physician services. However, a group shouldn't even consider moving to this type of system unless it has an excellent information system and competent coders. RVU-based systems are extremely complex. And they're not cut and dried; for example, the group will still have to determine the worth of non-RVU work, such as practice administration.

---

[2] In a relative value scale, each procedure or service is assigned a relative value, usually on the basis of CPT codes.

Several organizations provide data for developing RVU-based compensation systems. Again, geographic considerations are important; groups need to be careful to determine whether the RVUs are reasonable within a given geographic market.

Efficiency Bonuses

Physician organizations can reward two types of efficiency: *site efficiency* and *practice pattern efficiency*. Site efficiency bonuses motivate physicians to work collaboratively with the healthcare system (hospital, medical group, etc.) to keep costs down at the practice site by using the practice's facility and personnel resources in an efficient manner.

Practice pattern efficiency bonuses are earned by satisfying efficiency-supporting activities such as keeping length of stay within pre-established guidelines, adhering to clinical protocols and treatment guidelines, maintaining consistent referral patterns within pre-established guidelines, or conforming with preventive program goals consistent with those set forth by the National Committee for Quality Assurance (NCQA).[3] For physicians employed directly by a hospital, an efficiency bonus may be based on a comparison of what their hospitalized patients actually cost the facility versus what they were expected to cost.

Patient Satisfaction Bonuses

This includes any number of criteria addressing patient satisfaction via mailed satisfaction surveys, evaluating re-enrollment rates and enrollment retention, and physician-specific complaint assessment.

Quality Bonuses

This is an important determinant that physicians may embrace much more wholeheartedly than measures of productivity and efficiency. One way of rewarding quality is to maintain a database of clinical and functional outcomes on patients. This can be a complex and expensive task. Like other bonus systems, it may be wise to set goals for a handful of outcomes that are measurable and reward physicians for meeting or exceeding the goals.

Management Responsibility Bonuses

Management responsibility rewards physicians for time committed to management activities and leadership within the system or practice. Examples of such

---

[3] Or the Joint Commission for the Accreditiation of Hospital Organizations (JCAHO), for physicians practicing in a hospital setting.

commitments include serving as the organization's medical director, participating on a management committee, helping to develop medical management programs or treatment protocols, or overseeing business functions such as billing and collections. Because this bonus is related to "time served," it is typically rewarded as a lump sum stipend, on an hourly or per-meeting basis.

Other Incentives

In some cases, discretionary bonuses may be used in situations in which it is difficult to define and measure specific performance targets, or to recognize an individual physician's unique contribution. They are typically a fixed dollar amount and may encompass peer satisfaction, excess call coverage, an overall "good employee" award, and the like.

Selecting the performance criteria can be a painful job for practice management executives. One way to mitigate criticism is to include criteria that are being used by payors, saying that payors are looking at these benchmarks and physicians need to pay attention to them also.

In addition to individual benchmarks, a compensation model may include rewards for overall performance. These would include the following.

- Meeting group profitability targets
- Meeting prescribed clinical benchmarks, such as the Health Employer Data and Information Set[4] or the National Committee for Quality Assurance

Performance data should be shared fully with physicians to improve awareness and adherence to targeted performance measures. Payout schedules will differ by organization, but payouts become more meaningful if they are made more frequently (on a quarterly basis, for example). Annual payouts may not be frequent enough to encourage behavior, while monthly payouts tend to become an administrative burden. A balance should be struck based on the type of incentive to be paid (e.g., some incentives will require an annual data collection cycle) and what is appropriate for the practice setting.

With all types of incentives, reasonable compensation guidelines must be adhered to, and capping bonus potential must be considered. Under the glare of payors and regulators, healthcare organizations would be prudent to ensure that their compensation systems are reasonable for physicians and don't include excessive rewards.

Remember the saying, "Be careful what you wish for?" Directing physician behavior through incentives is admirable. However, managers developing compensation models need to consider how those models may change physician be-

---

[4] HEDIS has more than 100 different standardized performance measures that allow employers to compare different health plans.

BOX 5–2

"HOMEOSTATIS"/INCOME TARGETING

Whenever changes to a compensation model are contemplated, a physician organization must factor in behavioral changes that may occur when a physician's pay is ratcheted downwards. Such behavioral change methodology is already factored into Medicare's physician reimbursement system. HCFA has decided that for every dollar that fees are reduced, physicians will increase the volume and intensity of services to make up 50% of that reduction, and reimbursement levels are adjusted accordingly.

The desire of physicians to work harder to protect their compensation has been termed "homeostasis" or "income targeting." An article in the summer of 1998 issue of the *Journal of Health Care Finance* pointed out that for a hip replacement, Medicare pays the surgeon $2,000, but spends another $30,000 in costs as part of that procedure.[1] If Medicare cut the surgeon's fee to $1,000, the surgeon may try to make up the lost income by doing more procedures, each of which will result in an additional $30,000 in expenses. So, for every $1,000 in cost savings derived from fee cuts, the program may be spending an additional $30,000—not exactly the way a cost-reduction plan is supposed to work. In fact, this article concluded that cutting surgeon's fees for hip replacements by 50% would produce $1 billion in additional spending.[2]

Physician organizations should heed this phenomenon when adjusting their compensation schedules. Obviously, they can get around it if the physicians are also at risk under a capitation payment system. However, if physicians were previously being paid under a case rate or discounted fee-for-service system, the physician organization must proceed with caution. If the organization is trying to reduce medical costs by decreasing physician fees, it could well be courting disaster.

[1] Bernstein, J. (1998). Policy of Implications of Physician Income Homeostasis. *Journal of Health Care Finance,* Summer.
[2] Ibid.

havior under both the best- and worst-case scenarios. If physicians attempt to make up for reduced compensation by performing more procedures, they could blow the organization's budget sky-high (Box 5–2).

THE COMPENSATION PLANNING PROCESS

There are several considerations we have found helpful in establishing comprehensive compensation programs. These steps are designed to involve both physicians and those who will administer the programs (Human Resources, Office Manager). In addition, these steps ensure that an overall compensation strategy is established to serve as a guide to the development and ongoing administration of the system.

Compensation Philosophy

A compensation philosophy, or strategy, articulates management's and physicians' beliefs about pay. It details the targeted market position for base salary (e.g., do we want to pay at the "middle of the market"/50th percentile, or do we need to pay at the 75th percentile to attract and retain key talent and specialists?). In addition, the compensation philosophy details the strategy for incentive payment. Before putting any incentives in place, the physician group must decide what its goals are. Does the group want to encourage physicians to see more patients or do more procedures? Or is the goal to control hospital utilization or expenses within the office? Does the group want to encourage good "citizenship," in which physicians are motivated to work in committees on care pathways or developing formularies? Once it decides on the behaviors it wishes to reward, it can develop appropriate incentives accordingly.

A philosophy also details the ratio of fixed compensation (base salary) to "at-risk" pay (variable pay). Most groups set parameters for each benchmark. For example, a compensation package might consist of 60% from base salary plus a 5% seniority factor and 35% divided equally among four incentives: patient satisfaction, practice efficiency, citizenship, and clinical outcomes. This apportionment will, in large part, be determined by factors such as the targeted market for base pay, as well as organizational and cultural considerations.

Finally, the philosophy provides an ongoing framework for making compensation decisions that support basic conceptual and policy matters critical to compensation program design. "Gap analysis" methodology is often employed to identify the level of disparity between the present system and what is being sought in the future compensation system (Figure 5–4).

FIGURE 5–4

No Consensus on How to Base Incentive Pay among Medical Practices

- 19% use patient satisfaction surveys
- 14% use peer review
- 24% factor in administrative or governance responsibilities
- 15% consider service quality
- 10% include seniority

Source: 1998 MGMA Physician Compensation and Production Survey.

Physician Input

A compensation committee or physician advisory committee comprising representatives from among the physicians provides the organization with direct input from physicians who can provide specialized knowledge and insight about the compensation system's design. This input ensures that considerations that are important to physicians are included in compensation and incentive design. Incorporating physician input into the design process also supports a sense of "buy-in" and ownership into the process. Furthermore, it gives management an opportunity to educate physician leaders about compensation concepts and incentive plan options. In fact, a compensation committee can serve as a crucial conduit of information to physicians.

If a committee approach is not chosen, the organization may conduct interviews with a representative sample of physicians to solicit input in order to do the following.

- Develop a thorough understanding of current professional responsibilities
- Develop an estimate of the time spent within the major areas of responsibility as well as the amounts of time spent on specific duties like rounds, on-call, admitting, etc.
- Identify key quantifiable performance measures that might be used to gauge performance and improve productivity
- Discuss any concerns physicians may have regarding the current compensation system

Evaluate Alternatives

Alternative models of compensation programs should be created and evaluated based on the compensation philosophy and any information collected from the committee or from physician interviews. Because compensation is a personal as well as professional issue, physicians will key in on how any new model will affect their income levels. Therefore, any proposed compensation models should contain data on how the formula was decided on, implemented, and validated. The healthcare organization also must communicate how each physician's income level would change under various scenarios or benchmarks.

The alternatives should be financially practicable and legally sound. Additionally, the financial impact of implementing the program should be assessed, for example, bringing physician compensation levels in line with market rates, if appropriate.

Legal Considerations

Physician organizations that provide services to Medicare, Medicaid, or other federal program beneficiaries must be careful to structure compensation (particularly incentive compensation) in such a way that they do not violate federal anti-kickback statutes (see Chapter 7). Certainly, compensation plans in general should be cleared with the physician organization's attorneys. As practice management companies increasingly turn to expansion through ancillary development, physician groups must ensure that bonuses will not be construed as a remuneration for referring a patient whose care is covered by Medicare, Medicaid or another federal benefit program to a facility in which the physician has a financial interest.

In addition, HCFA has issued regulations that prohibit HMOs or health plans from making specific payments to physicians as inducements to reduce or limit medically necessary services to Medicare enrollees. Medical groups that pay physicians based on meeting certain efficiency targets that are dependent on under-utilization should keep this in mind.[5]

The following guidelines related to gains sharing programs—in which physicians receive bonuses as a way to share in the profits of an organization—were provided by Davis Wright Tremaine, Seattle.

- Pay fair market value.
- Identify objective, non–volume-related, measures of measuring physician performance. Focus on quality measures; avoid structuring compensation to be related to physicians' patient volume, revenues, or billings.
- Describe in detail the services provided by the physician.
- Document how the incentives will improve quality and increase efficiency.
- Set a cap on the amount of compensation that may be paid—again to ensure that pay is reasonable.
- Consider excluding data relative to Medicare or Medicaid patients from the incentive program.
- Consider involving a payor or insurance entity in the incentive program.
- If the incentive program is based on cost savings, make sure the savings are real, not illusory.

EXAMPLES OF PAYMENT SYSTEMS
Capitated System

A capitated payment system puts the physicians at risk for HMO contracts, encouraging them to treat patients in a cost-efficient manner and to nurture patient satisfaction. Physicians comp is based on the number of patients, so that the physicians are subcapitated—the capitation payment is split among them. One much-discussed system for compensating specialists is "contact capitation." Analogous to a school-choice voucher system, this model is kind of a "popularity

[5] Gainsharing and Physician Incentive Compensation, Robert Homchick, partner, Davis Wright Tremaine, Seattle, Wash.

contest" that rewards specialists who receive the most referrals. The logic is that specialists that receive the most referrals are highly regarded by the primary care physicians making the referrals. Specialists receive points every time a patient is referred to them. In some contact capitation systems, points are weighted by specialty and by severity of illness; in others, by specialty only.

One advantage to the system is that specialists receive the same number of points regardless of the mode of treatment employed, so there is no incentive to perform unnecessary procedures. One practice administrator noted that when his group switched ophthalmologists to contact capitation, the number of cataract procedures plunged 50% in one month. "With each specialty we switched, we achieved similar results," he said.[6] One specialist related that a hysterectomy under discounted fee-for-service paid him as much as $2,000, but under contact capitation he received only $227.[7] This may sound incredible, but it essentially compensates the physician for encounters rather than production.

As previously mentioned, when switching to such payment systems, a physician organization must be aware of the behavioral changes that may occur when a physician's pay is ratcheted downwards (see Box 5–2).

"Eat-What-You-Kill" System

In some offices, physicians are paid based totally on productivity. This generally is a system based on collections or revenue. Obviously, this works best in groups that are reimbursed primarily with fee-for-service or discounted fee-for-service systems (Figure 5–5).

---

[6] "Can contact capitation conquer costs?" by Neil Chesanow, Medical Economics, Sept. 21, 1998.
[7] Ibid.

FIGURE 5–5

Collections is the Most Common Productivity Measure Used by Medical Practices in Compensation Methodology

Productivity Measures

Net collections—62%

Gross charges—28%

Net or adjusted charges—19%

Patient encounters—10%

RVUs—15%

Source: 1998 MGMA Physician Compensation and Production Survey.

When A.J. Rosmarin was asked to take over as CEO of a 15-physician obstetrics/gynecology medical group, he found a group in which physicians were disgruntled because their incomes had withered dramatically over the previous three years. Under the group's existing compensation mechanism, all of the payments received on patient accounts each month were funneled into one account, then divided among the physicians based on the amount of gross billings they had generated. This system did not reward physicians whose receivables were collected more quickly than others, and moreover, overall collections were lagging far behind physician performance.

What's more, the group (which generated $10 million in revenues annually) had just one employee doing collections. Since collections were not being made in a timely manner, everyone was receiving less than they should have.

Rosmarin set up a new system, which he described as "you eat what you kill." Under the system, compensation is based on collections rather than billings, and physicians are incented to work hard and to help with collections.

Here's how it works. First, the expenses of the practice are divided among the physicians and subtracted from each doctor's collections for the month. Based on prior performance, each physician receives a "draw," or base salary each week. Assume that Dr. Smith's monthly draw is $20,000. If his collections for a particular month were $60,000, and his portion of the practice's expenses were $30,000, his earnings for that month were $30,000. However, he can only draw $20,000 of that out as salary. Each quarter, Dr. Smith's draw is adjusted based on his earnings for the prior three months. If he averaged $30,000 per month all three months, his draw would be raised from $20,000 to $30,000 for the next quarter. However, if he only averaged $10,000 a month, his draw would drop accordingly.

The system allows physicians who want to take a lot of time off to do so, but "they'll take a hit the next quarter," Rosmarin said.

Every doctor receives his or her own profit-and-loss statement, showing compensation and how it was determined. In addition, each physician receives a statement about how his or her collections are faring. "The physicians know the patients. It was amazing how aggressive they got. They knew when to push it and when not to," he added.

In addition, Rosmarin expanded the collections effort, adding five more employees to do collections.

"We just wanted to keep it simple," said Rosmarin, noting that he looked at several different compensation models prior to settling on this one. The group has both salaried physicians and shareholders. Physicians who join the group are salaried for three years. Then, they can buy into the group for a predetermined amount. Salaried physicians have the same expenses taken out of the compensation except that they don't pay for leasehold improvements.

In addition to the compensation model, Rosmarin started a reserve fund to pay for capital expenditures. One percent is held back from shareholders for the reserve fund. When the fund reaches $200,000, the excess is distributed to the shareholders.

Dental Compensation Systems

In most dental practice management companies, dentists are compensated based on either a percentage of collections or a percentage of revenues.

At Gentle Dental, dentists receive an average of 25% of collections as compensation. "We're not interested in buying a business in which the owner takes off," said Michael Fiore, the company's president and CEO. This compensation model rewards dentists for productivity and for catering to clients who will pay their bills. The more services they provide, the more they get paid. Gentle Dental also uses a sweetener—after subtracting practice expenses and Gentle Dental's management fee, any remaining profits are split with the dentists (75% Gentle/ 25% dentists).

If a dentist is paid based on revenue or collections alone, he or she may concentrate on pricey procedures that are costly to perform (e.g., procedures that utilize crowns, dentures and other prosthetic devices that must be custom-made in a dental laboratory). The physician earns higher compensation but the management organization bears the higher expenses associated with those procedures. To dissuade dentists from running up the expenses side of the ledger, Monarch Dental, which pays its dentists between 20% and 25% of collections, deducts a percentage of the lab fees incurred. For example, a dentist who receives 25% of collections will also have 25% of the lab fees deducted from his or her compensation. Monarch also makes use of sweeteners; for example, dental directors that oversee other dentists receive a small percentage of those dentists' collections and are eligible for profit-sharing from the office.

At Harbor Dental in Atlanta, dentists receive an average of 28% of collections. Harbor receives the other 72% to offset the expenses of the practice and the corporation. Bruce Broussard, Harbor president and CEO, points out that the typical dentist office has about 60% to 65% overhead costs, which is lower than the 72% collected by Harbor. However, the dentist also shares in the residual profits of the practice. Residual profits are figured by taking collections and subtracting the practice's operating expenses, the dentist's compensation and Harbor's return on investment (computed as 23% of the purchase price of the practice). What's left represents the residual profit, which Harbor splits 40/60 with the dentists (60% for the dentists and 40% for Harbor).

At Castle Dental, the dentist's income is based on a percent of revenues, rather than collections. As the dentist produces more revenues, the percentage steps up. In addition, the dentist receives a bonus each month and each quarter depending on whether his practice has met certain performance targets. However, the amount of the bonus depends on each center meeting specific patient satisfaction goals. Castle surveys patients for each center every month. Patient satisfaction must be in the 90% to 100% range to receive 150% of his bonus. It must be in the 80% to 90% range to receive 100% of the bonus. If it's below 80%, the dentist forfeits his bonus even if he meets other financial targets. The centers are ranked so that everyone knows how he or she compares in terms of patient satisfaction.

PricewaterhouseCoopers Tips for Compensation Models

- Choose incentives carefully to ensure that the practice management organization or health system doesn't end up rewarding behavior that benefits the physician not the whole organization.

- Use a maximum of four benchmarks for incentive compensation. Too many benchmarks won't drive the changes needed in the organization. Incentive-based systems shouldn't calibrate dozens of different benchmarks in an incentive/bonus pool. Pick three or four items in which to influence physician behavior—for example, patient satisfaction scores, length of stay, referrals out of the group, diagnostic tests per patient, inpatient days per thousand.

- Be wary of fraud and abuse pitfalls; consult legal counsel on changes to the compensation plan.

- Plan on it taking twice as long as you'd expect to get physicians to agree to changes in a physician compensation model. If a large group requires 75% of the physicians to approve a change in compensation structure, that change could take a year or more to accomplish.

- Drastic changes in individual compensation can be more trouble than they're worth. If certain physicians' income levels are out of kilter, deal with them through gradual corrections, if possible.

RESOURCES

The following are organizations that produce physician compensation and production data.

- American Medical Association
- American Medical Group Association
- Executive Compensation Services (Watson-Wyatt)
- Hospital and Healthcare Compensation Service
- Longshore & Simmons
- Medical Economics
- Medical Group Management Association
- Warren Surveys
- William M. Mercer

6

CHAPTER

The Give and Take of Risk Contracting

Sandy Lutz

Peter Gyorgy

The decision to enter into risk-based managed care contracting requires careful analysis and soul-searching for a physician group. Unless the organization has the proper infrastructure, information systems, and financial alignments, risk-based contracting can be a financial disaster.

Often, physician organizations have difficulty getting physicians to think of themselves as "businesses." A quick trip around the risk-contracting block will drive that point home in a hurry. There's no ambiguity in risk contracting. Failure to perform the appropriate accounting and actuarial calculations will produce a surge of red ink. If a management organization signs a bad managed care contract, they're going to lose money—it's just a question of how much.

The pitfalls associated with risk contracting are huge. So, why even consider it? Simply put, its profit potential is mightier than any other aspect of practice management.

Practice management companies go through an evolution of bringing value to their physicians. Initially, they gain savings from consolidation of certain administrative functions. But these excess expenses—what investment bankers call the "low-hanging fruit"—are quickly eliminated. After all, many groups have already benchmarked their performance against reports published by organizations like the Medical Group Management Association, and are operating relatively efficiently. There may be some additional savings that the practice management company can bring through consolidation, but it's not likely to be in the 15% to

30% range needed in order for the physicians to see ongoing value in the management fee they are paying.

How can a practice management firm continue to bring value in years two, three, and four? By focusing on building revenues. However, unless a practice management company is bringing in significant new revenues for the practices by developing ancillary services, the big jumps will have to come through risk contracting.

Here's how it works. Take $1 of managed care premiums. Of that, assume that physicians receive 30 cents, hospitals receive 45 cents, other providers take 10 cents, and the insurer keeps 15 cents for administration and profit. The higher up the "food chain" the physicians move, the more they can get of that dollar. If they are paid the entire dollar under a global capitation contract, then they can control how it's spent. If physicians are able to limit hospital utilization (and thus produce cost savings), then it may only need to pay the hospital 35 cents. The extra 10 cents moves into the physicians' pocket along with the 15 cents the insurer was collecting. (Of course, the physicians will have to spend more on administration, medical management, marketing and other costs.) The higher they move up the food chain, however, the greater the financial risks the physicians must assume.

Managed care contracting is a fact of business for physician groups (Box 6–1). The success factors of contracting are many.

BOX 6–1

THE COMPLEXITIES OF REIMBURSEMENT

Ninety-two percent of physicians were in practices that had contracts with one or more managed care organizations, up from 88% in 1996, according to the American Medical Association.

However, by signing on to more and more contracts, physicians increase their administrative headaches. For example, of those practices with managed care contracts, 52% have more than 10 contracts, according to a 1997 survey by the National CPA Health Care Advisors Association.

Physicians are notorious for signing multiple managed care contracts, with little analysis about how profitable they will be. The CPA Health Care Advisors Association survey also reported that 46% of physicians say overall profits have decreased since they began participating in managed care contracting.

The share of practice revenue from managed care contracts was 44.2% in 1997, up from 38.4% the previous year.

Interestingly, capitation revenues declined in 1997. The AMA reported that the percentage of practice revenue from capitated contracts dropped to 7% in 1997 from 8.4% in 1996.

RISK CONTRACTING BASICS

Physicians exhibit varying degrees of risk tolerance, which will be reflected in the degree to which their organizations are willing to participate in risk contracting. In some cases, the physician organization or practice management company will be willing to absorb all of the risk; in other cases, little (Table 6–1). Signing managed care contracts is nothing new to physicians. The American Medical Association reports that 92% of physicians now have managed care contracts. However, no two managed care contracts are exactly alike, and the degree of risk varies based on the contract terms.

Risk-contracting organizations that physician groups contract with include the following.

- Health maintenance organizations, which include staff, group, network, and independent practice association (IPA) models
- Preferred provider organizations
- Exclusive provider organizations
- Medicare and Medicaid risk plans
- Indemnity insurers
- Provider sponsored networks

The ways in which physicians are paid under risk contracting arrangements also varies. Here are some typical payment arrangements used in risk contracting, ordered from least risky to most risky.

- **Fee-for-service or discounted fee-for-service.** This is the traditional payment method. Payors usually want a discount, which may or may not be negotiable. Physicians may balance-bill under fee-for-service arrangements unless there are contractual prohibitions in place.
- **Fee schedule.** A fee schedule may include a cap or maximum fee. An example of this is Medicare's resource based relative value scale

T A B L E   6–1

Percent of Physicians with Direct Contracting Arrangements
(Ranked by Practice Size)

1 physician	8%
2–4 physicians	12%
5–9 physicians	12%
10–24 physicians	20%
25 or more physicians	31%

Source: AMA Socioeconomic Characteristics of Medical Practice 1997.

(RBRVS). The relative value scale uses a predetermined weighted value (called the "conversion factor") for each procedure or service performed. That conversion factor is then multiplied by a fixed dollar amount to determine the reimbursement amount. Modifications of RBRVS also are used as the basis of payment by some commercial insurers and managed care plans. For example, some insurers may pay physicians 150% of Medicare fees, while others may actually discount the Medicare rate to 80% or 90% of fees. Under these arrangements, physicians are usually prohibited from balance-billing for changes over the set fees.

- **Case rate or package pricing.** Bundled case rates refer to a reimbursement method that combines both the institutional and the professional charges for a particular procedure into a flat-rate payment. For example, a bundled case rate for hysterectomy would cover the charges from the hospital, the surgeon, the anesthesiologist, and the pathologist, as well as all preoperative and postoperative care.

Before its recent financial woes hit, Oxford Health Plans was experimenting with care rate pricing through a specialty division called Oxford Specialty Management. Gathering claims data from its own patient population, Oxford determined how much it was paying out per episode of care for patients with specific types of cases in 12 carved-out specialties (for example, in OB/GYN the teams developed cases for maternity, neonatology, hysterectomy, and infertility). Then, Oxford solicited bids from physician specialty groups that were interested in handling those types of cases. The physicians would be paid case rates for an entire episode of care, and it was up to them to manage the care. Oxford would pay the physicians on an installment basis: they would receive an initial payment, a secondary payment, and a final payment when the job was done. The kicker was this: the specialists' bids had to be at least 20% below what Oxford was currently spending on those patients' care.

Oxford was sending a message that, because the specialist is the purchaser of whatever inpatient hospital, lab, radiology, physical therapy, home healthcare, or consulting physicians services the patients require, they were at the "hub of the wheel" for practicing cost-effective medicine. It also forced the physicians to think about the continuum of care and gaining efficiencies as a patient moved through the care pathway. Therefore, groups could take risks, manage care, and still make a profit. To ensure that profit was not maximized at the expense of quality, Oxford put together report cards on the specialty teams so that enrollees could select these teams when they entered the health plan. This process required a lot of information and careful planning to make it profitable for the physician teams. However, it also increased quality because it made physicians accountable for their care from both a cost and quality perspective.

- **Capitation.** Under capitation, physician groups may receive a per-member, per-month fee to provide physician services to a defined population of health plan members. This rate will vary depending on the specialty and degree of utilization for that specialty. For podiatrists, it may be a few cents per member per month; for primary care physicians, it may be $40 per member per month (Figure 6–1).

- **Global capitation.** This is also a per-member, per-month payment; in accepting it, however, a physician group agrees to accept full risk for all professional, institutional, and ancillary services needed by a patient. That means if the patient is hospitalized, the physician group pays the hospital bill. If the patient requires outpatient rehabilitation services, the physician group makes the arrangements and pays the bill.

     Global capitation holds the promise of the most risk and the most reward. If a health plan's hospital utilization has been high, the savings from a utilization management program designed and followed by physicians under a global capitation payment mechanism can produce

FIGURE 6–1

Percent of Physicians with Capitated Contracts

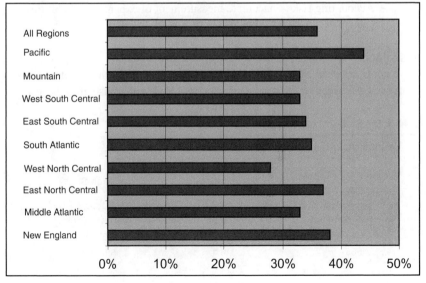

large rewards. If patient days were at 1,500 per thousand annually, and the physician group reduced that to 800 days per thousand, that translates into huge financial rewards for both the physician group and the health plan (Table 6–2).

Potentially, a physician could earn more under this type of payment arrangement than from a fee-for-service model. However, physicians must have a firm understanding of their practice patterns and services costs before entering global risk contracts because the risk—having to bear all costs associated with providing all care to a health plan patient—is significant.

Nature of Risks
Risk contracting entails numerous risks. These include the following.

- Underwriting risk—unfavorable morbidity, demographics, risk selection, statistical fluctuations, and technology
- Price level risk—unanticipated changes in subcontracted costs, fee and capitation levels, and nonnegotiated costs
- Utilization risk—inability to deliver anticipated utilization levels
- Environmental risk—impact of competitive, political, and regulatory pressures on the adequacy of pricing
- Marketing risk—membership shortfalls that affect fixed outcomes
- Legal risk—risks associated with quality of outcomes
- Accounting risk—inaccurate measurement of expenses or liabilities that can create problems with cost analysis and pricing

Risk Pools
Risk pools are used by managed care plans to share risk with providers and encourage cost-effective utilization of services. Risk pools also may be used to

T A B L E 6–2

National Averages for Hospital Utilization

Age	Discharges	Average Stay
<15 yr	38.2	4.6 days
15–44 yr	87.0	3.8 days
45–64 yr	117.2	5.3 days
65+ yr	346.1	6.5 days

Source: National Hospital Discharge Survey by the National Center for Health Statistics.

provide a financial cushion for incurred but not reported (IBNR) expenses or unusually costly claims.

Typically, a percentage of capitation payments is held back by the HMO and deposited into the risk pool. Withholds generally range from 5% to 25%. Risk pools can be either internal or external. An internal risk pool may be collected by a physician group and paid out if certain financial or clinical targets are met. An external risk pool may be collected by the health plan and paid out according to its own targets.

All providers—hospitals, physicians, labs, and outpatient centers—may be paid out of the same risk pool so it's important to determine how the pool will be distributed. One of the big savings in managed care contracts stems from reducing inpatient hospital days. How those savings are distributed through the risk pool will be an important part of negotiation.

Risk pools may be distributed either quarterly, semiannually, or annually. The contract should state when the risk pool is to be distributed. There has to be a lag time to make sure that all the claims have been paid. An appropriate time frame would be within 60 days of the operating year.

Medical Management Issues

Under managed care, physicians are a key component in controlling the utilization of services by a health plan's members. In most contracts, the physician organization will be required by the health plan to establish a medical management or utilization review function. They'll want to determine on the front end who is responsible for medical management. If it's the physicians themselves, then how are they paid for those services?

The building blocks of utilization management (UM) are peer review, in which physicians review each other, and clinical benchmarking. Reviews are typically performed in-house by physicians or nurses, although some managed care organizations are increasingly contracting with outside vendors called utilization review organizations. The American Accreditation HealthCare Commission/ URAC is an independent not-for-profit organization based in Washington, D.C., that accredits utilization review and utilization management organizations. The American Association of Health Plans provides a directory of these organizations.

Physician management organizations need to keep in mind that traditional utilization review methodologies may not be effective in reducing utilization because the group's traditional methods of reviewing utilization may have been developed in a fee-for-service environment.

If the physician group wants the health plan to delegate utilization management, that needs to be specified in the risk contract. Typically, the health plan or payor will want to conduct a site visit to determine whether the group is capable of handling that function before contractually agreeing to such arrangements.

If the physician organization wants the health plan to handle utilization review, the organization must look carefully at the plan's policies in this realm. Things to consider include the following.

- Physician responsibilities
- Types of reviews and approval/denial criteria
- Appeal process
- Grievance process
- Emergency admissions
- Role of the medical director
- Health plan specific ("non-standard") utilization review criteria

Contracting Tips

There's Strength in Numbers

As physician groups get larger, they tend to get more involved in risk contracting. Strength in numbers offers some degree of shelter from the barrage of managed care restraints. In recent years, some physicians have been "deselected" from, or denied participation in, managed care contracts, either for economic or quality reasons. Physicians often affiliate with health systems because they don't want to be locked out of managed care contracts. In fact, physicians are less likely to be dropped from those contracts when they're in larger groups. According to the AMA, only 3% of physicians in groups of 25 or more reported being denied contracts (Table 6–3). That percentage climbed as the group size decreased.

"Just Say No"

A desire to gain clout in negotiating with heavy-handed health plans also is fueling consolidation of the physician market into larger groups. "The contracts that major managed health plans are offering to physicians are becoming increasingly one-sided," said the late Ed Hirshfeld, vice president of health law for the American Medical Association, in an address to the American Health Lawyers Association in June 1998. "Some health plans have not stopped at the use of leverage to drive down costs. They have engaged in conduct that has been arbitrary, unfair and generally cavalier toward physicians. These health plans believe that they have enough economic leverage to get away with treating physicians badly."[1]

A few years ago, it was practically an anathema to turn down a managed care contract, but that's starting to change. Physicians in an IPA or group practice that is too large to be ignored have the power to reject a managed care contract.

---

[1] Hirshfield, E. (1998). Physicians, Unions and Anti-Trust. American Health Lawyers Association, June 28–20.

TABLE 6–3

Percent of Physicians Denied Contracts (Ranked by Practice Size)

1 physician	18%
2–4 physicians	14%
5–9 physicians	13%
10–24 physicians	10%
25 or more physicians	3%

Source: AMA Socioeconomic Characteristics of Medical Practice 1997.

If the reimbursement rate is too low or the managed care organization is financially frail, the physician group may be better off rejecting the contract or negotiating more favorable terms. Why sign a contract with a health plan that is slow to pay, provides too little reimbursement for no increase in volume, or provides no new market penetration?

Physician organizations can help physicians determine which contracts are worth signing. When First Physician Group in Irving, Texas (now part of PhyCor) was asked to sign a new managed care contract with a large HMO, it looked carefully at the contract terms. The deal contained a pharmacy cap: If the primary care physicians spent more on pharmacy than the contract allowed, those physicians would have to pay the additional costs themselves. Hundreds of area physicians, unable to determine whether the contract would make or break their income levels, signed on blindly. Yet, First Physician held back, taking time to pay a consulting company $50,000 to analyze whether that provision would be detrimental to its physicians. The consultants found that the group's physicians would lose some $300,000, collectively, if they agreed to the contract.

As a result, First Physician negotiated the pharmacy cap out of the contract. The contract ended up costing other area physicians millions of dollars. Those losses eventually led to a long legal battle and involvement by state regulatory agencies when physicians complained that they were having to pay for the drugs out of their own pockets.

"The problem isn't that risk is bad. It's the lack of structure in these relationships that's bad," said Robert Boyle, who was First Physician's CEO at the time. "Because of our size, we were able to spend the money to analyze the contract. Many smaller organizations couldn't afford to do that," he noted.

Before signing a risk-based contract with a health plan, consider these questions.

- Does the health plan give the group an opportunity to expand its market share?

- Could the physician group become an exclusive provider, thereby gaining more volume?
- Does the health plan have a history of prompt payment?
- Is the health plan expanding its market share, and how will that affect the physicians contracting with it?
- Is the health plan developing a Medicare product, and will the physician group be required to contract with that as well?
- How is the health plan pricing its service to employers?
- How will the health plan market its provider groups to employers?

Some groups recommend doing a survey of the market and the prevailing price scheme before taking on capitation risk. For example, survey physicians about how much reimbursement they're receiving from different payors. Go to the state's department of insurance and look at the budgets of HMOs and health plans licensed in the state. Analysis of those budgets and the plans' enrollment base can provide a quick estimate of per-member, per-month costs. Also, several software programs are available that are designed to help physicians with capitation contracts.

Watch Out for Contract Language
Managed care organizations may push voluminous legal contracts onto unwary physicians who are not savvy or informed enough to recognize the potential damage that can result.

In general, contract language is a powerful tool. Many terms (for example, *assignment*) have specific legal meanings. Those meanings usually are spelled out in the definitions section of the contract. If any of the definitions seem limited or unreasonable, the physician group should negotiate changes.

There should be no assumptions or ambiguities about what such terms mean, or misunderstandings may result. For example, if the contract blurs the terms *covered service* and *medically necessary service,* it may leave it up to the insurer—and not the physician—to determine what is medically necessary. Recently, physicians in Florida rebelled when a major insurer reportedly presented them with contracts giving itself unilateral authority to change material terms of the contract and to make determinations of medical necessity.

In some cases, contract terms may conflict with state laws. For example, a contract may indicate that the health plan and the physician group jointly own all data collected on a patient. However, some states dictate that medical records are owned by the physician; others (notably, the health plan) will require the consent of the patient to access that information.

Gag clauses also are illegal in some states. These clauses, which prohibit physicians from discussing with patients alternative treatments that are not covered by the health plan, continue to be included in many contracts. Typically, they're phrased in a way that prohibits a physician from implying that the care a patient is receiving is inferior because his health plan won't pay for it.

A rule of thumb: the bigger the health plan's market share, the more likely its contracts will have more restrictive convenants. Practice management organizations that contract with physicians must be alert for red flags. Table 6–4 is a chart of red flags to look for in managed care contracts.

Do Some Due Diligence

It's a wise move for physician groups to check out the financial, clinical and patient satisfaction ratings of health plans from which they accept risk.

Over the past year, physician groups have been stuck with unpaid bills from managed care companies that filed for bankruptcy. The financial status of health plans should be thoroughly researched before signing a contract, especially in recent times. According to a September 1998 report by Weiss Ratings, an insurance and financial ratings agency, the financial state of HMOs is grave. Weiss reported that 57% of all managed care companies lost money in 1997, and, nationwide, they suffered a combined loss of $768 million.[2] (See the Resources section at the end of the chapter for the Weiss Web site address.)

It's common practice for new or smaller health plans to cut their premiums to gain market share. Physicians groups should take extra precautions when contracting with these organizations. If the rates are too low, the reduced cash flow may affect the plan's services, administrative functions, or ability to pay down the road.

Several organizations provide report cards on managed care organizations that allow physician groups to get a clinical snapshot of the companies with which they're dealing. Perhaps the best known is the National Committee for Quality Assurance (NCQA), which accredits health plans and produces an annual report on quality indicators for these plans.

In 1998, for the first time, MEDSTAT Group, in conjunction with J.D. Power and Associates and New England Medical Center, released a report on how well physicians like the health plans they're dealing with. The consortium surveyed 9,000 physicians on their satisfaction with health plans in Atlanta, Lansing, Memphis, Greater New York City, San Francisco, and Southeast Michigan. Those types of surveys are likely to proliferate as physicians become more selective about their health plan partners.

Clean Claims

The expectation of payment is a given in contract law. When a physician group signs a risk agreement, it must agree to pay physicians within a certain time period, usually 30 to 60 days. In some cases, HMOs have been negligent in paying their providers within the prescribed period. In addition, some IPAs and practice

---

[2] "Weiss study finds combined $768 million loss," Modern Healthcare, Sept. 14, 1998.

TABLE 6–4

Red Flags in Managed Care Contracts

Contract Section	YES (Acceptable Language)	NO (Nonacceptable Language)
Amendments	■ Modifications in writing	■ Modifications without written consent ("as amended from time to time")
Arbitration/dispute resolution	■ Right to seek resolution ■ Costs paid to prevailing party ■ Useful for "any dispute related to agreement" ■ Arbitrator must be disinterested third party	■ Binding decision
Assignment	■ Assignment, delegation, or transfer in writing	■ Assignment, delegation, or transfer without written consent
Attorney's fees	■ Costs paid to prevailing party	■ Shared legal costs
Billing/claim submission	■ Reimbursement within 30 days ■ Right to bill members ■ Description of "clean claim" ■ Ability to extend required submission period ■ Notification of incomplete/pending claims	■ Inability to bill members ■ Claim form "acceptable to payor" ■ Immediate claim submission ■ Health plan not obligated to reimburse if hospital or physician group exceeds designated time period for claim submission ■ "Use of best efforts" in timely reimbursement ■ "Hospital or physician group will bill and health plan will reimburse the negotiated amounts"
Binding effect	■ Binding upon parties and successors/ assignees	
Certification	■ Termination if health plan's certification becomes impaired	

Red Flags in Managed Care Contracts *(continued)*

Contract Section	YES (Acceptable Language)	NO (Nonacceptable Language)
Amendments	▪ Termination if utilization review organization's certification becomes impaired	
Choice of law	▪ Laws of provider's state government	
Claims audits	▪ Notification of claims pending for review/audit ▪ Abide by hospital's or physician group's policies on reviewed/auditied claims ▪ Reimbursement of __% for audit/reviewed claims ▪ Notification if claims are pending beyond 30 days ▪ Reimbursement of hospital-incurred costs ▪ Retrospective denial will not occur if the hospital/physician has cooperated with the health plan's utilization review program	▪ Non-reimbursement of hospital/physician incurred costs for audits
Confidentiality	▪ Confidential information held in strictest confidence ▪ Definition of "confidential information"	▪ Confidential provision, if it favors health plan
Coordination of benefits	▪ Negotiated rates apply only to Primary Carrier	▪ Total reimbursement to not exceed the negotiated rate
Credentialing programs	▪ Cooperation with physician group's credentialing program	▪ Compliance with health plan's credentialing program
Eligibility/verification of coverage	▪ Prompt eligibility verification	
Entire agreement	▪ Exhibits, attachments, and amendments ▪ Supersedes all prior agreements ▪ Modifications in writing	▪ Modifications without written consent ("from time to time as deemed necessary")

Red Flags in Managed Care Contracts *(continued)*

Contract Section	YES (Acceptable Language)	NO (Nonacceptable Language)
Exclusivity/noncompete provision	▪ Notification of changes in provider network ▪ Renegotiation of rates if changes occur	▪ Contracting restrictions imposed on hospital or physician group
Grievance procedure	▪ Notification of changes to grievance procedure ▪ Opportunity to terminate contract	▪ Modification without notification or consent ("from time to time") ▪ Obligation to comply with grievance procedure
Indemnification	▪ No indemnification provision, or provision protecting hospital or physician group against health plan's negligence	▪ Unilateral indemnification provision protecting health plan
Insurance provisions	▪ Documentation of general and professional liability ▪ Designated dollar amounts ▪ Notification of reduction in coverage, expiration, or cancellation ▪ Terminated if coverage is not maintained	▪ No designated dollar amount ("adequate coverage")
Medical records	▪ Access to only medical and billing records related to covered services ▪ Authorization from member ▪ Reimbursement of copying costs ▪ No access to utilization management or quality assurance program reports ▪ No access to peer review committees' reports	▪ Access to "any" books or records
Medical staff membership and privileges	▪ No obligation to admit participating physicians who do not meet hospital's medical staff's credentialing requirements	▪ Granting of temporary admitting privileges ▪ Expedition of the admitting process for participating physicians

Red Flags in Managed Care Contracts *(continued)*

Contract Section	YES (Acceptable Language)	NO (Nonacceptable Language)
Most favored nations/more favorable agreements	■ No provision	■ The provider will give health plan a reimbursement rate no less favorable than it gives any other payor
Names and products	■ Approval of marketing materials prior to distribution	■ Distribution of marketing materials without group's approval
Notices	■ Notification in writing ■ Delivery in person or by certified or overnight mail	
Payor	■ Provider can terminate agreement with payor under certain conditions	■ No responsibility to ensure payors will meet their obligations
Precertification/ authorizations	■ Reimbursement if member makes mistake ■ No prior authorization for emergency services ■ Time period to notify health plan of admission	■ Authorization prior to providing service
Reimbursement	■ Reimbursement within 30 days ■ Reimbursement if member makes mistake ■ Minimization of financial risk ■ Annual renegotiation of rates	■ Restrictions on billing members ■ Notification prior to anniversary date
Reimbursement—pricing strategies and related provisions	Discount-off charges: ■ Negotiated rates applicable to covered services only ■ Nondiscounted physician charges Per diems: ■ Multi-tier per diem structure ■ Removal of high cost procedures ("carve-out") ■ Stop-loss on global or per case basis	■ Multiyear rates without renegotiation provision ■ "Cap" on outpatient rates ■ Limited time period to renegotiate rates

Red Flags in Managed Care Contracts *(continued)*

Contract Section	YES (Acceptable Language)	NO (Nonacceptable Language)
	▪ Exclusion of physician charges from negotiated rates ▪ Request to renegotiate rates ▪ Annual automatic rate increase ▪ Global outlier or stop-loss per case for outpatient package	
Silent PPOs	▪ Discounts will be extended only to members of the PPO who have cards identifying them as such ▪ All PPO members eligible for discounts will be subject to steerage mechanisms ▪ Types of entities that can be added to the network are identified in advance ▪ Provider receives timely notice when payors or employees are added to the network ▪ Any discounts applicable to a PPO enrollee will be disclosed at the time coverage is verified ▪ Sale or other unauthorized use of contract rate information is specifically prohibited	▪ Language that promises "best efforts" by the PPO to steer enrollees
Subcontracting		▪ Restrictions on the right to subcontract services
Survival	▪ Sections which continue after termination	▪ Termination only on contract anniversary date
Term, termination, and obligations thereof	▪ Termination without cause (provider's right) ▪ Termination for cause or material breach	▪ Termination after advance notice

Red Flags in Managed Care Contracts *(concluded)*

Contract Section	YES (Acceptable Language)	NO (Nonacceptable Language)
	■ Termination if health plan or payor files for bankruptcy	■ Continuation of services in accordance with contract terms
	■ Termination if health plan loses its license or certification	
	■ Reimbursement for charges after termination date	
	■ Continuation of parties' obligations after termination	
	■ Termination with defaulted payors	
Unforeseen circumstances	■ Protection if unforeseen circumstances prevent provider from fulfilling obligations	
	■ Definition of "unforeseen circumstances"	
Waiver of breach	■ Right to enforce obligations of other party	

management organizations also have been negligent about paying their physicians. Indeed, as a physician group becomes the risk bearer, it, too, may bear the wrath of providers if it drags its feet about paying claims.

There are two concerns for physicians as they enter risk contracts, one as the risk bearer and the other as the provider to a risk bearer. Because of the widely publicized cases in which HMOs were not paying their bills, some states have begun to legislate these reimbursements to provider groups.

For example, in Florida, managed care payors are assessed interest penalties if payment on "clean claims" takes longer than 35 days; however, the penalty doesn't apply to disputed claims. Recently, a major insurer in the state announced it was reviewing all office visit claims due to concerns that physicians may have been upcoding. Physicians, in turn, retorted that the insurer was merely trying to get out of making the interest payments.[3]

---

[3] "Doctors battle HMO in code war," by Gary Sheperd and Susan Lundine, Tampa By Business Journal, Sept 28, 1998.

Global Capitation

Physician organizations travel through an evolutionary process. First, they focus on operational efficiency. Next, they increase revenues through ancillary expansion or managed care contracts that have very limited risk. Meanwhile, they'll put information systems into place and begin sharing clinical and financial data. Only then should a physician organization consider taking on global risk-bearing contracts that potentially could sink the organization.

When an HMO enters into a global capitation arrangement with a physician group, it transfers its burden of payment and management to the physician group. In essence, the globally capitated medical group will function very much like an HMO. Running this type of business is very different from running a physician practice. It requires incorporating insurance functions such as underwriting and actuarial rate development into the practice's day-to-day operations.

A physician organization that wants to take on global capitation contracts should go through a thorough strategic planning process to determine if it's ready to make that leap. Groups will want to consider "Going Prepaid," a publication from the Medical Group Management Association that takes groups through a series of planning steps prior to making this complex decision.[4]

Utilization Management

Taking on global capitation relieves a physician group from having to deal with a utilization management regimen imposed by a third-party payor. At Kaiser Permanente, for example, a physician goes through fewer hassles in ordering a procedure than would a physician contracting with an HMO or IPA. However, the onus is on the globally capitated medical group not to go broke. Accepting full risk can be suicidal if a practice does not have excellent information systems and appropriate financial incentives to control utilization.

Regulation

In many states, assuming risk for services that aren't provided directly is akin to being an insurance company. Physician groups considering global capitation will need to research the insurance laws of the state(s) in which they operate to determine the level of risk they can take and the types of licensing required. In California, provider groups that take global capitation must obtain a Knox-Keene license (the state credentialing required of health maintenance organizations).

The reasoning behind the California law is that a provider group accepting global capitation should have the financial wherewithal to provide services for a large population of patients with sufficient reserves to cover unforeseen risks. For

---

[4] DeMarco, W.J., Garvey, T.J. (1986). Going Prepaid: A Strategic Planning Decision. Medican Group Management Association, September.

example, if a physician group accepted capitation for its services only and ran out of money, they could still provide services—they'd just be working for free. However, if the physician group had accepted global capitation and stopped paying a hospital from which it had purchased inpatient services, the hospital would likely stop providing services as well. That would leave patients in the lurch, something state regulators tend to frown on. That rationale underlies another California law prohibiting physician groups from accepting global capitation for hospital services unless the group owns a hospital.

The costs associated with licensure can easily exceed several million dollars, including statutory reserve requirements. Ongoing compliance with licensure regulations can also be expensive and time-consuming.

Pricing

When a group is functioning as an insurer of a risk, it must bear in mind that a natural rate cycle exists in the insurance business. Health insurance premiums rose at double-digit percentages in the early 1990s, then began to trim back. By 1996, HMO premiums actually dropped by nearly a percentage point, according to Sherlock Company's annual HMO rate survey. However, in 1997 and 1998 premiums began to inch up, and predictions are the upward cycle will continue for the next couple of years.

Understanding the underwriting cycle and its direction will benefit a physician group in its future contract negotiations. Here are Watson Wyatt Worldwide's predicted rate increases for 1999, by types of plan.

- 15% to 22%, prescription drug
- 12% to 15%, indemnity
- 9% to 11%, PPO
- 7% to 9%, point of service
- 5% to 7%, HMO[5]

These percentages vary by region and should not be expected to directly reflect increases in provider reimbursement. Physician groups should rely on their internal data when entering negotiations with a payor on a new or existing contract.

Subcontracting

When taking global risk, the physician organization, of necessity, will need to subcontract certain services it cannot provide, such as inpatient and ancillary services. In doing so, the physician group will have to determine how it will pay its subcontractors. This process raises many questions. What is the market's prevailing rate for these services? What's a realistic rate? Should these providers be

---

[5] "Health-care costs: it's deja vu all over again." *Business & Health,* September 7, 1998.

paid on a capitated, discounted fee schedule, per diem, or a case rate? What clinical standards should be set for these contractors?

Hospitals may be paid under a per-member-per-month arrangement or on a discounted charges schedule. However, the most common way to pay for subcontracted hospital services is per diem—a fixed amount per patient per day. Under a per diem arrangement, the hospital is paid a flat rate per day for inpatient care, including all required ancillary services. While sometimes an overall per diem may be negotiated, hospitals often prefer a negotiating handful of different per diem payments: one for the surgical unit, one for ICU, one for CCU, and another for obstetrics, chemical dependency, or psychiatric.

Per diems include all the costs associated with inpatient care, allowing the physician group to get a handle on hospital inpatient use. Because the hospital is the most expensive setting, physician groups will want to ensure they don't overuse this service setting. In addition, the costs involved in a hospital stay tend be the greatest in the first few days. Hospitals usually make their greatest profit margin on the latter end of a patient's stay, when the patient is recovering, demanding less care. That's why it's important to carefully monitor those stays. Per diems do not control output costs at the hospital.

Marty Stango is regional director and general manager of Heritage Southwest Medical Group in Dallas, an IPA affiliated with 320 primary care physicians and 1,200 specialists. Heritage contracts for full risk and provides credentialing, claims adjudication, and utilization management services to its physicians. Heritage has contracts with nine health plans. Its physicians can opt for the health plans they want to contract with, but they can't split plans. In other words, they can't say "yes" to a health plan's commercial product, and "no" to its Medicare product. Heritage has contracts with 50 other healthcare vendors, including hospitals, outpatient surgery centers, and laboratories.

Stango noted that in the Dallas/Fort Worth marketplace, contracting requires an understanding of referral relationships within a 200-square-mile area. The market of 3 million residents has distinct service pockets and few large multispecialty firms. No single medical group can cover the entire "Metroplex" area, which requires risk contracting to be a crazy quilt of relationships. Because residents often work in areas that are different than the ones they live in, the web of providers must stretch across many natural boundaries, such as major highways, rivers, or neighborhoods.

Physician groups that do risk contracting need to research practice patterns among specialists. Patient visits by specialist may vary by region. For national figures, see Table 6–5.

Stango has this advice for medical groups interested in global capitation.

- Make sure everyone understands the responsibilities being assumed and paid for.

TABLE 6–5

Patient Visits per 1,000 Population per Year

696	General practitioners/family practitioners
397	Internists
353	Pediatricians
226	OB/GYN
155	Ophthalmologists
145	Orthopods
110	Dermatologists
77	Psychiatrists
71	General surgeons
70	Otolaryngologists
56	Cardiovascular diseases
52	Urologists
32	Neurologists
279	All other specialists
2,720	All physicians

Source: The National Center for Health Statistics in the National Ambulatory Medical Care Survey. Based on data from 1995–1996.

- Get down to specific details when crafting your provider network, and understand the subpaths of care involving your providers. Who are the specialists? To which facilities do they refer? At which hospitals do they have admitting privileges? If you have specialists who admit to hospitals not in the network, it's going to mean additional payments for out-of-network providers. Also, if the primary care physicians have referral patterns with specialists who aren't in the network, that "leakage" will cost money.
- Have a clear payment policy for clean claims and define what constitutes a clean claim. Your providers should be paid in 30 days for clean claims, but they need to understand what "clean" constitutes.
- Have a clear understanding of co-pays and who's responsible for collecting them as well as handling coordination of benefits.

Disease Management
Global capitation allows a physician organization to take an evolutionary step toward being a disease management company. Chronic diseases take a huge bite out of the healthcare dollar—as much as 50% by some accounts. Yet, study after study has shown that carving out these members from the general enrollee popu-

lation and giving them preventive care tailored to their specific conditions results in documented financial savings for the health plan and improved health status for the patients. Kaiser Permanente and Aetna U.S. Healthcare are among the dozens of managed care companies that have initiated disease management programs within the last few years to reap the benefits of this cost/quality equation. Different types of disease management programs include asthma, HIV, chronic obstructive pulmonary disease, back pain, and other chronic illnesses.

In some cases, health plans initiate disease management programs as part of an accreditation process with the National Committee for Quality Assurance (NCQA), a group that compares HMOs based on selected indicators. The NCQA requires evidence of quality improvement for accreditation. It's part of a continuing cycle. Employers are demanding quality information. NCQA demands such information from health plans for accreditation approval. Health plans establish disease management programs to address quality concerns. Health plans establish practice guidelines and case management processes that physicians must follow to receive reimbursement.

In some cases, physician-driven health plans are also seeking NCQA accreditation, thereby setting up the disease management programs themselves.

Carve-Outs

The physician organization may want to subcontract or carve out certain services that other organizations may be able to perform more economically. Practice management companies are wise to determine what services they can profitably contract for and which ones are better left to specialty companies. Mental health and chemical dependency services are often carved out to specialty companies. Vision and dental services also are frequently carved out.

Another area that physicians may want to consider for carve-out is pharmaceutical benefits. There's a widespread presumption that because physicians are the ones who issue prescriptions, they can exert significant controls over pharmacy costs. Marty Stango of Heritage doesn't believe that's necessarily true. "The onslaught of direct-to-consumer advertising by pharmaceutical companies makes it harder for physicians to control those costs now than has been the case in the past," he said. He's referring to the fact that pharmaceutical companies have increased spending on consumer advertising to get patients to ask their physicians to prescribe certain name-brand drugs. As a result, drug spending continues to rise with no abatement in sight. In fact, U.S. spending on drugs is expected to double from $62 billion in 1996 to $171 billion in 2007, according to the latest estimates from HCFA. That statistic should be a warning to physician groups bearing risk—the costs are expected to escalate quickly, and it's going to be difficult to manage.

Both pharmacy benefit managers and HMOs receive rebates from pharmaceutical manufacturers to encourage them to recommend certain drugs. That's one way to mitigate the risk of rising drug costs. Although drug costs may rise as the number of prescriptions rise, the PBM or HMO offsets that rise with an increased rebate from the pharmaceutical company. Physician groups may not get that same type of deal when they're asked to bear risk in pharmacy costs, making it a much riskier proposition. However, large physician groups or practice management companies that develop national risk contracts may be able to cut the same deals as HMOs with pharmaceutical companies. In other words, they may be in a position to also receive rebates to include certain drugs in their formularies. Then, the question may be, do they want to be in a position to receive rebates for prescribing certain drugs?

Direct Contracting

Some risk-savvy physician groups bypass the risk contracting organizations and enter into direct contracting agreements with employers (see Table 6–1). The American Medical Association's annual survey reports that larger physician groups are more likely to be involved in direct contracting. Direct contracting may seem like an attractive avenue for sophisticated physician groups because it eliminates the middleman. However, the group also would have to be able to differentiate itself in the market place to snag the attention of large employers. Such differentiation is difficult without data to back it up. Even with such data, it may be difficult to get employers interested without a significant marketing effort. Direct contracting also requires volume to spread the risks, making it difficult for small groups of physicians to do it themselves.

The legal ability of provider groups to directly contract varies from state to state. For example, Minnesota recently passed a law allowing such contracting with cooperatives of hospitals and doctors.

The Balanced Budget Act of 1997 contained provisions aimed at encouraging providers to form special groups to engage in direct contracting with the Medicare program. This is discussed in the following section.

PSOs—Medicare's Offer to Shift Risk to Providers

Before President Clinton signed the Balanced Budget Act of 1997 (BBA), Medicare beneficiaries had two health insurance coverage options: the traditional Medicare indemnity coverage, and Medicare HMOs. The act created a new program, Medicare+Choice, to provide beneficiaries with new private-sector choices for coverage, including provider sponsored organizations (PSOs).

In essence, a PSO (or *provider sponsored network,* as they are sometimes called) is a globally capitated provider entity that is formed for the purpose of direct contracting with Medicare or other entities, such as employers. It's like an HMO with the middleman eliminated; in fact, Medicare will reimburse PSOs in the same manner as it reimburses HMOs—with monthly capitated payments for each enrollee. The Congressional Budget Office estimates that PSOs, when fully phased in, will enroll one million seniors, or about 2.5% of all Medicare beneficiaries. At the end of 1998, only a half dozen PSOs were operating.

PSOs are expected to have some of the same appeal to beneficiaries as HMOs—for example, providing alternatives that cost less or provide more benefits than traditional Medicare. Because PSOs will be run by providers who form their own organizations, they are expected to draw from the most reputable hospitals and physicians in local markets, which also will be appealing to seniors. This can be a double-edged sword, however. Medicare HMOs have tended to be popular with seniors who have fewer health problems and, therefore, aren't as wedded to their choice of doctors as chronically ill individuals tend to be. However, when an HMO-type organization that features those doctors is formed, the chronically ill beneficiaries may be delighted to find that their favorite physicians are part of a new PSO that will provide them more benefits and significant out-of-pocket cost savings. If PSOs are flooded with costly, high-acuity patients, this may result in adverse selection.

Physician groups need to carefully consider whether to become a provider sponsored network, as the effort will entail considerable expense, capital investment, and risk.

Capital Requirements

A PSO's capitalization must come from the providers themselves. Although a PSO can be entirely physician driven, it's wise to include a hospital in the ownership because of the capital they can bring to the organization. The required capital investment is significant—the start-up costs are estimated to run from $8 to $12 million and include the following.

- $1.5 million set aside for statutory reserves
- $6 to $10 million in operating capital for the first two to four years
- Consulting fees ranging from $600,000 to $1 million

According to HCFA, PSOs must be able to meet the following solvency requirements.

- *Tangible assets.* A provider group must have tangible assets of $1.5 million or more, half of it in cash, in order to start a PSO. All of a physician group's tangible assets—such as clinic buildings and equipment—can be counted toward meeting the requirements. (Once the PSO is up and running, the requirement drops to $1 million.)
- *Intangible assets.* If $1 million of the $1.5 million is in cash, HCFA allows 20% of the remainder to be in intangible assets such as capitalized management services agreements. If less than $1 million is in cash, only 10% of the remainder can be in intangibles.
- *Projected losses.* HFCA requires that the PSO have enough cash on hand to cover the first six months of projected losses. Realistically

speaking, however, start-up PSOs are likely to face up to four years of operating losses. That fact alone may be sufficient to convince a physician group that it wants to sit out this particular round of risk contracting. For those that decide to go forward, outside consultants can help with projections of losses.

The Application Process

If physicians decide to go forward, they are likely to need consultants to help them with the complexities of preparing the PSO application, such as the following.

- The application must include a map illustrating that a market's Medicare beneficiaries have access to the organization's primary care and specialist physicians. The ratio of Medicare beneficiaries to primary care physicians must be adequate for the market. The PSO must directly provide at least 70% of all healthcare services and items required by its enrollees.
- All network contracts and physician credentialing must be completed before the PSO can submit its application.
- A draft of the PSO's marketing materials must be included with the application. (HCFA provides a template to guide the PSO with preparation of these materials.)

It may be wise to hire a consultant as project manager for the application project and use the provider's own managers to carry out the various functions. Here's why: Before approving the application, HCFA will do a site visit to verify the organization's credentials. If an outside consultant has merely put together a turn-key program without local involvement or input, the HCFA surveyor will quickly catch on when asking questions of the local managers. For example, the HCFA surveyor may ask questions pertaining to information contained in the materials submitted. If an outside consultant wrote those materials with little input from the providers, it might be hard for the local provider to answer specific questions. That could result in a denial of the application.

The completed application can be filed on-line at HCFA's Web site.

Licensure

PSOs must also apply for a state license (Figure 6–2). If the state has more stringent PSO solvency standards than the HCFA requirements discussed above, or if the state fails to act on the PSO's license application within 90 days, the PSO may apply for a federal waiver from HCFA. Waivers are only available through October 31, 2002. If a waiver is granted, a PSO still must apply to HCFA for a federal license to operate a PSO. The application to file a waiver also is available at HCFA's Web site.

FIGURE 6–2

PSO Application Requirements

> **1.** Contracts with network participants
> **2.** Credentialing of providers
> **3.** Geo-access map

Hospital Sponsored PSOs

Most PSOs will be formed by hospitals, not physician groups. However, physician groups may be asked to join in the ownership of PSOs with local hospitals. In some cases—for example, when a hospital has a dominant market share and the PSO will be a major marketing vehicle—physician groups will find it advantageous to join the PSO.

If physicians join a hospital-sponsored PSO, physicians need to be sure that the financial risk is shared fairly among providers. The biggest savings in capitated contracts usually comes from cutting hospital patient days. Physicians need to be sure that the contract's financial incentives benefit outpatient as well as inpatient providers. The biggest mistake a hospital-owned organization makes in forming a PSO is protecting market share of inpatient bed days. However, bed days will likely decline, and the PSO's financial incentives need to be structured to recognize that outcome. A hospital sponsoring a PSO will have to expect a decline in bed days as care is managed more tightly for Medicare beneficiaries.

Other Issues to Consider

- Some critics question the financial feasibility of PSOs. While HMOs must have at least 5,000 enrollees to be allowed to contract with Medicare, PSOs are allowed to get in on the act with as few as 500 enrollees. That may not give them enough healthy enrollees to offset the costs of treating sicker members.
- Under the BBA, HMO and PSO rates will be held to a rate of growth that is below that of Medicare expenditures in the fee-for-service sector. Medicare's per-member-per-month rates traditionally have been set at 95% of what the government estimates it would have expended for that member under the traditional Medicare system. Due to the efficiencies inherent in the managed care programs, the government figured that health plans would be able to manage profitably at this amount. In fact, HCFA analysts believe that due to factors such as favorable selection, health plans could still be profitable at rates that were 10% less than

fee-for-service (FFS) expenditures. The problem is that under the BBA, it is estimated that the HMO rates will deteriorate to 89% of FFS expenditures by 2003 (Table 6–6). At that level, many HMOs and PSOs may encounter financial struggles.

- Physician companies also need to consider that a PSO is an insurance company. Becoming an insurance company involves dealing with a whole new realm of regulations. It also requires a change in mind-set: this is a whole new way of operating a business, requiring specialized expertise that goes well beyond medical management. Furthermore, physicians—who may regard insurers as adversaries—will have to get used to being on the other side of the payor equation.

- Physician groups also may want to consider whether they want to cross the tracks in terms of their reputation in the community. If a physician group carries high esteem in the community and HMOs are regularly slammed in the media, why would a physician group want to risk muddying its reputation?

Here are some questions physicians should ask before forming or joining a PSO.

- How will the capitation dollars be divided between physicians and other providers?
- How quickly can physicians refer patients to other physicians inside and outside the network?
- Do physicians have experience in managing populations?
- Are your patients—who may enroll in your PSO—going to drive up costs because they represent a more acutely ill population?

TABLE 6–6

Medicare+Choice Capitation Rates (Average Medicare Risk Enrollee)

	Year		
	1997	1998	2003 (est.)
Fee-for-service	$546	$565	$742
Capitated plans	$519	$530	$658
Ratio	0.95	0.94	0.89

Health Policy Economics Group, PricewaterhouseCoopers LLP.
Source: Based on data from the Health Care Financing Administration and the Congressional Budget Office.

AN EXPERT'S PERSPECTIVE: BILL GIL, SENIOR VICE PRESIDENT OF MANAGED CARE, UNIMED MANAGEMENT CO., BURBANK, CALIF.

In the risk-contracting sphere there are two different worlds: California and everybody else. California's mix of payors, the size of physician groups, and regulatory activity set it apart from the rest of the country when it comes to matters of risk contracting. California physicians typically contract with 15 different managed care plans; this means that they must keep track of 15 sets of referral, prescribing, and utilization systems to receive reimbursement.[6]

With 20 years of experience in risk contracting for physician groups, Bill Gil understands the evolution that takes place as managed care contracting ripples through a local market.

"The laws of economics in medicine are no different than in the restaurant industry or the automobile industry," said the UniMed executive, who is a frequent speaker on risk contracting at national conferences. "It makes physicians nuts when I say that because they say, 'No, healthcare is different.' But it's really not." Burbank, Calif.–based UniMed operates groups with about 6,000 physicians, including one of the state's largest independent practice associations, Huntington Provider Group in Pasadena.

Gil paints the following scenario of how risk-based contracting changes the economics of a local healthcare market.

Take a large metropolitan area where physicians are generally being paid on a fee-for-service basis. At the urging of employers who want to curb benefit costs, HMOs enter the market, and they're anxious to sign up as many providers as possible. As an incentive, the HMOs offer to pay physicians 150% of the Medicare fee schedule.

A few years later, the HMOs add Medicare products to their offerings. Because the area has traditionally enjoyed high Medicare HMO per capita rates and has had few controls on utilization, the per-member, per-month reimbursement allows HMOs to make a healthy profit margin off the Medicare business, say $50 per enrollee per month. So, to gain even more market share, they underprice their commercial HMO product, figuring they can make up the profit on the Medicare enrollees and step up overall enrollment. The commercial HMO product is now priced below the traditional indemnity product. More employers offer it, more employees sign up.

Soon, physicians see the winds of change. More and more of their patients are now enrolled in HMOs. These physicians, too, join the HMO momentum and begin signing more managed care contracts. As overall HMO penetration increases, so does the physicians' dependence on those contracts. Another phenomenon takes place. Overutilization is squeezed out of the system because

---

[6] Number of Managed Care Contracts per Practice, American Medical Association, Physician Marketplace Statistics, 1996.

physicians' practice patterns are closely monitored by the HMOs and physicians realize that their reimbursement will be higher if they don't overutilize services.

As the HMOs become more dominant, their leverage increases. When its time for contract renegotiations, they only offer physicians 100% of Medicare rates instead of 150%. Physicians don't like it, but these contracts have by now become the lifeblood of their practices. Without them, they could lose their patient base. As a result, the physicians become dependent on HMOs for patient volume.

During the next five years, the squeeze becomes a tourniquet. HMOs offer physicians less and less reimbursement. Physicians continue to sign the contracts even though their revenues are dwindling. Eventually, reimbursement slides to 70% or 80% of Medicare rates, and provider profits are minimal.

Physicians, like restaurants and auto dealers, become subject to the same factors of marketplace leverage as other businesses. "It's very rational, very logical," Gil explained.

The only way to survive in that climate is to discern which contracts are profitable and which aren't, Gil said. "Until recently, nobody was really negotiating on a cost-based approach," Gil said. "Although your per-member, per-month minimum might be $38, you'd take from $36 and up. Even if your dumpster price was $36 and the best they offered was $34, groups sometimes signed the contract anyway and slowly bled to death."

For years, physician groups were cavalier in signing managed care contracts because they didn't want to be left out. Risk-based contracting involved a lot of back-and-forth negotiating. But, inevitably, at 11:59 on the day the contract would expire, the parties would reach an agreement, Gil noted. "You'd take the last offer on the table," he said. "It didn't matter what the costs were. You figured you could subsidize one contract and make it up on others."

In California, "there was a feeling that doctors were always willing to take 10% less (than they had taken previously)," Gil said. Following the bankruptcies of some physician groups, the specter of financial disaster has made payors realize they can push too far. "We're seeing some of the HMOs act a little more responsibly about not pushing the groups into bankruptcy," Gil said.

He noted that physician groups are becoming more selective and strategic about who they contract with because margins have gotten so thin. "You're going to see more lines drawn in the sand than ever before," Gil noted. "Five years ago, you had enough margin that if you signed one or two bad contracts, it wouldn't matter." That's no longer the case. However, he pointed out that the same tight margins are impacting the health plans. "Sometimes, both of us are willing to walk away," Gil said.

In addition, "groups have started to realize that you can't wait two or three years to analyze whether a contract is a money maker or a money loser. Groups have to know what their costs are and if they're going to make money from the outset," he added. It's become incumbent on physician groups to understand their own cost structures and get them in line, he noted. "You don't want to sign a contract that

FIGURE 6–3

Contract Negotiation Tips from Bill Gil

- Know your data inside and out.
- Be disciplined. As Kenny Rogers would say, "You've got to know when to hold 'em, know when to fold 'em."
- Don't make threats if you don't intend to back them up.
- Don't attempt to negotiate if you don't have the authority to act. Don't be a fancy talker or just a messenger.
- Keep your eye on the ball—know how much every point is worth. If you can do quick calculations in your head faster than the party on the other side of the negotiation, you'll win some points.
- Remember, it's not the principle, it's the money. This is a monetary transaction. If you deal on that unemotional level, you'll get a quicker resolution.
- Payors or health plans may try to coax your group into signing by telling you that "all the other groups have signed." Don't believe them without checking it out.

loses you money, but, on the other hand, no one is going to hand you a contract that's above the market price. So, if the market price is $40 per member per month, and it would cost your group $42 per member per month, maybe you don't deserve the business. The market isn't going to subsidize anyone." Gil points to the market for new cars, saying, "Ford isn't going to drive up the market price for its cars by saying, 'But our costs are higher.'" (More tips from Gil are in Figure 6–3.)

The only products that are going to command a premium in the market are those with brand recognition, Gil said. In healthcare, a few highly regarded organizations—Mayo Clinic and Cleveland Clinic being notable examples—have brand recognition among consumers. The great wash of other providers are not going to be able to drive pricing up based on brand recognition. Consumers assume that quality is a given with their healthcare providers—they're not going to pay extra for it.

PricewaterhouseCooopers Tips for Risk Contracting

- Get everything you want in writing. Don't sign a contract now and work out the details later.
- Don't share risk with vendors who can't manage that risk. If they can't manage the risk, they'll end up having financial problems, which may impact your group and you may end up footing the bill.
- Ensure that the health plan or payor understands the data you need from it to comply with a risk contract and how data will be shared.

- Hire or contract with actuarial experts to review contracts to ensure their financial viability.
- Research your care partners' financial, clinical, and customer satisfaction status.

TABLE 6–7

Managed Care Contracting Provider Financial Strategies

Contract Type	Nature of Risk	Critical Variables	Provider Strategies
■ Discounted charges	■ Price	■ Contribution margin	■ Vary rate with volume (days or charges)
■ Per diem	■ Price ■ Intensity	■ Contribution margin ■ Volume of ancillary services per unit ■ Mix of days by unit	■ Vary rate by service ■ Vary rate by day of stay (front-load) ■ Exclude specific high cost services, products ■ Add stop-loss clause
■ Per case	■ Price ■ Intensity ■ Severity	■ Contribution margin ■ Volume of ancillary services per unit ■ Mix of days per unit ■ Length of stay	■ Exclude specific high-cost services, products ■ Increase rate for outlier days ■ Guaranteed level of payment
■ Capitation and percent of premium	■ Price ■ Intensity ■ Severity ■ Frequency	■ Contribution margin ■ Volume of ancillary services per unit ■ Mix of days by unit ■ Length of stay ■ Admission rate	■ Phase in services ■ Exclude specific high cost services, products ■ Set up contingency fund ■ Include revenue guarantee ■ Specify effective and termination dates ■ Consider buying reinsurance ■ Balance physician/hospital incentives

RESOURCES

www.urac.org—The American Accreditation HealthCare Commission/URAC accredits health plans and utilization management organizations.

www.ncqa.org—The National Commission for Quality Assurance accredits health plans.

www.weissratings.com—A service based in Palm Beach Gardens, Fla., that rates the financial health of insurers and HMOs.

www.hcfa.gov—The Health Care Financing Administration has applications online for PSOs.

http://www.hcfa.gov/medicare/mgdcar1.htm#operations—Operating guidelines from HCFA for Medicare+Choice organizations.

www.access.gpo.gov/su_docs—The Government Printing Office provides copies of PSO regulations.

7

CHAPTER

Fraud and Compliance: Doing the Right Thing

Sandy Lutz

Jo Ann Jany

Evelyn takes her son to see a pediatrician at the clinic where she works. The child has an ear infection, and after a five-minute exam, the pediatrician prescribes the usual antibiotic. As she leaves, Evelyn notices that her doctor coded the visit as a Level 5, the highest tier and most expensive office visit.

Evelyn knows the office visit was a perfunctory one that typically would qualify as a Level 1 or 2.

Is this fraud?

What should Evelyn do? Call the insurance carrier? Talk to the doctor or business office manager? Do nothing?

This scenario is one of several included in the integrity training at MedPartners, the nation's largest practice management company. In this scenario, Evelyn decides to talk to the business office manager, telling her the facts of the situation and that the bill was incorrectly coded.

She's done the right thing.

More employees and physicians at practice management organizations are participating in seminars in which they discuss these kinds of ethical dilemmas in the workplace. As the largest practice management company, MedPartners had one of the most comprehensive compliance programs.

Diane Nobles, compliance officer for MedPartners, advises other physician organizations *not* to play what she calls "the ostrich game." These groups can't pretend they don't know what's going on in their practice, she says.

MedPartners isn't alone, however, in realizing the importance of proactive compliance programs.

Because practice management is such a new industry, many of the lines are blurry in terms of fraud and abuse. Physician organizations must be proactive in implementing programs designed to curb fraudulent practices and stay attuned as the rules evolve and change.

Here's the bottom line: a comprehensive compliance program can prevent misconduct, avoid litigation, and mitigate penalties if employees are found breaking the law.

Although headlines about healthcare fraud have centered on hospitals, laboratories, and home healthcare services, physicians are increasingly becoming targets as well. The Office of Inspector General (OIG) in the U.S. Department of Health and Human Services alleged that the Medicare program lost $5.9 billion in improper reimbursements to doctors in 1997.

The agency also claimed that physicians made up the single largest segment of providers to receive overpayments in 1997. Overall, Medicare lost $20.3 billion in 1997 due to waste, fraud, abuse, and simple errors, HHS reported. That amounted to 11% of the entire cost of the fee-for-service reimbursements. The good news was that the percentage fell 3 percentage points from 1996.

How do such errors come about? About half the improper payments resulted from documentation errors, 26% from insufficient documentation, 14% from no documentation because of extenuating circumstances that are under investigation, and 4% from no documentation at all, the report said. About 37% of the errors were blamed on a lack of medical necessity, 15% incorrect coding, and 3% noncovered or unallowable services. The remaining 1% were due to other circumstances.[1]

Many physicians are simply not spending enough time documenting what they do, and that can be construed as never having performed the service.

Physicians and outpatient services accounted for 52% of the documentation problems, the report said, up from 47% in 1996.

To force doctors to spend more time on documentation, the federal government last year proposed new documentation guidelines for evaluation and management (E&M) services. Those services represent about 50 different Current Procedure Terminology (CPT) codes.

After an outcry from physicians, however, HCFA—in April 1998—delayed implementing these E&M guidelines, which are now undergoing significant revision.

Medicare spent $16.3 billion in 1996 on evaluation and management services done by physicians, and the agency clearly wants more detailed data on how those services are performed. "We're finding that there's no documentation," said HCFA medical officer Bart McCann, MD. "It's happening across all levels."[2]

---

[1] "Medicare audit concludes losses reduced," by Howard Fields, Heathcare News Server, April 24, 1998.
[2] "Indefinite delay on E&M," by Sean Martin, American Medical News, May 11, 1998.

Although HCFA officials said they will only pursue physicians who display "fraudulent intent" in their coding and documentation, without proper documentation, a physician organization may be hard pressed to prove the work was done. The feds have said they will pursue cases in which they see "suspicious billing patterns," "reckless disregard," and "failure to respond to appropriate education efforts." The question remains—what are the parameters for these terms?

In today's climate, practice management firms must conduct their businesses with the assumption that Uncle Sam, or his state counterpart, could at any point scrutinize any transaction, procedure, or reimbursement. The number of investigations keeps rising (Figure 7–1). Even the simplest medical procedure today can involve a complex group of referral relationships that also can be scrutinized in terms of fraud.

What is fraud?

- Billing for a service never rendered
- Billing for a more expensive service than that actually performed (known as "upcoding")
- Billing for services not approved
- "Unbundling" service charges to receive higher reimbursement
- Billing for unnecessary or complementary services or overtreatments
- Filing false claims
- Kickback arrangements

FIGURE 7–1

Number of FBI Investigations in Healthcare Keeps Growing

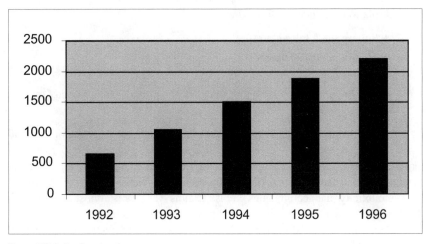

Source: U.S. Justice Department.

WHAT'S THE CHARGE, OFFICER?

Criminal Charges

Healthcare providers can be charged with numerous criminal violations that fall into one of the following categories.

- *The Anti-kickback Provision of the Medicare Act.* Under the Medicare or Medicaid acts, this provision prohibits any arrangement in which remuneration is solicited or offered in exchange for patients. It is punishable by a fine or imprisonment for up to five years, or both.
- *The False Claims Provision of the Medicare Act.* This prohibits making or causing to make false statements or representations on any Medicare claim. The penalty is the same as the anti-kickback provision.
- *Mail fraud/wire fraud.* This charge can be invoked because most Medicare and Medicaid claims are sent through the mail or wired.
- *Conspiracy.* This also can be tagged onto a fraud charge if more than one individual is involved in the fraud scheme. Same penalty.
- Other charges include money laundering, false statements, false claims, and the Racketeer Influenced and Corrupt Organizations Act (RICO).

Civil Charges

In addition to criminal penalties, a provider can be charged with civil violations of the False Claims Act. Damages include the difference between what the government paid and what the government received. In addition, the False Claims Act carries penalties of $5,000 to $10,000 per claim.

Violations include the following.

- Submitting a false claim
- Making a false statement
- Conspiracy
- Making a reverse false claim in which the provider failed to pay the government

False Claims Act cases are initiated either by a federal agency or criminal prosecutor; a private party, known as a *qui tam* case; a national initiative; or a criminal referral. In the investigation, a provider will be asked for a plethora of documents, and the discovery process alone will be extremely expensive. In addition, publicity that accompanies a False Claims Act case is almost certain to affect the share price of a publicly traded physician organization.

Qui Tam. Most False Claims Act cases now stem from qui tam complaints, which are individuals who know or suspect that a fraud is being committed. Once filed, it is up to the government to decide whether to intervene. If a provider can convince the Justice Department not to intervene, the litigation will be less expensive and extensive.

If the government intervenes, it likely will file an amended complaint, which the qui tam relator may join. Also known as "whistleblower" cases, these actions could reward a healthcare worker up to 25% of any money recovered by the government. Because these suits can reach into the tens or hundreds of millions of dollars, a whistleblower is looking at collecting a sizable bounty.

Whistleblowers can be anyone who is an "original source" of information. This can include nurses, physicians, billing and coding personnel, or competitors.

The potential rewards can be so lucrative that some law firms have advertised in such well-read publications as *USA Today* and the *Wall Street Journal,* telling healthcare workers that there are rewards for reporting Medicare and Medicaid fraud. These firms also have begun advertising on the Internet.

Such potential bonuses are having the desired effect for regulators. In 1991, only 14 whistleblower cases were filed in healthcare nationwide, according to HHS. By 1997, more than 200 were filed, the agency reported. One half of all government whistleblower cases now involve healthcare, according to the Deputy Attorney General.[3]

Once a qui tam case is filed, it's up to the federal government to decide whether it wants to join in the action. If the government decides not to join in, the cost of pursuing the case will weigh on the individual.

National initiatives. The government has pursued several of these, including the patients at teaching hospitals initiative, known as the PATH audits. Such initiatives start with the Justice Department or the U.S. Department of Health and Human Services. The PATH audits have yielded several six-figure settlements from teaching hospitals and prompted the American Hospital Association to intervene on hospitals' behalf.

Government investigations. These types of investigations often start with Medicare intermediaries that notice billing or coding problems.

Criminal referrals. Most criminal cases will be reviewed on a civil base, leading a provider to fight its case on two fronts.

Enforcement

The Health Insurance Portability and Accountability Act, passed by Congress in 1996, established new programs to rein in fraud and abuse. Essential elements included the following.

- Fraud and Abuse Control Program. This is a joint law enforcement effort to coordinate federal, state, and local law enforcement programs

---

[3] "AHA Members Urged to Watch Their Ethics," Reuters, Jan. 30, 1997.

regarding healthcare fraud. Between fiscal years 1997 and 2002, nearly $1 billion will be allocated from the Medicare hospital insurance trust fund to support the program. In addition, $434 million will be allocated from the general U.S. Treasury for specific use by the FBI. Congress created the Health Care Fraud and Abuse Control Account, which receives money from civil penalties, assessments, and fines. The money funds future fraud investigations, so the more successful the government is in its investigations, the more money it has to launch additional probes.

- Medicare Integrity Program. This permits HHS to contract with private entities to conduct the review and audit functions of Medicare Part A intermediaries and Part B carriers. Between 1997 and 2002, $3.4 billion will be appropriated from the Medicare trust fund for these activities.

- Revision of Civil Monetary Penalties. The penalty that can be collected for each instance of civil fraud increased from $2,000 to $10,000.

- Revisions to Criminal Law. Creates a section for federal healthcare offenses that allows criminal penalties to be imposed for specific types of healthcare fraud, embezzlement, false statements, the obstruction of a criminal investigation, and money laundering.

These laws have plenty of teeth. Convictions, penalties, and exclusions from government programs are on the rise (see Figures 7–2 and Figure 7–7).

THE STARK TRUTH

It's impossible to talk about fraud without mentioning the Stark rules.

Fraud and abuse laws in healthcare have long been championed by Democratic U.S. Rep. "Pete" Fortney Stark, former chairman of the House Ways and Means subcommittee that oversees Medicare. The Californian has long been a thorn in the side of healthcare providers, although his influence waned after 1994, when Republicans gained control of the House.

Stark was instrumental in initiating the ongoing investigation launched against the nation's largest healthcare services company, Columbia/HCA Healthcare Corp. He began pushing the HHS Inspector General's office to investigate the company in the late 1980s and kept the heat on for more than a decade.

When the first set of so-called "Stark rules" was issued 10 years ago, it sent a chill through the industry. After fine-tuning, however, the regulations ended up being applied only to clinical labs in which a referring physician has a financial interest.

The theory of self-referral legislation is that physicians who own equipment or facilities have an incentive to overuse them. For example, the first Stark regulations were prompted, in part, by an OIG report that showed doctors who owned or invested in clinical labs ordered 45% more lab work on patients.

Federal Agencies Increase Enforcement Activities

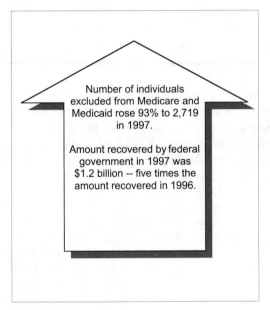

Number of individuals excluded from Medicare and Medicaid rose 93% to 2,719 in 1997.

Amount recovered by federal government in 1997 was $1.2 billion -- five times the amount recovered in 1996.

Source: HHS Office of the Inspector General.

In 1993, clarification rules for Stark I included a section referring to 10 "designated health services" and said the same self-referral language used for clinical labs would be used for these other services until the rules could be written.

Details weren't revealed, however, until January 1998, when the Stark II proposed regulations were published—over 79,000 words, consuming 70 pages of the *Federal Register.*

Those regulations, written by the Health Care Financing Administration, expanded the federal self-referral legislation to cover the following.

- Radiology, including magnetic resonance imaging, computerized axial tomography scans, and ultrasound services
- Radiation therapy
- Durable medical equipment and supplies
- Prosthetics, orthotics, and prosthetic devices and supplies
- Home healthcare services

- Outpatient drugs
- Physical and occupational therapy
- Parenteral and enteral nutrients, equipment, and supplies
- Inpatient and outpatient hospital services

This directly impacts physician organizations, some of whom boost their revenues through integrating usage of ancillary services. To meet the Stark rules, management organizations need to realize that these designated services need to be provided by the group practice, not the management company.

Needless to say, Stark II—although not yet approved—complicates fraud concerns for physicians. In fact, in a letter to HCFA about Stark II, the Medical Group Management Association (MGMA) referred to the 60 pages of fine print commentary that accompanied it, saying it could "become the 'lawyers and accountants relief act' of the next millennia."

MGMA wrote HCFA, noting several problems in the new rules. One overriding concern to the trade association—and its physician group members—was that the rules seemed to set up increasing road blocks to the integration that so many physician practices are working toward. "Stark remains a serious impediment to integration and managed care contracting," wrote MGMA president and CEO, Thomas L. Adams. He noted that on one hand, the government is smoothing the way for integrated networks to contract at risk with Medicare and Medicaid. Yet, on the other hand, the government is telling physicians that those at-risk arrangements may break the law when used in a fee-for-service model. "The same financial and clinical relationships that are developed to serve Medicare and Medicaid risk contract enrollees are often used to serve some Medicare fee-for-service patients, particularly those in commercial managed care plans, but with secondary Medicare coverage. Thus, the exception that protects those financial relationships in the case of prepaid enrollees is of little value if those relationships don't fit nicely into one of the other Stark law exceptions."

The Stark II regulations are aimed at group practices, particularly "clinics without walls" in which physicians work at various locations but share the costs and profits of expensive equipment.

Under Stark II, a device, such as an x-ray machine, must be located on the same premises as the referring physician, and the technicians must be directly supervised by the referring physician, or a member of his group.

Some exceptions in the proposed rules benefit physician management organizations. For example, in-office ancillary services are exempted, although those services must be furnished personally by the referring physician, one in the same group practice or an individual supervised by the physician in the same group practice.

Another benefit to physician management organizations: the rules prohibit some of the below-market-value deals that have enticed physicians to join hospital networks instead of physician companies. In the same vein, physician management organizations must be careful if they're leasing space or equipment from a hospital to ensure that the rent is consistent with fair market value.

For now, Stark II regulations are in the proposal stage. However, physician management organizations must realize that these rules are a framework for laws that will govern their work in the future.

AN OUNCE OF PREVENTION: COMPLIANCE PROGRAMS

A compliance program provides the proverbial "ounce of prevention," giving physician management organizations an infrastructure to identify and eliminate possibly fraudulent behavior. Practice management firms should have a corporate culture that deters fraudulent activities and ensures that employees and physicians know that there are consequences to such activity.

While compliance programs are a fairly new concept to many physician groups, they are becoming more standardized in corporate America. Some 86% of 240 companies surveyed have formal compliance programs, according to a 1996 Survey of Corporate Compliance Practices by PricewaterhouseCoopers.

The PricewaterhouseCoopers survey reported that healthcare companies were more likely to adopt compliance programs after 1994. In fact, of the 30 industries survey, healthcare had the largest group—24%—adopting such programs after 1994.

Compliance programs cut across several areas that are important to physician group operations. For example, a strong compliance program will integrate with financial auditing to ensure proper coding and reimbursement. It also strengthens a physician group's risk management and quality control.

Leo E. Sands, chief compliance officer for American Oncology Resources, said the compliance program he instituted in 1998 incorporates many of the same initiatives as the accreditation process AOR is going through for Joint Commission on the Accreditation of Healthcare Organizations. "There's a nice cross-pollination," between the programs, Sands said. "Documentation on one side feeds the other."

The OIG has issued model compliance plans to help guide healthcare organizations. Not surprisingly, hospitals are more likely than physician organizations to have codes of ethics (Figures 7–3 and 7–4).

While those plans can provide guidance, it's best to tailor a compliance program to the complexities of the practice management business.

A physician group that is dragging its feet about establishing a corporate compliance program need look no further than the penalties that could be handed down in a fraud conviction. Criminal or civil penalties can be imposed on the corporation and individuals involved. The federal sentencing guidelines establish a complex, but mandatory formula for imposing fines in criminal cases. A base

F I G U R E 7–3

Physician Executives Who Say Their Organizations Have Business Codes
of Ethics

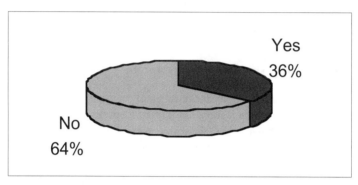

Source: PricewaterhouseCoopers, Hospitals & Health Networks.

F I G U R E 7–4

Hospital Executives Who Say Their Organizations Have Business Codes
of Ethics

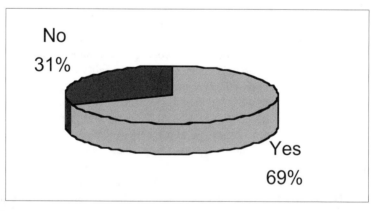

Source: PricewaterhouseCoopers, Hospitals & Health Care Networks.

level is determined, then adjusted depending on aggravating or mitigating factors.
In terms of fines, the amount is determined by calculating a base fine, which is altered depending on the corporation's "culpability" score.

The government took the carrot-and-stick approach to incentives here. The
stick delivers a system of consistent and adequate punishment to punish corporate
crime. However, as a carrot, it wanted to offer corporations the possibility of low-

ering its penalties if it put in place an "effective" compliance program. The key word here is "effective." The government will determine those that work well and those without substance.

With an effective program, a corporation's culpability score is reduced, which potentially can save millions of dollars in fines.

The following are the factors that the sentencing guidelines set out as part of an effective compliance program.

- Establish compliance standards, procedures, and policies.
- Assign oversight responsibility to an individual high in the organization's structure.
- Conduct effective training and educational programs.
- Utilize monitoring and auditing to detect noncompliance and improve quality.
- Develop effective lines of communications for reporting violations and clarifying policies.
- Enforce standards through well-publicized discipline guidelines and procedures.
- Respond appropriately and immediately to detect offenses and prevent further offenses through systemic changes and corrective initiatives.

The sentencing guidelines also set out the following "relevant factors" for an effective compliance program.

- Size of the organization. Generally, the larger the physician organization, the more formal its compliance program should be.
- The likelihood that certain offenses may occur because of the nature of its business. If there is substantial risk that illegal activity could occur, the responsibility for having an effective compliance program increases.
- Prior history. Organizations with past problems should be more aware of the problems that can occur and have programs in place to handle them. For healthcare companies that have settled fraud investigations with the federal government, a compliance initiative is typically required as part of the settlement agreement.

In addition to possible fines and jail sentences, physician organizations convicted of criminal fraud can be excluded from the Medicare and Medicaid program for five years or more.

Baseline Audit

The first step toward building a compliance program is a baseline audit. Where is the practice right now in terms of compliance issues? Does a written code of ethics exist? What kind of training program is available? What is the process for reporting violations? What risk issues exist for this organization?

Some organizations may want to perform an ethics risk assessment, which identifies and prioritizes the pressure points and incentives that give rise to the biggest ethics risks. This type of assessment can be done by an outside consulting firm to provide preventive strategies and the diagnostics of an ethics and compliance program.

It also gives the physician group a starting place and a way to measure future progress as well.

A management company often is a collection of physician practices, each of which will have a history of their own accounting and billing. Historical accounting records must be reviewed, and this may involve building an electronic database in order to analyze and retrieve the relevant information.

Obviously, a physician group must start out on the right foot by putting together a structure that doesn't invite fraudulent practices. Issues that must be considered include the following.

- Evaluate incentives and compensation structures for physicians. Physician contracts need to be scrutinized and benchmarking practices must be assessed to determine whether they encourage fraudulent practices.
- Link technical data of billing and coding with related accounting and compliance filings.
- Install software that can detect upcoding, unbundling, or other billing abnormalities.
- Review financial relationships with physicians, especially in light of recent advisory opinions by the OIG.

Code of Conduct

Another early step is to write a code of conduct. Although it may be tempting to simply replicate another practice management company's code, practice management firms will do well to tailor the code to their own particular business.

The code should encompass relevant federal, state, and local regulations. Obviously, this would include fraud-related laws, but also should include topics such as sexual harassment and copyright laws.

Each employee should receive a copy of the code of conduct, which should include the following elements.

- Ethical principles
- Detailed explanations of the laws
- A hotline phone number (hotlines will be explained later in the chapter)

- Statement that whistleblowers will not be subject to retaliation
- Explanation of how investigations are handled

The code may be prefaced by a letter from the CEO or compliance officer and a company "mission and values statement." Many healthcare organizations already have one of these. If not, this is a good time to develop one because the mission statement can give credence to the code.

By way of example, American Oncology Resources' code of conduct includes different sections that address issues such as quality of care, conflicts of interest, protection of proprietary business and patient interests, and billing, coding, and records integrity.

In conjunction with writing the code, practice managers will want to write down the procedures and policies that employees and physicians must follow in the jobs they do. For example, some physicians traditionally granted courtesy discounts or waived co-pays for fellow physicians, a practice now considered illegal. Written policies should also address other financial practices, such as self insurance, bad debt, and financial hardship.

The code should be distributed to each employee, who should sign a form indicating that he or she understands and will comply with it. Physician management organizations shouldn't assume that only certain employees in certain departments are liable to commit fraud. Any employee can witness fraudulent activities.

MedPartners' code is a 27-page booklet that includes written policy statements on business conduct, patient care, treatment of employees, financial and professional records, compliance with the law, company property, confidential information, conflicts of interest, marketing practices, government requests, and community commitment.

MedPartners also distributes to employees a small, wallet-sized card that includes the Ethics Helpline telephone number and the TRUST decision-making model (Figure 7–5). Other practice management companies may want to consider producing such a card as an easy reference tool for employees.

A Compliance Officer

During the last few years, many physician groups began to appreciate the importance of a compliance officer to the operations of its physician clinics.

Christopher Ideker joined Medaphis Physician Services Corp. as compliance officer in 1997. Atlanta-based Medaphis provides a range of services for 17,000 physicians in 47 states, including data input, medical coding, billing, cash collections, and accounts receivable management. About one-fourth of the nation's physicians use an outsourcing company like Medaphis for these services.[4]

---

[4] Medaphis S-1, March 6, 1998.

The TRUST Ethical Model

MedPartners employees are advised to think about ethical situations by using what MedPartners calls the TRUST ethical decision-making model.

- **Think** about the situation.
- **Recognize** motivations.
- **Understand** company policies and applicable laws.
- **Satisfy** the "Headline Test"—how would this look if the media or your family found out about it.
- **Take** responsibility for your actions.

Upon his appointment as compliance officer, Ideker immediately began focus groups to document the company's procedures. The focus groups included 20 employees, three consultants, and two attorneys to determine where the risks were and what controls were in place to overcome the risks.

Ideker, a certified public accountant formerly with Pricewaterhouse-Coopers, put together an 18-person compliance department and $4.5-million budget for the first year. After the first year—1997—the compliance budget will probably shrink to $3 million, Ideker said.

He got the company's board and management to agree to the program, although implementation included significant disruptions to everyday business. Ideker recommends getting support from the board, chief executive officer, chief financial officer, vice president of human resources, and vice president of marketing. "They will become your biggest supporters if properly convinced," he noted. (Other tips from Ideker are in Figure 7–6.)

One segment of the plan was core competency training for coders. Certification for employees who do coding is emerging as a new standard in the industry, and as part of its compliance program, Medaphis decided to require that its coding supervisors complete one of the three coding certification programs.

The company agreed to pay for the coding certification training and pay the supervisors a bonus if they passed. The bonus was larger in 1997 than 1998, creating an incentive to go through it sooner rather than later.

In addition, Medaphis upgraded the skills of front-line coders by designing an 80-hour coding class that became a requirement as well.

In addition to this investment in training, Medaphis purchased a $1.75-million information system that can detect billing abnormalities and might spot fraud before it happens.

Ideker also urges practice management organizations to hire experts in this field. For example, he recommends retaining an experienced attorney who has both healthcare knowledge and white-collar crime experience. The compliance

FIGURE 7–6

Minefields to Plan For

- Getting a buy-in from middle management may be more difficult than from top management. It falls on middle managers to find the time for training their workers and implementing the program.
- When a billing problem is found, it may be difficult to rectify it. Some payors don't have procedures in place for refunds. Medaphis found that some payors deducted from future bills; others simply returned the refund checks.
- Implementing the plan may be more difficult in a decentralized environment. Since many PPMs are decentralized, recognize those challenges and design the plan with those problems in mind.

Source: Christopher Ideker, Medaphis.

program must have an adequate regulatory library, he added. Medaphis has five employees in its regulatory group that keep up with changes in this area. It also may be wise to consider contracting with industry consultants with knowledge in the field, he said.

Medaphis' physician clients are extremely interested in preventing fraud. In 1997, Medaphis took that one step further by teaming with the Graham Company, a Philadelphia-based insurance broker, in 1997 to develop an exclusive insurance product that will pay for losses (civil fines, penalties, and multiple damages) incurred by a physician for any actual or alleged breach of duty, misleading statement, omission, or act in billing his or her professional services.

At MedPartners, Diane Nobles assumed the job of compliance officer when her firm, Caremark, merged with MedPartners in late 1996. Because Caremark had settled with the federal government over a fraud charge a year earlier, the Illinois company was required to have a compliance program, ethics classes, and hotline as part of its settlement agreement.

Nobles used the merger as an opportunity to expand MedPartners compliance initiatives. She successfully convinced MedPartners' board to agree to fund a substantial compliance program in 1997, which expanded the department from herself to 25 individuals.

Because of MedPartners' growing size, Nobles realized that MedPartners must have a top-notch program: "We're not a small physician practice in Iowa. We're MedPartners, and everyone in government knows who we are. The level of scrutiny is different," Nobles said.

MedPartners had grown very quickly through acquisition, and a compliance program had not been developed prior to the Caremark merger. Acquiring multiple firms also presents on-going compliance challenges. This isn't unusual for a fast-growing physician management organization, where other priorities push the details of compliance aside. "It's very unusual for a practice management company to be organized as we are," Nobles said.

Nobles has responsibility for five areas: due diligence, setting standards and policies, compliance audits, training and education, and enforcement.

Around those tasks, MedPartners' compliance department is divided into four departments.

1. Coding, billing, and reimbursement
2. Quality and regulatory services—issues with the Food and Drug Administration and the Drug Enforcement Agency, CLIA laboratory certification
3. Education—ethics training, hotline, program development
4. Environmental health and safety—hazardous waste disposal and liability, Occupational Safety and Health Administration issues

If a physician group isn't big enough to support a dedicated compliance officer, it may want to consider having a senior-level executive take on those duties. In hospitals, the OIG has suggested that the compliance officer not report to the general counsel because they don't want the same person in charge of compliance and enforcement. Physician groups should consider that advice in designating individuals for their programs.

As physician groups consider whether to have a dedicated compliance officer, the following are some responsibilities for that position.

- Conduct baseline audit of compliance
- Design and implement compliance program
- Distribute fraud alerts to physicians and employees
- Document compliance training and sign-in sheets
- Oversee and document hotline activity
- Work with general counsel and human resources director on compliance issues
- Document any investigations that take place
- Handle and document disciplinary procedures

Ethics Training

To ensure that employees understand the company's procedures and standards, practice management companies must design training programs. The earlier-mentioned scenario with Evelyn is part of an hour-long integrity training session that is required for all MedPartners employees once a year. New MedPartners employees must go through the compliance program training within the first two months.

"People solve their own problems," explained Mary A. Bennett, director of education and program development for MedPartners, about the real-life situations that are presented and discussed in the sessions.

MedPartners employees are encouraged to know the law and regulations affecting their jobs, know where to go for support, and be proactive. "Don't just sit on an issue, hoping it will go away," the trainer tells employees during these sessions. MedPartners hopes to give employees the tools, and perhaps the courage, to take a stand in their everyday work environment.

MedPartners' integrity training tells employees that they are the conscience of the corporation. It is each employee's responsibility to know the laws and regulations related to their job and know what to do if an ethical dilemma arises. In the training video, MedPartners managers explain that integrity is defined as "the consistency between your ethical standards and your behavior."

More than 500 MedPartners managers are trainers for the sessions. Although there's some debate in the industry about whether to use employees or outsiders as trainers, Bennett believes employee managers make the best trainers.

Other advice from Bennett on designing an ethics training program includes the following.

- Sessions should last at least one hour. Anything less than that is not worthwhile.
- Live, interactive sessions work best and keep people's interest.
- Don't make it a one-time event. It may take three years of ethics training to get the values fully ingrained in the corporate culture.

For MedPartners' 1998 ethics training, Bennett adopted themes from *How Good People Make Tough Choices,* a book by Rushworth Kidder. The book stresses looking at ethical situations through four themes.

1. Truth versus loyalty
2. Individual versus community
3. Short term versus long term
4. Justice versus mercy

For example, under the "justice versus mercy" theme, one scenario involves a nurse who breaches confidentiality to tell a cancer patient's daughter about the availability of free care. Should the nurse's supervisor fire her?

Bennett recommends that practice management companies allow their compliance programs to evolve as the company matures. What starts out as a compliance program should eventually mature into an ethics program that teaches values on a visceral level and empowers employees to make tough choices, she noted.

Although a practice management firm can require employees to go through the ethics training, it may not be able to do the same with physicians because most physicians are not employees of the practice management firm. "We offer the training to physicians as business education," said MedPartners' Bennett.

AOR makes appeals to its physicians, telling them, "This is in your best interest as a doctor," Sands said. Then, the training materials are specifically tailored to their needs.

Columbia/HCA Healthcare Corp., which underwent a massive ethics initiative in 1998, uses videotapes featuring physicians to deliver its message about a new compliance program. Columbia's code of conduct can be viewed on the Internet (see Resources at the end of the chapter).

Be prepared for the attitude by physicians and employees that they don't need ethics training. Some may even be insulted by the suggestion that they need to be taught how to make good decisions. Unfortunately, good ethics don't come naturally.

Here's evidence: A recent survey of 30 young managers who graduated from Harvard's MBA program found that most had performed unethical acts.[5] The report said that the MBAs admitted to being pressured to act unethically to meet expectations of their organizations. More importantly, the survey found that corporate ethics programs, codes of conduct, mission statements, and hotlines can make no difference. Instead, corporations need to weave ethics into their overall operation, not make it a stand-alone function. Physician organizations and health systems need to ensure that their training is consistent with what the company is trying to accomplish. This may involve transforming the company culture and communicating that transformation in the training sessions.

Coding

When talking about fraud, the first issues that come to mind are coding, billing, and reimbursement.

MedPartners' Dan Untch heads up billing and coding compliance, a hot button in any discussion of compliance and fraud. His department spends about 50% of its time on audits at MedPartners clinics. The other 50% of the department's time is spent in regulatory policy development, assisting clinics with Medicare audits and postaudit follow-up with the clinics. In addition, the department monitors changes in coding, billing and reimbursement through a variety of publications including the *Federal Register.* The *Federal Register* is published daily, reporting on proposed and final rules developed by HCFA.

Untch also edits a quarterly newsletter, "Coding Educator," that updates the clinics on changes in the industry. Both the CPT book *(Current Procedural Terminology)* and the ICD-9-CM *(International Classification of Diseases, 9th*

---

[5] "Business ethics: A view from the trenches," California Management Review, January 1995.

Edition, Clinical Modification) publish additions, deletions, and revisions on an annual basis. A recent issue of their newsletter included a full page filled with new ICD-9 codes for 1998 and another that listed invalid ICD-9 codes.

Other changes in billing are reported in the newsletter also. For example, in 1998, Medicare made changes in the billing for nonphysician practitioners, such as nurse practitioners and physician assistants, allowing them to bill directly. That affected many of the MedPartners clinics and the bills they mail out.

Because coding has become so specialized, many practices use some kind of coding software. However, in late 1998, the HHS inspector general's office said it was looking into the use of automated encoding software in billing Medicare for physician services.[6]

Auditing

In determining whether a compliance plan is effective, the government will analyze how it functions. It's not enough to put a compliance program into place; executives must monitor it on a regular basis.

At MedPartners, compliance audits are conducted throughout the year at practices large and small. Typically, the larger practices are audited regularly and smaller ones are audited on a random basis or when a problem is indicated.

Each group in MedPartners' compliance department dispatches two- or three-person audit teams that go in the field. For example, in Bennett's group, auditors make sure that employees have gone through the training and have signed sheets testifying to that.

Many physician organizations aren't large enough to conduct such audits on their own, so they contract with their outside auditors. This type of partnership can work hand in hand with the compliance department.

One single-specialty practice management company extended the responsibilities of its auditors, PricewaterhouseCoopers, to include random audits for compliance purposes. In that way, the auditors can work closely with compliance to ensure that standards and policies are being carried out appropriately.

Audits typically cover four main areas: policy, billing, contracts, and marketing materials. Auditors also can assess the risks. These include the following.

- Past violations
- New regulations
- Acquisitions
- New management
- High employee turnover
- Expanded operations

---

[6] "HHS plans to add doc, DME probes," by Kristen Hallam, *Modern Healthcare*, Oct. 19, 1998.

These factors apply to all corporations, but practice management companies—by their nature—embody several of those risk factors. They are expanding organizations that are making many acquisitions and encounter numerous new regulations.

Outside auditors can help establish systems that are designed to detect improper conduct and ensure that reports are made to top management on a timely basis. As well as ensuring that the company has reliable financial reporting, auditors are able to look at the efficiency of the operation.

If a practice management company or health system is accused of fraud, regulators will want to know if regular audits were conducted during the time period of the unlawful activity.

Due Diligence

Physician groups often make acquisitions, which will require due diligence into past activities that may have the potential for fraud.

MedPartners integrated compliance audits into the due diligence process. The compliance department sends a checklist to the targeted practice of compliance procedures to determine where the practice is in terms of meeting MedPartners' standards. Nobles' team also conducts an on-site audit and interviews the practice's top officers.

"If you don't look at all, that's the worst of all positions," Nobles said. If there is a problem, the government is not going to buy the argument that the problem occurred before the practice was acquired, she pointed out. "You want to create a trail that you made a reasonable effort to look at what's going on," she advised.

A physician group may want to engage "forensic" accountants and other consultants to ferret out whether the physician practices have in the past engaged in billing or coding that could be interpreted as fraudulent by regulators.

Nobles mentioned these red flags to look for in proposed acquisitions.

- No ethics policies in place
- Lack of staff knowledge in proper coding and billing requirements
- Excessive third-party insurance denials
- Aberrant patterns of physician billing—one physician accounts for a disproportionate share of billings; this could signal upcoding by that physician or other physicians using his or her provider number
- Lack of physician interest and sensitivity to issues in coding and billing

A full compliance audit of a clinic may not be completed until after the acquisition is completed. Because of confidentiality issues, the clinic may not be able to release certain medical records that contain information about billing practices.

Corporate Hotline

A physician organization should establish a pathway for employees who have questions about compliance issues or simply want to report a problem.

A corporate hotline gives an organization the opportunity to head off problems before they worsen. Large physician groups should assume that without a hotline, a disgruntled worker who notices fraudulent activity could decide to "blow the whistle" by filing a qui tam action. Obviously, the organization would rather be notified first.

MedPartners' hotline receives about 100 calls a month. Not surprisingly, hotline calls usually spike in the winter and spring months when the ethics training is in process because workers think more about the choices they make on the job.

Two MedPartners compliance department workers handle all hotline calls. Callers are asked to provide the name of the facility and business unit they work in, but are not required to give their names. They're encouraged to handle the problem locally, but if that's not possible, hotline workers will contact managers and field staff themselves. In some cases, an on-site investigation is conducted.

Healthcare organizations often find the vast majority of hotline calls are human resources issues—complaints about bosses or coworkers.

AOR contracts with an outside service for its hotline, and Sands said a rule of thumb is that a hotline generally will receive one call per 1,000 employees per month, implying that it's not cost effective to bring the effort in-house in organizations with less than 5,000 to 6,000 employees.

Investigations and Disciplinary Procedures

Physician group executives must coordinate an investigation if there is a possible problem. This may include retention of outside counsel who can structure an investigation so that it can remain confidential. However, the practice management firm may eventually have to disclose the results of that investigation.

If a practice management company or health system finds what's determined to be "credible evidence of misconduct," it must be reported to the appropriate federal agency within a reasonable amount of time. Although the Office of the Inspector General has not identified what qualifies as "reasonable" for physician companies, the agency has specified that it not be more 60 days for hospitals and labs in both of their model compliance plans.

No matter how bad its bark, a compliance program is nothing without a strong bite. Disciplinary procedures must be established well in advance and be strictly observed. That sends a message to employees that the physician organization is serious about compliance, and that it maintains consistent enforcement.

Management Incentives

Many healthcare organizations that manage physicians have begun to include compliance goals in bonus programs for managers. If managers don't complete the compliance goals, they won't receive bonuses, regardless of financial performance.

In addition, employees' completion of ethics training is frequently a part of their evaluations.

AOR's Sands said the company's bonus structure for managers has compliance goals. If they don't meet those goals, managers can lose their whole bonus.

Measuring Up

The following are some questions that physician management organizations can ask themselves to determine the success of their compliance program.

- Can employees recite the company's 800 hotline number or identify where it's posted?
- Is the hotline answered in a timely manner?
- Is the record of the call disseminated in a reasonable time frame to the appropriate persons?
- Has disciplinary action been taken against employees identified to be engaged in inappropriate conduct?
- Is the program being monitored to determine whether denials are related to compliance or medical necessity issues?
- If overpayment, refund, quality of care, or legal issues are detected, are corrective actions adequate in scope and timeliness?

SO, WHAT'S THE COST?

Compliance programs can cost from $100,000 to several million dollars. When drawing up a budget, consider the following.

- How much government business does your practice do?
- How many different kinds of government business does your practice do? For example, some practices also have home healthcare businesses. That type of business entails an additional layer of government regulation and scrutiny.
- What is the risk and what will it take to manage that risk?

FIGURE 7-7

The Feds Are Serious About Fraud

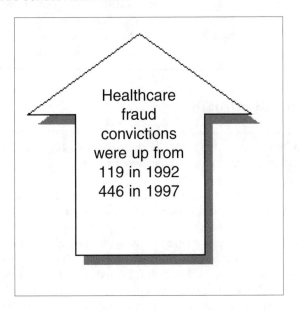

Healthcare
fraud
convictions
were up from
119 in 1992
446 in 1997

Source: FBI.

Practice management companies soon realize that the cost of compliance programs goes far beyond the training seminars, consultants, published materials, videotapes, and compliance personnel. The effort also takes a considerable amount of time from top and middle managers, who must be involved and shepherd the project along.

Another cost to be considered is the possibility of lower revenues. If physicians were aggressively billing the government or private payors in the past, a compliance review may diminish reimbursement.

One way to rationalize the cost is that a thorough compliance program is likely to be far less costly than a government investigation. Any government investigation is likely to drag on far longer than anyone likes, and those costs will mount as time passes. Many of the large Medicare fraud investigations have lasted a year or more. And, remember that failing to cooperate with a government investigation may prompt regulators to broaden a healthcare fraud investigation into one of obstruction of justice.

Federal investigations tend to draw attention from other sources, which effectively multiplies the cost. Many executives don't realize the cost of an investigation mounts with outside consultants and counsel, space for investigative staff and documents, getting copies of seized documents and medical records back, disruption of executive staff and physicians, as well as staff time in accounting and billing.

A federal investigation that makes its way into the newspapers is often followed by lawsuits from commercial payors. Shareholder suits often follow if the company is publicly held and news of the suit negatively impacted the stock price. At this point, a healthcare provider is fighting an expensive battle on a number of fronts.

A WORD ABOUT DENTISTRY

Much fraud is couched in terms of Medicare and Medicaid, and that may lead dentists to believe they don't need to be concerned. However, in 1998 Valley Forge Dental began instituting a compliance program that mirrors many being implemented on the medical side.

"We have felt that given some of the events that have happened over the years in the publicly traded healthcare companies, we should create a compliance program while we're still a private company," said Joseph J. Frank, president and CEO of Valley Forge Dental Associates, King of Prussia, Pa. The dental practice management firm has practices in Colorado, Florida, Georgia, Maryland, New Jersey, Ohio, Pennsylvania, and Virginia. "Even though the payor mix in dentistry is remarkably different, it's better to do it sooner rather than later," said Frank.

While physicians receive an average of 40% of their payment from Medicare and Medicaid, dentistry is generally not covered under the Medicare program. Medicaid reimbursement is limited to pediatric cases, meaning the percentage of payment from government programs is very small.

Frank and his management team believe, however, that both indemnity and managed care payors will become more diligent about payment practices and policies, making fraud a concern for dentists. Managed care makes up about 20% of reimbursements for dentists.

"Education is really necessary," said Jeanne Marie Welsko, Valley Forge's vice president of human resources. Because dentists traditionally haven't dealt with compliance programs, they need to understand the importance of such a program.

Senior management from operations, finance, and human resources have designed the program, and the company's chief financial officer will be overseeing the program as the corporate compliance officer. Many of the compliance functions—training and hotline—will fall under Welsko's responsibilities.

AN EXPERT'S PERSPECTIVE: PAUL DEMURO, PARTNER WITH LATHAM & WATKINS

Compliance programs that seek to curb fraud are a thorny issue for practice management companies because of the complicated structures of these organizations and their relationships with physicians.

"It is a much more difficult situation than in any other industry," said Paul DeMuro, who has worked with numerous practice management organizations as a partner with Latham & Watkins in Los Angeles and San Francisco. "The nature of the relationship between the management organization and the doctors is somewhat unique. This industry presents myriad regulatory issues, most of which do not have simple answers, but are incredibly interesting," he added.

For physician organizations going public, DeMuro recommends that they get good advice all along the way. "We're not comfortable in advising anybody unless one of the Big 5 firms has already been in," DeMuro said. "The accountants have to agree if they're going to consolidate revenues. You're better off having the accountants argue with the SEC for you."

One of the interesting questions is how to ensure physicians understand all of the federal and state regulations. Some attorneys argue that only in states like Florida, Virginia, and others—where it is possible to employ physicians—can management companies require doctors to implement a compliance program.

To get a compliance program buy-in from the doctors, DeMuro suggests that practice management companies include an agreement to adopt the compliance program in the management services agreement or when the physicians are employed, in their professional service or employment agreements.

The practice management firm can agree to develop a compliance program and the physicians' professional corporation can agree to implement it under the direction of the management organization. However, the management company may only be able to suggest that the physicians adhere to its compliance program. The physicians, through their professional corporation, may decide to adopt their own compliance program, for example.

Health systems and management organizations can get around such problems by writing or amending the management services agreement to say that the professional corporation will implement the compliance program "as proposed by the PPM," DeMuro suggested. That makes the compliance program a contractual obligation of the physicians' professional corporation, he added.

Although many physician management organizations have not had a compliance program, he believes that is changing for the better. "A number of investors in control, like venture capital firms, are in the position to just tell the CEO, CFO and professional corporation, 'We are going to have a compliance program.' Then, it happens," DeMuro said.

However, for publicly traded management companies, "until (Wall) Street requires that they have a compliance program, it is often viewed as a cost item by executives," he noted. He's heard all the excuses for not having one (Figure 7–8).

He also advises practice management companies to be sure to implement the terms of its compliance program as part of an acquisition agreement when buying a new practice.

DeMuro recommends that an officer of the corporation be responsible for monitoring compliance, and that such a person report directly to the board of directors.

F I G U R E 7–8

Top Excuses for *Not* Having a Compliance Program

- It is not budgeted.
- We can get a copy of someone else's plan and copy it.
- We do not want to have to change our activities to conform to it.
- We do not want to spend a lot of money.
- Nobody can agree on what kind of compliance program to have.
- Somebody already looked at all of our agreements and they're in compliance.
- We will only look bad.

Source: Paul DeMuro.

"Many compliance officers do dual duty although we suggest it not be the chief financial officer or an in-house counsel. A lot of times it works well to have the risk manager or internal auditor perform the function." However, if the company can afford it, a separate compliance officer who oversees the compliance program is preferable. Obviously cost is an issue. For example, a radiology management organization may generate more dollars and be able to afford a compliance program more than a primary care or multispecialty organization, DeMuro said. However, the primary care or multispecialty organization probably needs the program more because the number of billing codes are so much greater, making the risk higher.

DeMuro added, however, that compliance officers are in high demand. He recently heard of a search being conducted for one offering a starting salary of $250,000 although starting salaries are normally much less.

He also advises that a baseline audit be conducted in which all of the agreements with physicians, laboratories, other ancillary providers and suppliers, health plans, and other contractors are examined to ensure they are within the scope of applicable law and regulation. If there is a particular billing irregularity, the management organization probably should retain a billing consultant—under the direction of the attorneys for attorney-client privilege purposes—to examine it. For example, if a management company is having problems with billing for services under the Medicare hospice program, a billing consultant in that area may understand it best.

Frequent problem areas include the following.

- Courtesy discounts for physicians or waiving co-payments for physicians
- Any payment that can be construed as inducing referrals
- Double billing
- Research payments to physicians
- Loans to physicians

DeMuro says a strong compliance program also may head off potential whistleblowers.

However, a strong compliance program that urges employees to know what the law is and take responsibility for what goes on around them can mitigate these suits. DeMuro notes a physician management firm could claim: "Sally knew and did not report it. We did the best we could as a corporation. When we discovered the problem, we disciplined Sally." He also urges physician groups and health systems to conduct an exit interview in which a departing employee is asked about any potentially fraudulent activities. An employee who was reticent to talk about such activity while employed may feel more comfortable talking about it on the way out the door.

If a practice management company discovers a problem, DeMuro urges them to conduct an investigation before turning it over to the regulatory agency. "Do not just turn it in and say, 'Do whatever you want to us.'" He notes that the practice management firm will want to determine what the potential liability is. By working with a knowledgeable accounting or consulting firm—for example, a Big 5 firm—the management organization can find out what the problem is, how much, if anything, might be required to return to the programs."

PricewaterhouseCoopers Tips for Compliance

- Top-down support for a compliance program is essential. All top officers and the board of directors must voice support for and integrate compliance into the company's daily operations.

- Tie in financial rewards to compliance targets. Often, compliance guidelines run counter to profit objectives. If meeting financial targets are the only road to bonuses, compliance will become a distant second in priorities.

- Don't install a complex compliance program without an infrastructure to support it. Ongoing audits of the compliance function are necessary.

- Don't take "Everything is OK" as an answer or excuse. In fact, that type of response should be a red flag that controls are not tight enough.

- Compliance must start early. Before acquiring a practice, conduct a compliance audit to determine how diligent the practice has been in following ethics standards, particularly in billing and coding.

RESOURCES

Internet

        www.columbia-hca.com/ethics—the Columbia/HCA code of conduct.

        www.corporatecompliance.com—Corporate Compliance newsletter

www.carswell.com/records/CPG.html—Compliance programs and corporate sentencing guidelines

www.hcfa.gov—Health Care Financing Administration

www.dhhs.gov/progorg/oig/—Office of Inspector General

Paper

Corporate Compliance Officer newsletter by Opus Communications, Marblehead, Mass.

8
CHAPTER

Antitrust and Other Legal Issues

Sandy Lutz

At a recent physician practice management conference, one attendee voiced his sentiment about the government's role in antitrust actions: "It seems like they're there to protect managed care," he commented. Physician groups may sympathize with those sentiments. As managed care payors grow larger and exert more market control, it's often hard to understand why a handful of physicians can't share pricing strategies.

As physicians and physician groups organize physician network ventures, they come under increasing scrutiny from government regulators. For networks such as IPAs and PPOs, the setting of prices is integral for managed care contracting purposes; however, agreements that fix prices or allocate markets among competitors are illegal under antitrust law. Physicians must therefore be aware of the ways they can work together, particularly when contracting with payors. Fortunately, guidelines are available from the U.S. Department of Justice and the Federal Trade Commission (FTC), the two government agencies that administer the antitrust laws.

As consolidation has swept the industry, power plays among providers and insurers have become common. In many cases, insurers viewed the mergers of large medical groups as a threat to their power base and alerted federal antitrust regulators of activity that they viewed as anticompetitive. "Where there are very large multi-specialty group clinics . . . and very large single specialty groups with, say, 50 to 75 physicians in a larger metropolitan area, the FTC may want to take a closer look," Bob Leibenluft, the FTC's assistant director of healthcare told the American Health Lawyers Association in the summer of 1998.[1]

Payors and providers have adversarial roles in contracting, and that can easily flow over into antitrust issues. Sometimes, however, payors believe that proposed medical group mergers will lead to lower prices. In those cases, "it's going to be a lot harder for the agency to challenge it, and I think we probably wouldn't," Leibenluft said.[2] After all, the agency's proviso is to protect competition, and as such it would consider what the payor says.

Leibenluft, who has since left the agency for private practice with Hogan & Hartson in Washington, D.C., noted that antitrust situations are highly dependent on the individual facts of each case. Because healthcare is a local market issue, providers shouldn't assume that what the agency blesses in one market will be approved into another. "It really depends on the particular market we're talking about," he said. In this sense, "market" refers to product as well as geographic markets.

SAFETY ZONES

Antitrust attorneys often reference a 1995 case in which the federal government sued Danbury (Conn.) Hospital, the Danbury Area IPA, and HealthCare Partners, a physician hospital organization in which the hospital and physicians owned equal shares. The government alleged that the hospital formed an alliance with nearly all of the physicians on its staff to halt or delay the development of managed care plans in the area. The government contended that the arrangement limited competition and would cause an increase in healthcare prices in the community.

In 1996, the U.S. Justice Department and the FTC jointly issued antitrust guidelines on physician network joint ventures. These describe the agencies' antitrust analysis of physician network joint ventures, set forth antitrust safety zones that provide guidance about types of ventures that the agencies will not challenge, and present illustrative analyses of several hypothetical physician network joint venture situations.

The safety zones are a "shortcut" employed by the agencies to define certain categories of ventures that are not likely to be challenged. Using a few factors that are relatively easy to apply, the agencies define a category of ventures for which they will presume no anticompetitive harm exists, absent extraordinary circumstances. Ventures that do not fall within one of the safety zones must be analyzed on a case-by-case basis.

The antitrust safety zones differ for "exclusive" and "non-exclusive" physician network arrangements. In an exclusive venture, the network's physicians are

---

[1] "Federal enforcers are looking at group practice mergers that may threaten competition, but no recent actions have been taken," by Sarah A. Klein, American Medical News, July 20, 1998.
[2] Ibid.

restricted in their ability to individually contract or affiliate with other network joint ventures or health plans. In a non-exclusive venture, on the other hand, the physicians may affiliate with other networks or contract individually with health plans. For groups that share risk, the safety zones are as follows:[3]

- Exclusive networks—Absent extraordinary circumstances, the agencies will not challenge an exclusive network whose physicians share substantial financial risk and constitute 20% or less of the physicians in each physician specialty with active hospital staff privileges who practice in the relevant geographic market. In relevant markets with fewer than five physicians in a particular specialty, an exclusive physician network joint venture otherwise qualifying for the antitrust safety zone may include one physician from that specialty, on a non-exclusive basis, even though the inclusion of that physician results in the venture consisting of more than 20% of the physicians in that specialty.

- Non-exclusive networks—Absent extraordinary circumstances, the agencies will not challenge a non-exclusive physician network whose participants share substantial financial risk and constitute 30% or less of the physicians in each physician specialty with active hospital staff privileges who practice in the relevant geographic market. In relevant markets with fewer than four physicians in a particular specialty, a non-exclusive physician network joint venture otherwise qualifying for the antitrust safety zone may include one physician from that specialty, even though the inclusion of that physician results in the venture consisting of more than 30% of the physicians in that specialty.

The agencies will judge whether a network is exclusive or non-exclusive based on how the network operates, rather than what it professes. For example, to determine whether a network is non-exclusive, the agencies will seek to determine whether the following occurs.

- Viable competing networks or health plans compete in the area.
- Physicians actively participate in those networks.
- Physicians receive "substantial" revenue from other networks or contracts.
- Physicians were leaving other contracts or networks.
- Physicians were not colluding on pricing or other "significant terms" of managed care contracting.

A key requirement for qualification for an antitrust safety zone is that the network physicians share "substantial financial risk" in providing all the services

---

[3] Statements of Antitrust Enforcement Policy in Health Care, Issued by the U.S. Department of Justice and the Federal Trade Commission, August 1996.

that are jointly priced through the network. This isn't because such risk sharing is a desired end in itself, but rather that risk sharing normally is a clear and reliable indicator that a physician network involves sufficient integration by its physician participants to achieve significant efficiencies. Furthermore, risk sharing provides incentives for the physicians to cooperate in controlling costs and improving quality by managing the provision of services by network physicians. The government "is saying to doctors that it may be OK to get together to jointly negotiate, but you need to integrate in some way," Leibenluft said. However, "if you're integrated, the government will still look at the ability of the group to raise prices with the presumption being that that ability is enhanced for a group with a very large market share."

The types of risk-sharing arrangements contemplated include, but are not limited to the following.

- Agreements made by the venture for its physicians to provide services to a health plan at a "capitated" rate.
- Contracts in which the venture's physicians are paid a predetermined percentage of revenue or premium by a health plan to provide certain services.
- Financial incentives by the venture to encourage the physicians as a group to achieve specified cost-containment goals, such as withholds or bonuses based on meeting specific cost or utilization targets.
- Contracts in which the venture's physicians are paid case rates.

RULE OF REASON ANALYSIS

Risk-sharing network arrangements that do not fall within the mathematical parameters of the safety zones aren't necessarily illegal, the agencies said, if they can demonstrate that they are creating efficiencies and not being anti-competitive. In addition, networks in which physicians don't share financial risk wouldn't necessarily be illegal either, as long as the ventures had programs that demonstrated clinical integration. Some examples of ventures that would not fall within the safety zones include the following.

- The venture comprises over 30% of the physicians in a number of relevant specialties in the geographic market.
- The physicians in the venture do not share substantial financial risk.
- The venture negotiates and enters into both capitated and fee-for-service contracts on behalf on its physicians.

A determination about the lawfulness of ventures that fall outside the safety zones must be made on a case-by-case basis according to general antitrust principles. If the setting of prices is considered to be integral to the venture's use of the network arrangement (as opposed to constituting "naked price fixing"), the venture would be analyzed under the "rule of reason." A rule of reason analysis determines whether the formation of the venture may have a substantial anticompetitive effect, and if so, whether that potential effect is outweighed by any procompetitive efficiencies resulting from the venture. The rule of reason analysis takes into account characteristics of the particular physician network joint venture, and of the competitive environment in which it operates, that bear on the venture's likely effect on competition.

If the analysis indicates that formation of the venture would not likely hamper the ability of health plans to contract individually with area physicians or with other physician network joint ventures, or enable the physicians to raise prices above competitive levels, or otherwise be anticompetitive, there is no need for further detailed evaluation—the agencies would not challenge the joint venture. Physician groups that compete should realize that some topics are off limits for discussion (Figure 8–1).

The following steps are used in analyzing whether a network is anticompetitive under "the rule of reason."

1. **Define the relevant product and geographic market.** The agencies evaluate the competitive effects of the venture in each relevant market in which it operates or has substantial impact. In defining the relevant product and geographic markets, the agencies look at the substitutes for the services in question that are, as a practical matter, reasonably available to consumers.

2. **Evaluate the competitive effects of the physician joint venture.** The agencies examine the structure and activities of the network to determine whether the network is likely to have an anticompetitive effect. Key areas of concern are whether the venture could raise the prices for physician services charged to health plans above competitive

FIGURE 8–1

Competing Medical Groups Should *Never* Discuss the Following with Each Other (Absent a Legitimate Joint Venture)

- Prices
- Customers with whom they do business
- Geographic service areas
- Products or services they will or will not offer
- Costs, margins, negotiating strategies, or future business plans
- Other sensitive business information

Source: Hogan & Hartson

levels whether the venture, could prevent or impede the formation or operation of other networks or plans, or whether the information shared by the partners could be used by the network's physician participants to set prices for services they provide outside the network (termed *spillover*). Ventures that are structured to reduce the likelihood of spillover are less likely to result in anticompetitive effects. For example, if a network uses an outside agent to collect and analyze fee data from physicians for use in developing the network's fee schedule (and thereby avoids the sharing of such sensitive information among the network's physician participants) this may reduce the agencies' concerns that the information could be used by the network's physician participants to set prices for services they provide outside the network.

3. **Evaluate the impact of pro-competitive efficiencies.** This step requires an examination of the venture's likely pro-competitive efficiencies, and the balancing of these efficiencies against any potential anticompetitive effects. The greater the venture's potential anticompetitive effects, the greater the venture's probable efficiencies must be in order to offset them. In assessing efficiency claims, the agencies focus on net efficiencies that will be derived from the operation of the network and that result in lower prices or higher quality to consumers. The agencies will not accept claims of efficiencies if the parties reasonably can achieve equivalent or comparable savings through other means that are significantly less anticompetitive.

4. **Evaluate collateral agreements.** The final step examines whether the venture includes collateral agreements or conditions that unreasonably restrict competition and are unlikely to contribute significantly to the legitimate purposes of the venture. The agencies will examine whether the collateral agreements are reasonably necessary to achieve the efficiencies sought by the joint venture. For example, an agreement between physician participants in a physician network joint venture regarding the prices they will charge patients who are not covered by the health plans with which their network contracts plainly is not reasonably necessary to the success of the joint venture and is an antitrust violation.

Leibenluft pointed out that this process is "very complicated. If the agencies have to bring a 'rule of reason' case, it's a very daunting thing to do."

The guidelines also provide examples of how the agencies would apply these principles to specific physician network joint ventures, and differentiate between ventures that would fall within the safety zones; ventures that do not fall within the safety zones, but would not be challenged; and ventures that would be challenged as *per se* illegal.[4] One example provided is a physician network joint venture involving clinical integration, but no financial risk on the part of physicians. Another is a physician network joint venture in which the physicians had both risk-sharing and non–risk-sharing contracts. Both of those examples got the green light.

However, the guidelines also give the example of an IPA in which physicians were not sharing risk, although each had contributed $2,000 to join the organization. The group actively blocked health plans from contracting with them unless they met the group's specific contracting guidelines. Even though these physicians contracted individually with managed care plans, they would only do so if the health plans offered the terms set by the IPA. The agencies deemed this unlawful because the physicians were using the IPA as a vehicle for collective decisions. In spite of the physicians' investment of $2,000, the government agencies said there was not enough financial risk to prevent the organization from being anticompetitive. After all, the agencies reasoned, such capital contributions can be used to finance a cartel.

Details of such ventures and how the agencies view them will be of interest to physician organizations that are signing contracts with managed care organizations. Both agencies have Web sites loaded with examples of antitrust cases in healthcare, with details about the providers involved, including the following examples.

- In July 1997, the government said it would not challenge a move by 40 physicians in Rutland, Vermont, to form the Vermont Physicians Clinic even though the clinic represented more than 30% of some specialties in the area. The agency pointed out that "managed care plans and other third-party payors had expressed no concern that Vermont Physicians Clinic would cause substantial anti-competitive effects, and were enthusiastic at the prospect of a joint venture because they believe that the Clinic will provide competition to the managed care panel of physicians formed by the only hospital in the Rutland area."[5]

- In September 1998, the Justice Department said it would not challenge the merger of a primary care physicians organization and a multispecialty physicians organization in Scranton, Pennsylvania. The merged network will include about 39% of the area physicians who are

---

[4] If the agencies finds certain types of conduct, they will not go through the "rule of reason" process. Those types of conduct are:
  - "Naked" price fixing—physicians agree to raise their rates all at once.
  - Group boycotts—an unintegrated physician group agrees that it won't take a managed care contract and no one in the group is allowed to negotiate separately
  - Market divisions—a medical group says we'll talke this half of the city and your group take that half and we won't compete with each other.
[5] U.S. Justice Department press release, July 30, 1997.

internists, family practitioners, or general practitioners, and 28% of the area's pediatricians. The multispecialty organization already included more than 50% of some specialties in the area, but that has not caused competitive harm, the department found.[6] The agency also determined that each physician specialty could be considered as a separate relevant product market.[7] "However, in this case, as in many markets, it appears that family practitioners, general practitioners and internists are considered to be good substitutes and can be viewed as participants in a single service market," the agency said.[8] However, pediatricians and other specialists were considered separate service markets.

MESSENGER MODELS

Some physician groups, particularly IPAs, have set up "messenger model" arrangements to contract on behalf of their physicians. In these, an agent or third party obtains fee information individually from physicians and gives that information to purchaser. For example, an IPA might determine that a group of physicians would be willing to accept $40 per member per month and take that information to a managed care plan. The managed care plan might respond that it will pay $39 per member per month. The IPA then would return to the physicians and make the offer, which the physicians could accept or reject individually.

The IPA can offer objective information about contractual terms because the agencies view dissemination of such information as pro-competitive. For example, if an IPA tells its physicians that Managed Care Organization A is paying $38 and Managed Care Organization B is paying $41, that is merely giving physicians information they can use to make a definitive choice. However, if the IPA's lawyer issues a statement to the physicians saying, "Don't ever sign a contract at less than $40 per member per month," then the federal agencies are likely to investigate, Leibenluft said.

OTHER LEGAL ISSUES—PERCENTAGE ARRANGEMENTS

At least half of the states have some form of "corporate practice of medicine" laws that prevent nonphysicians from establishing and operating corporations that employ physicians and render medical services. Because of these laws, practice management companies that are not owned by physicians cannot own physician practices or be equity participants in physician practices. In some cases, the

---

[6] U.S. Justice Department press release, Sept. 15, 1998.
[7] Correspondence from Department of Justice to Christopher Casey, Scranton, Penn., Sept. 15, 1998. www.usdoj.gov\atr\public\busreview\1941.htm
[8] Ibid.

practice management firm has a physician hold the shares of the professional corporation in trust for the practice management firm. This is a complex structure that may not be appealing or politically favorable to physician groups. That's why many choose an affiliated physician group structure instead.

The affiliated group practice structure, however, is not without problems of its own. Most management services agreements state that the practice management firm will be paid for its services based on a percentage of revenues or profits from the physician group. Yet, the Office of Inspector General (OIG) has indicated that such arrangements may pose problems.

These types of management fees are common among practice management organizations because they give physicians an incentive to participate in the success of the organization. Most equity-model practice management organizations take either a fixed percentage of physician revenues or a fixed percentage of practice income. Many practice management organizations have favored this over an employment model in which the physicians simply draw a salary. In states with a corporate practice of management prohibition, a management arrangement may be the only option.

A physician wrote to the U.S. Department of Health and Human Services' OIG to request an opinion on a proposed management services contract between his practice and a practice management company. The physician asked whether the contract, in which a practice management organization would be reimbursed for its costs and paid a percentage of net practice revenues, would constitute illegal remuneration as defined by the anti-kickback statute of the Social Security Act.

In an April 15, 1998, Advisory Opinion, the OIG concluded that the physician practice management company in the proposed arrangement may be violating the federal anti-kickback statute, based on the information provided. The OIG said that a percentage-fee arrangement is problematic for the following reasons.

- It may include financial incentives to increase patient referrals because it will be based, in part, on providing marketing services. In addition, the physicians may be required to refer patients to specialist networks as part of their contractual arrangements.

- It may contain no safeguards against overutilization.

- It may include financial incentives that increase the risk of abusive billing practices, such as upcoding. The percentage arrangement may induce the practice management organization to upcode to increase revenues because doing so inherently increases its fee.

The Advisory Opinion (No. 98–4) states that these percentage-based arrangements do not qualify for one of the federal anti-kickback statute "safe harbors" because compensation is *not* an aggregate amount, fixed in advance, as the safe harbor regulations require. However, D. McCarty Thornton, chief counsel to the Inspector General, said in the opinion that such arrangements must be analyzed on a case-by-case basis.

The advisory opinion doesn't reflect a blanket prohibition on these fee arrangements, according to Jerry Sokol, a partner in the Miami office of McDermott, Will & Emery. He points out that the opinion is based upon the specific facts presented and is only applicable to the requesting physician. Sokol said that although the opinion does provide valuable insight into areas of government concern, the Inspector General has always expressed a concern with marketing services that involve percentage fees. Sokol believes that there should be a focus on the type of marketing and the specific payment arrangement in order to determine if there is really a payment for referral concern. Nonetheless, until there's further guidance, practice management organizations may want to consider having the marketing services provided within the practice and not by the practice management organization.

In addition, practice management organizations should be aware that the OIG is concerned when practice management organizations engage in network development with required referrals within the network, and provide billing services when a percentage compensation is involved. Sokol advised that practice management organizations have utilization review and control functions so that questions of overutilization and abusive billing are being handled in a proactive manner. However, he pointed out that with healthcare moving toward capitation, concerns about overutilization are minimized and there really should be a focus on underutilization. The legal context of percentage arrangements "is currently a gray area on the federal level, and I doubt that practice management organizations are going to jump to change their arrangements until there's more definitive clarification," he added.

Legal experts noted that the OIG opinion closely resembled a declaratory statement in which the Florida State Board of Medicine in October 1997 found that a percentage management fee based upon practice revenue violated a Florida fee-splitting statute. That issue involves Magan L. Bakarania of Tampa, Fla., and whether he could join a practice that had an arrangement to pay a percentage of its practice net income to PhyMatrix Corp., a publicly traded practice management organization based in West Palm Beach, Fla. The Florida board said the arrangement amounted to fee-splitting, which is illegal in the state.

PricewaterhouseCoopers Tips for Management Fee Arrangements and Antitrust Situations

- Consider restructuring their arrangements with physicians, allowing them to fall back to flat fees if the percentage fees are deemed to be illegal.

- Expand the "risk factors" section of their disclosures to shareholders to include a discussion of this matter.
- Ensure that their contracts have the flexibility to change as regulators continue to draw and redraw the boundaries under which practice management organizations operate.
- Retain professional legal advice before merging practices in cases in which the combined entity exceeds safety zones.
- Don't exchange too much information in pre-merger negotiations.

RESOURCES

www.doj.gov

www.ftc.gov/bc/health.htm

Figure 8–2 is an example of a letter from the FTC that provides an illustration of what a provider may receive. Similar examples are available on the agency's Web site.

FIGURE 8–2

Example of an FTC Letter

United States of America
Federal Trade Commission
Washington, D.C. 20580
Bureau of Competition

John Doe, Esquire
Doe & Company
700 Main Street
Anytown, State 99999

Dear Mr. Doe:

This letter is in response to your request for a staff advisory opinion on behalf of ABC Specialists, P.C. ("ABC"). ABC is a for-profit corporation composed of physicians who are board-certified or board-eligible in hematology/medical oncology ("hematologist/oncologists"). Established to develop and manage the provision of hematology/medical oncology ("hematology/oncology") services through a network of providers in the area surrounding Anytown, ABC will negotiate and enter into contracts with

Example of an FTC Letter, Continued

third-party payors under which its members ("participating physicians") will provide such services to the beneficiaries of those payors' health plans. As explained more fully below, neither the formation nor the operation of ABC appears likely to violate any law enforced by the FTC.

ABC will be managed by a board of five directors, three of whom will also serve as officers. These officers will serve one-year terms and may serve up to three consecutive terms. With the assistance of an independent contractor, ABC will market its network services, primarily on a capitated basis, to third-party payors, including health maintenance organizations and possibly self-insured employers. Each payor's capitated payment will cover all physician services rendered to its beneficiaries under its contract, and participating physicians will share the risk that the cost of providing services to a payor group will exceed that payment. However, drug therapy, a critical aspect of the treatment of certain hematology/oncology patients, initially will be provided on a modified fee-for-service basis. ABC estimates that drug therapy may account for approximately 30% of its volume of business, but has been unable to obtain data on utilization patterns or costs per patient for drug therapy. ABC asserts that it lacks sufficient experience with protocols for drug therapy to establish capitated rates for such therapy at this time.

ABC intends to develop and implement quality assurance and utilization review programs in order to ensure the provision of necessary and appropriate care and minimize the risk borne by participating physicians. For example, a "Continuous Quality Improvement" committee will develop and administer practice parameters. ABC will monitor individual participating physicians' practice patterns through a medical management information system, and will provide training to assist physicians in fulfilling their responsibilities under the payor contracts. ABC also intends to offer group purchasing benefits to participating physicians for billing services, insurance, medical equipment, and other supplies.

ABC's Board of Directors will calculate a reimbursement formula for physician services based on McGraw-Hill relative value scale standards. Each month, ABC will set aside approximately 20% of the monthly capitated payments to pay expenses, management fees, and incentive compensation to physicians who meet certain cost-saving, utilization, and quality-of-care standards set by the Board. The company will distribute the remaining proceeds, on a pro rata basis, to participating physicians who provided services to beneficiaries during that month. ABC also intends to

Example of an FTC Letter, Continued

set aside a minimum of 20% of the monthly fee-for-service payments, which will be disbursed to participating physicians on a pro rata basis if applicable performance standards, established during negotiations with third-party payors, are met. ABC has not yet determined the details regarding forfeiture of withheld amounts.

ABC will consist primarily of hematologist/oncologists from a nine county area, identified in your letter as ABC's primary service area, that encompasses Alpha, Beta, Gamma, Delta, Epsilon, Zeta, Eta, Theta, and Iota counties. It will also include physicians from an area, identified in your letters as ABC's secondary service area, that encompasses Kappa, Lambda, and Mu counties. There is currently one specialty hematology/oncology network, as well as health maintenance organizations and other managed care entities, providing hematology/oncology services in this area.

ABC is owned by shareholder-physicians who are qualified to provide hematology/oncology services, meet specific practice guidelines, and who agree to comply with ABC's quality guidelines, procedures, and protocols. Participating physicians will make an initial capital investment of $2,000, contribute $100 towards the cost of a management information system, and execute a $3,000 demand promissory note. ABC may also contract with non-shareholder hematologist/oncologists as necessary to provide full geographic coverage or to meet other payor demands.

Participating physicians will provide their services to ABC on a non-exclusive basis. Participating physicians may not decline to participate in agreements negotiated by ABC, but may participate in other provider organizations. The five directors are precluded only from simultaneously serving as officers or directors in other single-specialty networks that provide hematology/oncology services on a risk-sharing basis. This restriction is intended to protect against the possibility of disclosure of confidential information to competing, single-specialty hematology/oncology networks.

ABC currently represents thirty-five participating physicians, accounting for fewer than 30% of the hematology/oncology specialists in the area in which it intends to operate. Participating physicians currently account for 27.34% of the hematology/oncology specialists in the area identified as ABC's primary service area, and 25.93% of those in the area identified as its secondary service area. ABC is currently accepting applications from additional physicians; however, the network will restrict additional participation to ensure that its current market share is not substantially increased.

Example of an FTC Letter, Continued

Based on your description of the proposed operation of ABC, as summarized above, the proposed course of action does not appear likely to violate the antitrust laws. ABC appears to fall within the definition of an antitrust "safety zone" for non-exclusive physician network joint ventures established in Statement 8 of the 1994 Statements of Antitrust Enforcement Policy and Analytical Principles Relating to Health Care and Antitrust ("the Statement"). The safety zone applies to "non-exclusive physician network joint venture(s) comprising 30% or less of the physicians in each physician specialty with active hospital staff privileges who practice in the relevant geographic market and share substantial risk."

It appears that ABC will operate as an economically integrated, non-exclusive physician network joint venture composed of fewer than 30% of hematologist/oncologists in the relevant market. The Statement identifies as a recognized form of economic integration the acceptance of capitation contracts. ABC will contract on a capitated basis for physician services and participating physicians will share substantial financial risk that costs for a payor group will exceed the capitation payment for the bulk of the services rendered.

ABC has not yet determined important details surrounding the proposed use of a discounted fee schedule in conjunction with a 20% withhold for drug therapy, and it is not clear from the information currently available whether participating physicians will share substantial financial risk for the provision of drug therapy. Nonetheless, to the extent that participating physicians will collectively agree on the prices for drug therapy, such agreement appears to be ancillary to the main purpose of the joint venture, and subject to a rule of reason evaluation. Under the circumstances, including the present difficulties of including the cost of drug therapy in a capitated rate and the importance of providing drug therapy to certain hematology/oncology patients, the proposed use of a discounted fee schedule, for a transitional period as the network develops the requisite data to formulate capitated rates for this therapy, appears to be reasonably necessary to the joint venture's primary purpose of providing capitated physician services to hematology/oncology patients. The price restraint appears to be of no broader scope than is reasonably necessary to further that purpose. Furthermore, the network is not likely to give rise to market power in the

Example of an FTC Letter, Concluded

provision of hematology/oncology services. In short, the fee-for-service component of the network appears to be ancillary to its primary purpose and justifiable under the rule of reason.

It also appears that ABC will be composed of 30% or fewer of the hematologist/oncologists who practice in the relevant geographic market. Although it is not clear from the information that you have provided whether the relevant geographic market is the stated eight county primary service area or some smaller area, it does not appear critical to determine its precise limits: ABC'S share of participating physicians is less than 30% both in the area you define as the primary service area and in Alpha County, the county in which the vast majority of hematologist/oncologists appear to practice.

Finally, it appears that ABC will operate as a non-exclusive venture. The Statement defines a non-exclusive venture as one that does not impose any "significant explicit or implicit restriction" on the ability of participating physicians to participate in other provider organizations or to contract with payors directly. ABC's limited restraint on officers and directors merely precludes them from simultaneously holding offices in other single-specialty networks that provide hematology/oncology services on a risk-sharing basis. It is a narrowly tailored provision that does not preclude officers or directors from participating in other types of provider organizations or from contracting with payors directly.

For these reasons, the formation and operation of ABC, as proposed, would not appear to violate any law enforced by the Federal Trade Commission. This letter sets out the views of the staff of the Bureau of Competition, as authorized by the Commission's Rules of Practice. Under Commission Rule § 1.3(c), 16 C.F.R. § 1.3(c) (1994), the Commission is not bound by this staff opinion and reserves the right to rescind it at a later time. In addition, this office retains the right to reconsider the questions involved, and with notice to the requesting party, to rescind or revoke the opinion if implementation of the proposed program results in substantial anticompetitive effect, if the program is used for improper purposes, if facts change significantly, or if it would be in the public interest to do so.

Sincerely yours,

9

CHAPTER

Valuations: A Changing Vision in the Beholder's Eye

Sandy Lutz

Allen Hahn

One practice management firm that was recruiting physicians in the Southwest during the mid-1990s flashed a chart during presentations that was an instant audience grabber. Titled, "The High Cost of Selling Out," the chart showed how $1.5 million worth of stock—presumably the average price for a physician practice—growing at 15% annually for four years and 8% annually for 11 years would amount to more than $6 million in 15 years. In comparison, it showed a signing bonus of $600,000—presumably the average being paid by local hospitals for physician practices—would net $432,000 after taxes. At an 8% compounded rate of return, this would amount to $1.37 million in 15 years. The difference between the two numbers was startling, and a big selling point for the practice management firm.

The numbers were fictional, but grounded in truth—at that time. More importantly, the chart was meant to show physicians how selling out to a management company would return more value than selling out to a hospital.

"A lot of physicians want to make sure they're dealing with a company that's going to be public," one former management company executive would tell prospective sellers.

During the 1990s, bidding wars ensued and valuations rose higher and higher, rooted in few facts and gobs of hype. With a plethora of buyers—public and private companies as well as eager hospitals—the bidding wars heightened the value of physician groups. However, the bottom fell out when two large bidders fell by the wayside in 1998—MedPartners and community hospitals. MedPartners' furiously fast purchases of physician groups and other management companies goosed prices during 1996 and 1997. The company's $2.5 billion purchase of Caremark International in 1996 was the largest single transaction of a physician practice management company. It would have been eclipsed by the $8-billion purchase of MedPartners itself by PhyCor, a deal that fell apart in early 1998.

Hospitals began buying physician practices to create integrated delivery systems. At the time, it seemed like a good strategy. For example, Philadelphia was viewed as one of the best markets for physicians wanting to sell. "Every physician practice that goes on the market has five or six bidders for it," complained Todd Sagan, head of practice acquisitions at Temple (University). "Most of the deals are being driven by a worry that if we don't do it, someone else will."[1]

Yet, the red ink that stemmed from this overindulgence gave hospitals financial cramps. Most didn't know what to do with the practices they bought. The practices began to bleed red ink, in some cases threatening the systems' otherwise pristine bond ratings.

Some physicians sold their practices just as they were reaching their peak in their productivity. Once they reviewed their bulging bank accounts, they asked themselves, "Why am I working this hard now?"

In one such case, a hospital system's practice management company bought a strong OB/GYN practice started by a respected practitioner in his late 50s. The practice was a true family affair. The doctor's wife was the nurse, and his son also was a physician in the practice. They contracted with a long-time friend for accounting services. Not long before selling out, the lead physician decided to expand and hired four new residents, who were on guaranteed salaries.

So, the hospital bought the practice for an eight-figure sum that went primarily to the lead physician and his son because the new residents weren't yet partners in the venture. About a year later, the founding physician decided to retire. So did his wife. So did his son. That left the four new physicians who hadn't been there long enough to gain any patient loyalty. Much of the patient base eked away.

As this story illustrated, a fatal flaw to many practice acquisitions was excessive up-front payments to physicians with no guarantee of return.

Add to that the pock-filled track record of publicly traded management companies in 1998, and the valuation for group practices and practice management companies fell dramatically. Unfortunately, stocks don't always go up. Hundreds of physicians were burned when they sold their practices for stock that plummeted in value.

---

[1] "Hospitals That Gobbled Up Physician Practices Feel Ill," by George Anders, Wall Street Journal, June 17, 1997.

In the latter half of 1998, the CEO of a large group practice in Texas was asked why the group decided to sell to a one particular practice management firm. The answer was succinct: "They wanted to buy us." It was a buyer's market and sellers just had to take what they could get. Unfortunately, this particular group had venture capital financiers who wanted their money back. For groups that had to sell because they were running out of capital or their venture capital backers wanted out, the valuation was disappointingly low.

Because fewer organizations were bidding for physician practices, leverage swung away from physicians and toward the acquirers. In fact, some large practice management companies walked away from deals in which prices had been negotiated a year earlier and market factors made the transaction an economic boondoggle.

It would be easy to have a Chicken Little mentality about prices for group practices and practice management companies. Yet, consolidation of physicians into larger groups will continue and the number of transactions among buyers and sellers is likely to rise in coming years. The reasons for joining larger groups—freedom from administrative hassles, managed care contracting clout, and the need for capital—haven't gone away. As figures from Irving Levin Associates demonstrate (Table 9–1), the momentum to consolidate grew considerably in 1997. In 1998, the growth rate and the purchase prices were declining. However, as with all cyclical markets, 1998 may have been merely a breather during which to digest the consolidation already underway.

BALANCING ASSETS AND LIABILITIES

In the typical scenario, a practice management firm acquires the non-clinical assets of a physician's practice and signs a long-term management services agreement with the physicians. Most physician practices have very few tangible assets unless they own outpatient centers, laboratories, or capital equipment. That means the valuation will hinge on the intangible value of the practice, which includes the value assigned to the management services agreement.

TABLE 9–1

Physician Group Transactions

	1996	1997	% Change
Deals announced	242	275	14%
Physicians	19,950	26,700	34%
Total purchase price (billions)	$4.50	$4.45	−1%

Source: Irving Levin Associates.

The intangible value will be based, in part, on the history of the group practice being acquired. Some acquirers look back as far as five years into the practice's revenue history, staffing levels, salaries, other expenses, and third-party reimbursements. The most recent year's results, however, will be the most critical.

Getting a good handle on the value of a practice's assets can be difficult if the physicians don't want their staff to know that they're considering a sale. Most practice management firms employ an executive who heads acquisition efforts, but that individual usually has a title like "chief development officer" or "vice president of development." Business cards with those titles don't sound so threatening to a group practice employee as one that includes the words "mergers" or "acquisitions."

Often, a group's biggest asset is its accounts receivable, which the acquirer may or may not choose to purchase. If the acquirer buys the AR, it usually is discounted, depending on the age of the accounts. The discount deepens for older accounts.

There are pros and cons to buying AR (Figure 9–1). From a tax perspective, purchasing the accounts receivable places the tax burden on the physicians. The old professional corporation is usually using the cash method of accounting for tax purposes, which means there is zero basis in the accounts receivable. When the stock of the old PC is acquired, the tax burden of the zero basis accounts receivable will likely fall on the shoulders of the management organization. To prevent, this the management organization can purchase the accounts receivable and the old PC will recognize the income. The old PC then can bonus it out to the physicians. However, it's important that the parties to the transaction know who will bear the tax burden on the collection of the receivables.

Physicians may want to sell AR so they don't have to worry about collecting it. However, the practice management firm needs to be sure they understand how collections will be handled by the new management company. In some

FIGURE 9–1

A Lesson in Purchasing Accounts Receivables

One practice management organization purchased each physician group's accounts receivables when they joined the group. To entice doctors to join the group, they told the physicians that if they ever left the organization, they could take same amount of AR with them when they left. In other words, they wouldn't lose anything. When the organization began to falter, several physicians left and took AR with them. That undermined the organization's financial base as physicians draining its biggest asset. Shortly thereafter, the company filed for bankruptcy.

cases, physicians have been dissatisfied with the way collections were handled, especially if physicians weren't aggressive about following up with patients in the past. Billing for services is a tangible part of what physicians do, and separating them from this function can disrupt the efficiency of the practice. For that reason, many practice management firms leave the billing and collections function in the practice.

What about liabilities? In the past, few groups had any debt, but that has started to change. As physician organizations move into a second cycle of consolidation they tend to have more debt. Their growth has been fueled by venture capitalist funds, banks, or other institutions that have financed their growth, and those debts will factor into the group's valuation.

VALUATION METHODOLOGIES

In valuing physician or dental groups, one size does not fit all. Just as the models of practice management companies vary widely, so do the ways they value practices.

When asked about how much they pay for physician groups, practice management executives typically rattle off a range of multiples. "We pay six to eight times," they'll say. That divulges very little information, however, because the multiple is of a cash flow figure that includes a wide range of assumptions. By and large, management organizations don't want to disclose their exact formulas for valuing physician groups or dental groups. As with buying a car, there's an art to the negotiation process.

There is no cookie-cutter formula for valuing physician groups or practices because the variables include the group's potential for growth, how mature the local managed care market is, how cohesively the group works together, and how soon the group will be able to conform to the new organization's culture and financial forecasts.

Two basic methodologies for valuing business are integrated to generate the multiples: the market approach and the income approach. The income approach has two techniques: discounted cash flow and capitalization of excess earnings.

Market Approach

The market approach is a method of determining an asset's fair market value (Figure 9–2). Of course, the buyer and the practice itself will have their own assumptions about fair market value. Fair market value assumes that the practice is being purchased for the highest possible value based on current market conditions. That value may be augmented by a strategic value, which takes into consideration how a practice will benefit the new physician acquirer. For example, practice management firms often pay a premium for group practices that give them a toehold, or more, in a competitive market. Buying a premiere group in a

FIGURE 9–2

Legal Definition of Fair Market Value

The price at which the property would change hands between a willing buyer and a willing seller when the former is not under any compulsion to buy and the latter is not under a compulsion to sell, both parties having reasonable knowledge of the facts.

market that has not yet consolidated could give the practice management firm the momentum to attract other practices at lower prices. In their pitches to investors and physicians, practice managers have a litany of examples showing how they bought a group practice and expanded it by adding other physicians in the community. Ideally, this is the goal of practice management companies. They must have both internal and external growth. If external growth dries up—which started happening in mid-1998—then the management organization can only derive growth by organically expanding those practices it already owns.

In some communities, a practice management firm's acquisition of a large practice is the ignition key for the steam roller of physician consolidation because a management organization that paid a strategic premium value for the first group practice can offset that cost by paying lower prices for additional groups.

Buying physician practices has evolved into a sophisticated analysis during the past 10 years. In the early days of practice management companies, reaching an acquisition price was an inexact calculation. In many cases, acquirers were working with very little information to model into a valuation. One development executive talked about how it was either feast or famine at the groups they were courting. In some cases, physician groups had just a few pieces of paper that listed the group's financial results, forcing the practice management company to extrapolate those figures into a pro forma spreadsheet and valuation. In other cases, physicians shipped boxes and boxes of general ledgers and other documentation, requiring hours to sort through and summarize into meaningful data.

W.L. Douglas Townsend Jr., managing director and CEO with the investment banking firm of Townsend Frew & Co., Durham, N.C., noted that in the early years of physician acquisitions, companies had limited financial information about the clinics they were buying. The clinics were "price takers" because the financial projections were built based on what the management organizations developed.

When the market was booming and Wall Street was awarding lofty multiples to management company stocks, clinics began to hire their own bankers to develop financial projections that would translate into a sales price and future compensation formulas. Competitive bidding developed. The brokers performed an assessment of the practice and massaged it for dissemination. In some cases, practice management companies had to take that spoon-fed information, coupled with their own research about the local market, to arrive at a valuation. The practice management organization or health system might or might not be offered an opportunity to meet with the physicians themselves before making an opening bid on the practice.

As in an auction of prized paintings, bidding got out of hand. Some hospitals and practice management companies ended up paying premium prices based on unrealistic growth curves. Although valuations are generally well thought-out calculations, they're only as good as the assumptions built into them. If the assumptions call for adding more and more physicians and ancillaries and signing multiple managed care contracts—in other words, aggressive growth—the valuation was going to be higher. Many practice managers valued groups based on projections of how the group would grow. Since practice management companies were operating in a nascent industry, growth projections could be almost unlimited.

The market approach for valuing physician groups can be extremely volatile because it stems from actual transactions. It is easily caught up in momentum that moves in one direction or the other and can miss vital valuation clues, such as clinical reputation, synergies within the group, and corrections in market movement. Be careful when considering historical acquisition prices. Last year's prices for physician practices may be unreasonable considering the current state of the market. In a market that hits the skids, fair market value may be the liquidation value—what the practice is worth if it was shut down.

Income Approach

Discounted Cash Flow

Discounted cash flow, a common business valuation technique, is the most customary way to value physician practices. It is a sophisticated analysis used to quantify projected operating assumptions and consolidate them into an evaluation of a physician's practice. Although discounted cash flow analysis is an extremely useful technique, realistic estimates of value are derived only through proper application of operating and financial assumptions. Studies have demonstrated that discounted cash flow analysis consistently produces higher estimates of practice goodwill than other valuation techniques.

One reason the discounted cash flow method has been popular for valuing practices is that the IRS wants to see that type of analysis when it investigates transactions with not-for-profit hospitals. Because not-for-profit hospitals have been aggressive buyers of practices, physicians were accustomed to seeing those types of valuation analyses. When tax-exempt organizations purchase physician practices, they have to be careful of private inurement issues. The tax-exempt organization cannot use its assets for the private benefit of individuals, such as physicians. By obtaining a credible valuation of the practices it's buying, the hospital can demonstrate that it didn't overpay the physicians to encourage them to refer patients. In discounted cash flow analysis, the weighted average cost of capital is used as a discount rate for valuing the practice.

Capitalization of Excess Earnings

Another method of valuing practices is by converting the practice's earnings into an estimate of goodwill value by dividing normalized earnings by an appropriate capitalization rate. Value is derived based on historical or current performance of the practice.

One variation on this method is to value a practice based on a multiple of EBITDA. EBITDA stands for earnings before interest, taxes, depreciation and amortization. The problem is many physician practices don't have any EBITDA. Any left-over earnings are usually paid out to physicians in compensation.

For that reason, most practice management companies calculate a pro forma estimate of what the EBITDA of the practice would be under the management organization. The pro forma takes out the practice's expenses, which include physician compensation and the management fee. Because both of those are negotiating items with the management organization, the EBITDA is going to be negotiable. The EBITDA also fluctuates depending on the cost savings brought to the practice by the management organization. For example, if the management organization estimates that it will save the practice 10% on supplies, 30% on malpractice insurance and 25% in back office expenses, that would buoy the EBITDA level.

Once a pro forma EBITDA level has been decided on, the next determinant is the multiple. During the past five years, multiples have soared and fallen, sometimes reaching 10 to 12 times EBITDA, but in 1998 EBITDA multiples fell to 3 to 5 in many cases. The EBITDA multiple is much like a capitalization rate. For example, many management organizations were paying about six times EBITDA, which translates into a 16% capitalization rate. However, as management organizations came to have negative cash flows and disgruntled physicians, the business became riskier and the capitalization rate moved higher.

Another way to look at the purchase price is as a multiple of the management fee, because that's what the management organization is really buying. The practice management company's revenues will flow from the management fees collected, not the overall revenues of the group. In some cases, the management organization tells physicians that they're paying them, say, five times the projected management fee. In other words, it's a wash for the physicians over the first five years. The physicians may be able to rationalize the deal by saying that they're getting all the advantages of the management organization—capital, management expertise, group purchasing, information systems—free, at least for the first five years (or whatever the deal calls for). Examples of management organization deals are included at the end of this chapter.

Not coincidentally, five years is also the life of a typical non-compete agreement. However, physicians need to keep in mind that most management services agreements have a life of 15 to 40 years. That's why physicians, especially younger ones, need to be sure they're looking beyond the five-year financials of the deal. They need to be convinced that the transaction is going to make sense 15 to 25 years into the future. A sale may be far more appealing to a physician in his 50s than one in his 30s or 40s because the older physician won't be there for the life of the contract.

To make the transaction more palatable to younger physicians, a management organization may want to alter the distribution of sale proceeds. Some physician groups are structured so that each physician owns one share. In other groups, however, a disproportionate number of the shares will be in the hands of the older physicians who formed the group. Other physicians may have bought in later, but at a reduced equity percentage. As an incentive to retain younger physicians through the life of the management services agreement, the share distribution could be altered. After all, the younger physicians will bear the economic burden of a long-term management contract with the management organization for many more years than older physicians, who may retire in five to 10 years.

Discussion of how many shares each physician is going to get can easily explode into a quarrel, however. In some cases, dissension about the allotment of shares has overshadowed nearly all other aspects of a group's sale. Buyers should pay close attention to those disagreements because they may portend future problems with the way a group works together. The ability of the group to work as a cohesive unit represents a lot of the value in the group itself, and if strife over valuation and share allotment takes on a life of its own, the practice management firm may be better off walking away.

Although these are the two most common ways of valuing group practices, there are plenty of variations on this theme. For example, some practice management firms keep it simple by paying physicians or dentists one times trailing 12-months revenues. Obviously, such transactions lack the planning and analysis to make them successful in the long term.

THE FORMULA

The most common acquisition formula is equal parts of stock, cash and notes that mature over three to five years (Table 9–2). The price paid may depend on whether the company is private or public, and if public, how its stock is trading. When the management company stocks were flying high, these groups were more than willing to trade equity because shares were trading at 30 times earnings. If they bought a physician group at 20 times earnings, they had a spread of 10 points in arbitrage. Unfortunately, that formula works against companies whose stocks subsequently plummet. For example, as physician company stocks tanked to 5 or 6 times earnings, they couldn't get the same arbitrage spread.

TABLE 9–2

Acquisition Characteristics of Practice Management Deals

	1997	1998
Cash	35%	38%
Notes	19%	34%
Stock	46%	28%
Vesting	0–6 years	5 years
Management agreement	80%	81%
Term (average)	31 years	31 years
Fee % gross (median)	21%	20%

Source: Cordova Capital/*Modern Physician.*

In addition, a physician company probably won't want to use a lot of its stock in an acquisition if it believes the stock is undervalued. Stock is a form of currency in these transactions and physician companies will want to use the stock advantageously. Trading stock for physician practices is a good deal for the physician company if the stock is trading at a high multiple and it doesn't take as many shares to buy the practice. However, using several thousand shares of undervalued stock to purchase physicians will not benefit the company. It will end up diluting earnings per share unless the group's profits are immediately additive, which doesn't happen very often. It often takes a couple of quarters, at least, to integrate practices so that they add to overall profits.

In an acquisition, physicians or dentists often do not receive the cash, stock and notes in one lump sum. Typically, the practice management company sets earn-outs in which a portion of the purchase price is held back and paid back over the next two to five years. In some cases, the practice must reach certain targets, such as pre-determined EBITDA levels, to receive the additional consideration.

At American Oncology Resources, CEO Dale Ross preaches consistency with his physicians in the company's deal structure. Oncologists in affiliation discussions with AOR generate between $1 million and $1.5 million in annual revenue and typically take home between one-fourth and one-third of revenue. AOR purchases the assets of the physicians' practice for five times forward EBITDA.

In the acquisition, AOR typically pays 40% cash, 40% notes and 20% stock. Sometimes, however, physicians want the stock portion to be larger, and in some cases as much as 50% of the price has been paid in stock. The stock is delivered in increments of 20%, 20%, and 60% in the third, fourth and fifth years, respectively. Physicians are free to trade the stock once they receive it.

By delivering the stock in portions over a period of years, physicians remain tied financially to the practice management company. It also helps stabilize the stock price. Physicians may be tempted to sell their shares as soon as they can. If physicians start dumping shares, it will reflect poorly on the practice management firm. The sale of these shares will be tracked by brokers and research analysts who may view it as a lack of confidence in the physician company.

In general, physicians may need to be counseled about how and when to buy and sell their stock. Obviously, the practice management firm can't tell physicians when to sell or buy shares. However, a little investment advice will be appreciated. For example, one physician company executive described how several physicians were burned and blamed it on the company. They had received stock options that could be sold a year after the IPO. When the options vested, the physicians exercised them. They had to pay taxes on the gain, but instead of selling the stock right away, they held on to it. In the subsequent months, the stock's price plummeted and the physicians were left paying taxes on gains that they never realized.

A BUYER'S DUE DILIGENCE

Valuations must be based on proper due diligence of numerous factors, both economic and non-economic, in the practices. Factors to consider include the following.

- *Financial records.* Proper planning is the key. The acquirer must have access to reliable data at the practice. This must include the most recent financial statements and corresponding trial balances. In addition, the acquirer will want to research related entities owned by the physicians, such as labs, billing companies or outpatient centers. What are the existing lease obligations and payor contracts? Have payors in the region been slow to pay?

- *Operating systems.* The health system or management organization should review the practice's accounting and financial reporting systems. How are claims handled? What systems are set up for utilization management and credentialing? Getting a handle on these systems will help in a projection of how well the transition will be into the new organization. Are the systems compatible with the acquirer's? If not, how much will it cost to buy new ones or convert? How long will it take to accomplish that?

- *Existing policies and procedures.* What are the practice's existing policies and procedures, and can they be integrated into the buyer's?

- *Business philosophy and culture.* The health system or acquiring physician group must be sure that the physicians support the purchase of the practice and will unite with the new organization to work together as a team. Numerous acquisitions have imploded because there was no long-term commitment to the organization. Attitude may be hard to quantify, but may be the most crucial variable for long-term success. While doctors may be in favor of the transaction, they may not have worked through the issues of how this will change their practice as it goes forward. Also on the non-economic side, the management organization needs to consider the level of managed care penetration in the practice's market and how that has contributed to the practice's culture. This, too, may be difficult to quantify, but the acquirer will have to make some assumptions about how managed care will affect physician reimbursement and whether the practice is structured to accept contracts with partial or full risk. If the market is moving quickly toward capitation, the acquirer must evaluate the practice's readiness. For example, the acquirer will want to analyze the practice's utilization patterns (inpatient days per thousand enrollees, lengths of stay) and compare them with high managed care areas.

In terms of details, due diligence efforts also must focus on both balance sheet and income statement issues. Some highlights follow.

Balance Sheet

- *Accounts receivable.* Obtain an accounts receivable aging schedule and review actual versus estimated collections. Also, review the bad debt allowance and the level of contractual allowances.
- *Property and equipment.* Obtain related party fixed asset listings and review the future minimum lease schedule for capital and operating leases.
- *Goodwill and management service agreement intangibles.* Review the amortization schedule, keeping in mind the SEC is discouraging amortization periods of more than 25 years.
- *Debt.* Obtain the schedule of future obligations, looking for significant terms such as balloon payments.
- *Accounts payable and accruals.* Have expenses been properly recorded? Search for unrecorded liabilities and review period-end cut-off procedures.

Income Statement

- *Revenue.* Carefully look at the sources of revenue and the percentage that comes from commercial, Medicare, and Medicaid. Is the revenue mix appropriate for the practice? Would the loss of a few key payors compromise the practice's viability? Review revenue by procedure coding to determine whether its being recorded properly.

- *Payroll expenses.* Obtain physician salary and benefit information as well as office and administration payroll expenses for the past 12 months.

- *General and administrative expenses.* Review expenses by vendor in detail. Also, review insurance policies and determine whether there are any malpractice claims filed or pending.

THE PHYSICIAN'S EYE VIEW

Physicians, too, must weigh the credibility and durability of the practice management organizations and health systems with which they're considering affiliating (Figure 9–3). A start-up practice management firm often bids more for a group practice because it's trying to build up to a critical mass. An established company may not bid as much because they don't have to. Is the extra cash worth the risk of affiliating with a fledgling organization?

In addition, future compensation is a crucial element in the valuation because it will affect the management fee paid. As practice management organizations evolve, they're paying physicians less up front in exchange for a lower management fee.

FIGURE 9–3

Questions Physicians Should Ask Themselves Before Selling

- Is this the organization you want to work for in the long term?
- Are you willing to sacrifice some of your own autonomy for the good of the organization?
- Have you researched this organization and talked to other physicians who work there?
- How are physicians involved in clinical policy making?
- Has the practice management firm developed a business plan for your practice?
- Who makes operational decisions for the practice?
- How will affiliating with this organization change the day-to-day operations of your practice?
- Have you obtained an independent valuation, and are you satisfied with it?
- Does the management organization have the capital to expand local operations?
- Are the cost reductions planned by the management organization exaggerated?

Practice management organizations differ in the way they include compensation in the valuation formula. Some include it in expenses, while others take it out later.

One of hurdles practice management organizations must overcome is that when a management fee comes out of the practice's income stream, the physicians end up making less money. Only if the practice grows will the physicians receive more in compensation. That's why a business plan from the management organization is crucial as the physician group decides its future.

Rather than giving physicians all of the cash up front, some acquirers have arranged terms to pay it out over three to five years if the practice meets certain productivity or profitability goals. Ongoing compensation terms must be determined as well. By charging a management fee of 15% to 25%, practice management companies are taking away compensation that previously would have gone in the physicians' pockets. Unless the practice management firm improves overall profits, the physicians will ultimately be disgruntled.

Now, most physicians are interested in future compensation as much or more than how much the management organization is going to give them for their practice. In today's market, the only way a practice management organization or health system can convince physicians to sell is by demonstrating how they can bring operational benefits that would translate into higher compensation for the physicians. Physicians want to know how much they'll make in the future, and that depends on how much value the management firm can bring to the clinic. Yet that value remains elusive.

Investment banker Douglas Townsend noted that in a recent "auction" of a multi-specialty clinic, his firm queried bidders about that value by asking them to provide data on other clinics affiliated with their companies.

The questions were: "Since affiliating with the management organization, what was

- the increase in number of physicians?"
- the percentage of primary care physicians?"
- the increase in capitated lives?"
- the change in overhead ratios?"
- the growth in revenue?"

Of those organizations providing answers, only 29% percent answered the question on the increase in the number of physicians, and 14% answered the question about revenue growth. None answered the questions on the percentage of primary care physicians, the increase in capitated lives, or the change in overhead ratios.

Not much to go on, huh? Yet physicians need those types of information. In fact, Townsend believes that a practice management organization that can demonstrate operational value will pay lower prices up front, but deliver higher compensation down the road. On the other hand, those that can't demonstrate operational value to their physicians will pay more up front, but deliver less on the back end. The latter model is unlikely to endure in the long term.

"A physician management organization must convince physicians of their weaknesses by proving their strengths," Townsend added.

TAX STRATEGIES FOR BOTH BUYER AND SELLER

Many physician management organizations emphasize the tax advantages physicians reap by selling their practices. Since most physician practices are operated so that profits are distributed as earnings, they're taxed at the highest rate—38%. However, if a physician sells the practice, the income from the sale is taxed as a capital gain, an 18% reduction in taxes.

Physician management organizations will want to set up a tax structure that will do the following.

- Get the best financial account results
- Provide a tax deductible basis in assets acquired
- Minimize state tax liability
- Address business issues, such as assumption of liabilities and corporate practice of medicine laws

There are three common types of tax structures: asset purchase, stock purchase, or tax-free transaction. Table 9–3 provides a brief rundown of pros and cons on all three.

Timing

The acquisition process can take from a few months to years. All kinds of internal and external factors can delay the deal. For example, if the practice is using a lawyer who is not accustomed to working with practice management companies, the process can drag on much longer because of unfamiliarity with the inherent regulatory and legal details.

The time line for buying practices will extend proportionally to the industry's volatility. When physician consolidation was on a straight line up, closing deals could take as little as three weeks. When uncertainty about the industry clouded the market, deals began taking longer and longer. Physicians and dentists are getting more diligent about researching prospective acquirers and calling in their advisers to scrutinize the transactions.

In addition, some specialties may make decisions faster than others. Cynthia Dotson, chief financial officer of an OB/GYN company, MediSphere, said the

Text continued on page 201.

TABLE 9–3

The Three Major Types of Tax Structures

Asset Purchase		
	Pros	**Cons**
Management organization	■ Tax deductible basis in assets acquired equals fair market value. ■ Amortization/depreciation of intangibles and other assets. ■ No liabilities, or selected liabilities, can be assumed. ■ Different types of consideration can be used. ■ Tax associated with accounts receivable of a cash basis professional corporation is paid by the physicians' professional corporation.	■ Physicians may argue for increased purchase price because of the higher ordinary income tax rate as compared to capital gain tax rate.
Physicians	■ Possible deferral of gain if the transaction qualifies for installment sale reporting (this will depend on the type consideration received and the assets sold). ■ Different types of consideration can be used.	■ May involve two levels of tax. ■ Will pay ordinary income/short-term capital gains for the MSA.

Stock Purchase		
	Pros	**Cons**
Management organization	■ Different types of consideration may be used. ■ Possible stock purchase can be treated as an asset purchase for an S corporation.	■ No step up in basis of assets acquired. ■ Assumption of liabilities. ■ Tax associated with accounts receivable of a cash basis PC may be assumed by management organization. ■ PC must be converted into an entity that can be owned by management organization.

The Three Major Types of Tax Structures (continued)

Stock Purchase		
	Pros	**Cons**
Management organization cont'd		■ Transfer of medical assets (patient records, medical contracts, pharmaceuticals, etc.) to new PC can generate gain to acquired PC.
Physicians	■ Long-term capital gain to shareholders/physicians on stock (must meet holding period, etc.). ■ Only one level of tax. ■ Possible deferral of gain if transaction qualifies for installment sale reporting (depends on type of consideration received). ■ Different types of consideration can be used.	■ Formation of new PC required ■ Difficulties in distributing purchase price different from relative shareholdings ■ Transfer of medical assets (patient records, medical contracts, pharmaceuticals, etc.) to new PC can generate gain to acquired PC.

Tax-Free Transaction		
	Pros	**Cons**
Management organization	■ Different types of consideration can be used. ■ Different forms of a tax-free transaction are available. ■ Typically requires higher percentage of management organization stock in the consideration mix.	■ No step up in basis of assets acquired ■ Assumption of liabilities in certain tax-free transactions ■ Must meet various complex tax-free requirements of Internal Revenue Code ■ Tax associated with accounts receivable of a cash basis PC may be assumed by management organization ■ PC must be converted into an entity that can be owned by management organization ■ Transfer of medical assets (patient records,

The Three Major Types of Tax Structures *(concluded)*

Tax-Free Transaction		
	Pros	**Cons**
Physicians	■ No tax to shareholders/ physicians on stock received ■ Generally, capital gain to shareholders/physicians on nonstock consideration received (must meet holding period, etc.) ■ Only one level of tax ■ Different types of consideration can be used	medical contracts, pharmaceuticals, etc.) to new PC can generate gain to acquired PC ■ Formation of new PC required ■ Difficulties in distributing purchase price different from relative shareholdings ■ Transfer of medical assets (patient records, medical contracts, pharmaceuticals, etc.) to new PC can generate gain to acquired PC ■ Must meet various complex tax free requirements of Internal Revenue Code ■ Lack of liquidity of management organization's stock ■ Higher percentage of management organization stock in consideration mix

physicians in that specialty are conservative and just don't make quick decisions. "OB/GYNs are trained to wait," she said, nothing the nine-month cycle of the birthing process. "They're not risk takers and they're not overly aggressive."

VALUATION IN REVERSE

Messy divorce proceedings between practice management companies and their physicians scream from the pages of industry magazines and newsletters. Over the summer of 1998, the bottle-rocket growth of the practice management industry sputtered and its market capitalization snapped in half.

Just as Wall Street's expectations for management companies were not met, so have expected results failed to materialize between some physicians and their management organizations. Now some physician organizations are shredding apart, prompting questions about how the separation of physicians from their practice management companies will play out. Similar questions are arising at many hospital-based health systems that are divesting or restructuring physician practices.

This spate of separations doesn't signal a wholesale divestiture of physicians from practice management companies or health systems. Many health systems and other physician groups are still actively acquiring practices and physician consolidation continues. However, this evolutionary phase does warrant close attention. While disbanding these relationships may cause anxiety for those involved, bystander physician groups and other health systems that purchase physician practices may be able to benefit from the experience of their industry brethren.

Valuation

Methods of valuing practices during a company's go-go growth phase may not be valid when those deals unwind. The publicly traded practice management sector had a market capitalization of $8 billion in April 1998, but by August it had sunk to $4 billion due to numerous write-offs, management changes and scaled-back growth expectations. Cash-constrained companies are less apt to be acquirers, and not coincidentally, fewer buyers means lower prices. In addition, many hospital systems have curtailed their feeding frenzy of physician practices after red ink from those operations started leaking onto their otherwise healthy balance sheets.

In short, prices have fallen substantially. "Many buyers overpaid for these groups when they bought them," said Paul DeMuro, a partner at in the law firm, Latham & Watkins.

In a typical scenario, a management company acquires the non-clinical assets of a physician's practice and signs a long-term management services agreement with the physicians. The acquisition price is determined, in part, by forecasting how well the physician's practice will do under the management of the acquirer. The difference between the value of the practice's hard assets and the acquisition price is accounted for as goodwill or capitalized management agreements.

When market supply and demand changes or growth prospects shrink, as they have in the past six months, so do the valuations. So when the management organization decides to transfer, terminate, or sell that management services agreement, it is unlikely to realize the same value that it recorded on its books when market conditions were much more competitive or optimistic. As a result, some management companies have recognized losses on the management services agreements for practices that they plan on divesting.

In some cases, separation terms are spelled out in these agreements between the management organization and the physicians. For example, some organizations agree that they'll sell the practices back to the physicians for the book value or the unamortized value. Some agreements require that the physician practice repurchase the assets to protect the company from realizing a loss. However, those types of separation terms are included to cover contracts that have run their full term (25 to 40 years) or to organizations that have defaulted on their commitments, noted Mitchell Kornblit, a partner with Shattuck Hammond, a division of PricewaterhouseCoopers. Although these separation terms exist in MSA contracts, they usually don't apply to an unanticipated termination of the arrangement, he said. In fact, health systems and/or management companies usually haven't signed "prenuptial agreements" with their physicians that address what would happen if a separation occurs before the contract runs out.

In addition, amortization schedules may vary greatly. If the management organization wants to make it difficult for the physicians to repurchase their practices, the amortization schedule may reflect very little amortization in the early years of the agreement. That unamortized value, then, may be too much for the physicians to finance. In that case, the management organization or health system may be asked to loan physicians the capital to buy back their practices.

Some acquirers see opportunity in the numerous divestitures of physician practices by hospitals, practices, and large practice management organizations. In many cases, hospitals systems are buying practices divested by publicly traded physician companies, and vice versa. However, valuations can be problematic if those practices are purchased at a high multiple to future earnings. Not-for-profit hospitals that sell practices back to physicians need to be aware that the transaction could raise inurement as well as private benefit, intermediate sanction, anti-kickback, and Stark II questions. That's particularly true if the practices were bought by the hospital at a premium price and sold back at rock-bottom price, allowing the physicians to be viewed as having a financial gain. Certain attention must be afforded to practices that have accelerated the amortization and the write-off of goodwill and covenants not to compete.

Jerry Sokol, a partner in the Miami law office of McDermott, Will & Emery, pointed out that the divestiture by management companies of physician practices can be accomplished in two ways.

1. A transfer of the management company's interest in the practice back to the practice, which is accomplished by simply terminating the management services agreement.
2. Selling or transferring the management company's interest in the practice to a third party, such as another management organization. That can be accomplished by simply assigning the management services agreement to the third party.

With regard to terminating the agreement, many management services agreements spell out the terms of the unwind upon termination. These terms typically include what the practice must pay back to the management company upon termination. The problem, however, is that most management services agreements do not allow the management organization to unilaterally terminate the agreement "without cause." Therefore, the parties will likely need to negotiate a "reduced" unwind price in order for the management organization to unilaterally terminate the agreement.

With respect to a sale/transfer of the management services agreement to a third party, the critical provision here is the "assignment" provision of the agreement. If the agreement allows for an assignment by the management organization without the physicians' consent, then the management organization could potentially assign its interest (i.e., its right to the management fee) to a third party without the physicians' consent. In this scenario, the purchase price paid to the management organization by the third party would likely be the third party's perceived value of the future management fee. If the agreement does not allow for assignment without the physicians' consent, then it is likely that the physicians will seek some form of compensation in return for their consent to the assignment.

Incurring a loss on the divested practice may be just part of the overall separation cost to a management organization. In a divorce of spouses, one often has to pay alimony to the other. The same is true in a management organization breakup. To get away from a medical group that the practice management company doesn't want, it may have to pay to exit the employment contract with physicians.

Contract Expectations

A separation discussion may develop if the management organization or the physicians didn't live up to the terms of the management services agreement. In one well-publicized case, certain physician groups stopped paying the management organization its management fee, charging that the management company had not lived up to its promises. Recovering the several million dollars in receivables from physicians proved problematic, and the management organization ended up writing off much of those fees.

Management organizations need to protect themselves from the beginning—when the acquisition documents are written. For example, a frequent complaint made by management organizations is that once the physicians are put on salary, their productivity slides. If the physician practice is not performing well under the new management, the physicians may believe the management organization is at fault. The management organization, in turn, may believe the physicians are at fault for not working as hard as they had agreed.

These dilemmas can be avoided if the management services agreement includes specific responsibilities of each party. These may include the following.

- Productivity benchmarks for the group or for each physician
- Revenue and/or fee income requirements

- Support services that the management organization must provide to the practice
- Level of capital investment that the management organization must provide to the practice

Non-Compete Clauses

Typically, physicians sign an employment contract upon sale of the practice that includes a non-compete clause of three to five years. The non-compete will restrict a physician from practicing within a certain geographical area, which is negotiated at the time of the contract. Depending on the market, this area could range from as little as two miles to as much as 50 miles.

During 1997, the SEC began to require that publicly traded physician companies included a discussion of non-competes in the section of their registration statements that addresses risk factors. The concern is that non-competes may not be enforceable in some states, noted Latham & Watkins' DeMuro. For example, one company noted in its prospectus that it is not possible to predict whether its interests will be enforced by the courts "as the type of protectable business interest that would permit it to enforce such a covenant."

Unfortunately, physician companies are such a new industry that there haven't been enough judicial precedents to determine how the courts will rule on physician non-compete agreements.

Amortization

Traditionally, management organizations have signed management services agreements with their practices for 30 to 40 years, and many companies amortized the intangible value of the practices over a similar term. In 1997, however, the SEC began restricting new publicly traded management organizations to amortization periods of 25 years of less (even when the contract term is much longer), and in 1998, the SEC issued informal guidance instructing all practice management organizations to similarly reduce their amortization periods. The SEC cites concerns that industry characteristics and trends do not support an amortization period of more than 25 years and that, in fact, amortization over 5 to 10 year periods is probably more appropriate.

The subject of practice management company break-ups has implications beyond that of individual companies or their stock prices. If breaking off and transferring these management services agreements becomes an intrinsic part of this business, it could impact the way the SEC views practice management organizations from an accounting standpoint. For example, if the contractual term specified for MSAs begins to evolve to shorter and shorter life spans, the SEC may press management organizations to shorten their amortization period.

Bankruptcy

Some management services agreements state that the agreement will terminated if one of the parties files for bankruptcy. However, bankruptcy isn't an automatic out, DeMuro said. Once the acquirer is in bankruptcy, it's up to the trustee, who will appointed by the court in cooperation with the filing organization, to decide whether the company should accept or reject the contracts. Unprofitable agreements are more likely to be rejected, which would free the physicians to re-establish their own practices or join other groups. However, it also may release the management organization from having to continue to pay the physicians under the terms of their multi-year employment contracts. If a practice's contract is not rejected, the practice will continue to be part of the management organization even through its bankruptcy reorganization.

Although the bankruptcy reorganizations of two large provider organizations have rocked the industry, it's too early to know how physician contracts will be treated by bankruptcy courts.

The Next Step

Once a practice management organization and its physicians separate, it's not uncommon for those same physicians to rebound into a relationship with another practice management company or physician organization. Many physicians sold their practices to reduce administrative requirements, gain market clout in contracting and align with larger entities to protect referrals. Those are still valid reasons for affiliating with a larger organization.

Before these relationships are severed, it's important for physicians to review their strategic options going forward. Ideally, physicians must find organizations that understand their needs and with which they are willing to be in partnership for the long haul.

AN EXPERT'S PERSPECTIVE: MITCHELL KORNBLIT, PARTNER, SHATTUCK HAMMOND, NEW YORK

Mitchell Kornblit, an expert in healthcare valuations at Shattock Hammond, notes many practice management companies bought practices based on what he calls SEBITDA— "someday" EBITDA. Since the practice didn't have any operating cash flow, the management company may have projected the cash flow based on unrealistic expectations, he said.

Those values were based on optimistic feelings. "There's a lot of projection because a lot of these companies believe they can add value to the groups," he added. "What happened in the practice management sector is these doctors agreed to give management companies their business and income going forward.

Then, the business failed to grow because of managed care and other factors. When the revenues didn't grow, and the pot of money didn't get bigger, the physicians said, 'We have less money.' But they forgot about the million dollars they were given to buy the business."

The expectations by both the physicians and the management companies were unrealistic in many cases, and those expectations were formulated into the valuations. If the management organization thought that the physician group was going to grow at 15% a year, that was figured into the valuation. "You can't grow a medical group practice that quickly," Kornblit said. "It takes time to get new physicians, new members into health plans. If you're building in 15% a year for five years, you're saying that business is going to double every five years. You can't get that kind of growth organically, and you can't get it that quickly."

When practice management stocks were flying high, it was easier to round up physicians because acquisition prices were high. These organizations "would say, 'We think we can make net income of $1 million, our stock is trading at 20 times earnings, so if we pay at 10 times, we won't be hurt by it. A lot of deals were made that way," Kornblit said (Table 9–4).

While those days are gone, at least for a while, some basics remain. "There's nothing unique about valuing medical groups," Kornblit said. "The big change comes in how the income stream goes to the doctors after the acquisition." Doctors need to understand that there will be a fundamental change in how the practice's income is distributed. After the management company buys the practice, there's going to be less money for distribution to the physicians. The only way that pot of

TABLE 9–4

Top Ten Physician Medical Group Deals in 1997

Target	Acquirer	Price (millions)
InPhyNet Medical Management	MedPartners	$442
EmCare Holdings	Laidlaw	$402
Talbert Medical Management	MedPartners	$187
Health Partners	FPA Medical Management	$185
Vivra Specialty Partners	New company	$84
Advanced Radiology	American Physician Partners	$83
10 Massachusetts Blues Plans	MedPartners	$75
HealthCap	FPA Medical Management	$60
Foundation Health	Talbert Medical Management	$60
Aetna Professional Management	MedPartners	$57

money is going to increase is if the business is expanded, and the physician and practice management company have to work together to make that happen.

PricewaterhouseCoopers Tips for Valuing and Acquiring Physician Groups

- Understand why the physician and dental group wants to affiliate with the practice management company. If money is the only motive, walk away.
- Make sure the contract language is clear to all parties. Avoid overly complicated formulas with unrealistic financial targets.
- Don't rush into a deal. Take time to proceed with the proper due diligence.
- Consider the worst case scenario. If physicians fail to perform or the practice management company files for bankruptcy, what are the consequences and options? Include those in the agreements.
- Hire experts in accounting and legal services to structure the deals so you don't run afoul of federal, state and local regulations.

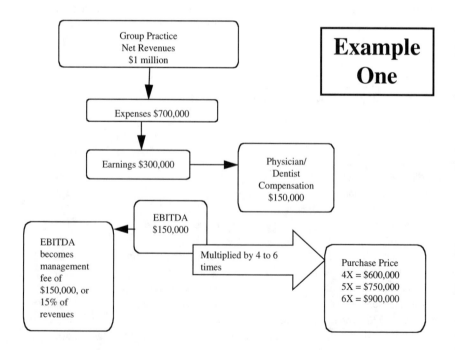

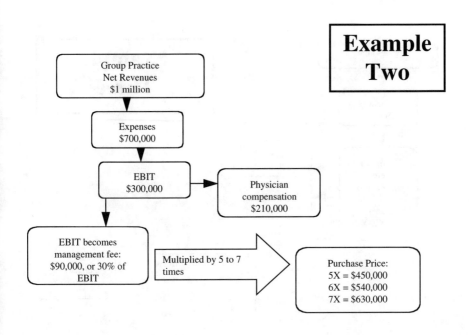

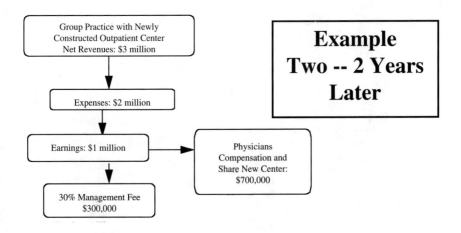

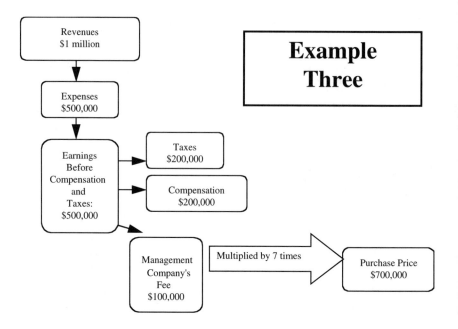

10

CHAPTER

Leadership: Who's in Charge Here?

Sandy Lutz

Jack Castle Jr. fondly refers to his father as "Dr. Jack." The father and son are a team that cobbled together Jack Jr.'s financial and operational experience and Dr. Jack's dentistry background into a practice management chain with nearly $50 million in revenues in 1997.

Together, they embody a theme that runs through practice management companies. Success typically stems from a team approach. Leadership implies a single person, but that's not the winning formula for a complex medical business with many moving parts and divergent constituencies.

"Dr. Jack"—Jack Castle Sr.—went to dentistry school on the G.I. Bill "but always wanted to be an entrepreneur," his son said. He built a hospital in Houston, which he sold to a hospital chain, American Medical International in 1980. In 1981, father and son researched various businesses they could undertake together and came up with retail dentistry.

Do you really want to scrimmage with physicians or dentists or bankers or accountants all day long? Pick your poison. If one of those is not what you're really good at, then you must find a leader who is.

A finely tuned physician organization is one that can draw on the right resources at the right time. Just like the body's immune system responding to different infections, a physician organization needs talented leaders who can respond to financial and clinical challenges. When one aspect gets out of balance, the physician organization gets sick.

Sounds simple, doesn't it? Yet, the delicate balance of leadership in physician management organizations is not easily achieved. Unfortunately, few physicians have been a part of a large group practice or practice management company that was a success. However, in the wake of many of today's failed physician organizations is the flotsam of inadequate leadership. Too often, physician executives have not been the top managers in their fields. They were physicians who had tired of clinical practice or business executives that saw an industry ripe for the picking.

The classic problem in these organizations can be summed up as follows. The leaders are either physicians who don't have sufficient business skills or business executives who can't work with physicians.

Let's face it. Most of us humans are limited to a certain set of skills in which we can be experts. It's rare to find the physician who also excels in business matters or a business executive who can lead physicians. Other industries encounter similar struggles: Software companies started by computer geeks. Restaurants opened by gifted chefs. Sooner or later, those talented entrepreneurs must acquire business skills or relegate some of their organizations' power to equally talented business leaders.

Yet, leading physicians companies seems to be one of the most vexing challenges in the business world. Why? Physicians are notoriously independent and leading them almost always prompts the tired analogies of "herding cats" or "hauling frogs in a wheelbarrow." What's more, physician companies struggle with some of the same questions as other for-profit healthcare companies: How do you maximize the bottom line without cutting into patient care, and how do you counter the perception that one compromises the other? If improperly addressed, those questions can shake the faith that physicians have in their leaders.

Finally, the practice management industry has foundered in part, because it's lacked role models that exhibit strong leadership traits. Leadership problems are bound to emanate if physician organizations can't answer this basic question: *Who's in charge?*

Practice management companies typically start as one or more large group practices that hire a CEO to lead the organization. At that point, the physicians may feel like that CEO is working for them. Yet, the CEO, whose job is to lead the group, may feel like the physicians are working for him or her. Who is right?

Without the power to hire or fire the physicians, the CEO's job may seem emasculated. "I will never work with physicians again," said one former practice management company CEO who talked about continuous battles over who was really in charge. Although the CEO was hired to run the company, he spent much of his time trying to deal with dissatisfied physicians who were trying to sell the company out from under him or jump ship to another practice management firm.

Physicians are accustomed to being in charge of their practices. Even after selling their practices, some may still think they're in charge of the practice, both clinically and administratively. Physician organization executives have a bounty of stories about how power struggles emerge after deal has closed. It's not unusual to hear of business office employees who are fired by the physician organization's managers and then later rehired by the physicians themselves. "Why can't we keep Sheila on the payroll?" the doctors moaned. "We're paying you that huge administrative fee."

Finally, physician organizations are in a battle for talent with other businesses that are far more attractive to young managers. For example, healthcare has a dearth of leaders who have strong information systems skills. Those talented individuals are more often attracted to other technology-savvy industries like banking, telecommunications, and Internet-related businesses.

LEADING PHYSICIANS

Arthur Greenberg, MD, a medical director with a primary-care practice management organization in Dallas, said that practice management organizations must help physicians practice better medicine more efficiently. Some practice management organizations have been satisfied with simply rolling up a bunch of practices, then letting the physicians do what they want. That model will fail, he predicts. It "reminds me of bookies who take a few percentage points off the top and don't care what you do afterward," Greenberg said.

To lead doctors in today's business world means to help them overcome old habits. For example, "We in medicine have operated under the illusion that every patient is unique," Greenberg noted. However, part of the value in practice management organizations is bringing some standardization to treatment processes. Physicians often balk at this, calling it "cookbook medicine," and saying, "You don't know my patient."

Yet, if physicians have input into the statistically validated protocols, they'll often see the value and validity of using them. "None of this has to be reinvented," he said, noting that medical specialty societies and associations have produced numerous protocols and other measures.

Putting protocols together with the necessary technology, and bringing that to the physicians is "the power of practice management organizations," says Greenberg. "Computers can do algorithmic analysis better than any human brain." When caring professionals apply those analyses in patient care situations, it breeds success, he said, adding that "computers can't lay on hands."

About leadership, Greenberg believes that physicians first need to realize that "we're all in this together." Next, "you have to make it easy for them to follow the path," he said, citing the availability of palm/hand-held computer technology that gives physicians the information at the point of service, what he calls "just-in-time learning."

Greenberg believes that the key to motivating physicians is compensation structures. Most physicians want some type of performance-based compensation because they're inherently competitive achievers, he said, adding: "They were the type of students that wanted to get the A in chemistry."

F I G U R E 10–1

Top Five Strategic Goals of Group Practice Executives

1. Information Technology
2. Commitment to Mission
3. Measuring quality of care/outcomes
4. Developing breadth of physician networks
5. Availability of qualified senior managers

Source: PricewaterhouseCoopers and *Hospitals and Health Networks* magazine, 1998.

He sums up the difference between physicians and business executives this way: "Physicians are used to making important decisions with very little data. They tend to be impulsive, and fly by the seat of their pants," Greenberg said. "Business types like lots of data. They always say, 'We need more data.' They'll have spreadsheets up to the ceiling."

Balancing those two tendencies is key to leading any physician organization. "The ideal management team is a physician who can schmooze the doctors coupled with a professional business manager," Greenberg said. He stressed that physicians must be part of the leadership team. "If you want to talk to doctors and win them over, you need a fraternity member."

Developing physician leaders in the ranks is crucial to managing these organizations. "Leadership isn't always inherent," said Barton Wald, MD, medical director at UniMed, the practice management division of UniHealth. "In today's complex medical business model, physician leaders need to have significant financial and management skills in addition to a charismatic leadership style. They also need a strategic understanding of the business." UniMed operates groups with about 6,000 physicians, including one of the state's largest independent practice associations, Huntington Provider Group in Pasadena, Calif. In 1998, UniMed had 60 physician leaders attend a governance seminar at UCLA. "Formal educational and development programs are necessary to developing good leaders," Dr. Wald said. Michael Linn, UniMed's president and CEO, also noted that physician compensation models need to include incentives for participation in and effectiveness in governance.

Linn agreed with Greenberg that leading physicians requires that the physicians understand the organization's interdependency. "What so many of the practice management organizations have done is separate the physicians from the outcomes of the business," Linn added. "You need to keep the physicians fully engaged. Loyalty is created because you create value for the physicians." To assist with that, UniMed has designed a Master Physician Organization that will allow it to take risk-based contracts as a single organization. The physicians' professional corporation will retain autonomy, however. The structure will give UniMed the clout to negotiate with large health plans on a more equal basis, Linn said. "The health plans have wielded tremendous power" in California, he said. "How big a hammer you wield in contract negotiations makes a difference."

Physician organizations and their leaders often underestimate the time and skill it takes to work together. Getting a multi-specialty group to work cohesively is very labor intensive. Cooperative efforts have to be put forth by physicians as well as management. For example, it may be difficult to get physicians to put in those efforts if the practice management organization's compensation system rewards productivity in terms of fees or revenues. In such cases, the physicians won't be induced to carve out time to help develop the practice management organization.

LEADING DENTISTS

Michael Fiore, the co-chairman, CEO, and president of Gentle Dental, noted that dentists, too, have concerns about business leaders who aren't dentists. "It's more effective if I have a partner who is a dentist," he says. Steven Matzkin, the company's co-chairman, president and chief dental officer, had been chairman and CEO of Dental Care Alliance, another DPM, prior to its merger with Gentle Dental in 1998.

Fiore sees a clear delineation between the dental practitioner and the business practitioner. "I will never be able to look in somebody's mouth as well as they do, and they will never be able run a company as well as I do," he says. As a former hospital system executive, he also observes that doctors and dentists have different ego levels. "Dentists have a more realistic view of their role," he noted.

Fiore has learned that being able to work with dentists as a team is key to leading a successful company. He recounts an earlier physician group acquisition experience prior to joining Gentle Dental. "I had this nagging feeling that they weren't going to be team players," Fiore said. The intuition was correct. The physicians were at loggerheads almost immediately with the company management. It was an experience he'd rather not go through again. He's learned to trust those feelings now whenever Gentle Dental does an acquisition. "I will walk away from a group that I don't think we can work with effectively," he added. "A lot of the mistakes that practice management organizations have made have been because the acquisitions made no sense."

SEEKING BALANCE

Practice management companies and their physicians must be willing to delegate decision-making authority to the experts. "I've promised them (the physicians) that I won't try to do total knee replacements," said Robert Yeager, president of OrthoLink, a Nashville-based practice management organization that specializes in musculoskeletal diseases and treatment. On clinical decisions, physicians need to have "95% of the decision-making authority," he said. But on business decisions, "physicians have to be willing to step back."

Many practice management organizations attempt to strike a balance by establishing joint policy boards on the local level. Here as in many other areas, PhyCor set the industry standard. The PhyCor model is to have a joint policy board comprising three physician representatives and three PhyCor representatives. The policy board is jointly responsible for strategic planning, budgeting, fee setting, capital expenditures, staffing and insurance. PhyCor then handles capital development, management, accounting and information systems. In some cases, the practice management organization also handles most of the managed care contracting. Meanwhile, the physicians take the lead in medical protocols and compensation allocation.

Other practice management organizations have embraced this model because it clearly delineates the responsibilities of each organization and its leaders. If done properly, it also enables the management company to demonstrate the values it brings to the physicians organization. Duties such as accounting, information systems, raising capital, and managed care contracting are the ones that physicians usually want to get out of—that's why they turned to a management company in the first place.

However, practice management leaders must ensure that they bring in competent managers who can deliver results in those areas. It's one thing to promise information systems or managed care contracting clout, and another to have the individuals who can actually perform those functions. For example, some practice management organizations have promised to help physician groups develop ancillary services, but they haven't the people in place who know how to develop and operate them. "A lot of times what's missing at practice management organizations is the middle management level," said Danguole Spakevicius, president and CEO of FemPartners, a privately held practice management company in Houston specializing in women's healthcare. FemPartners' affiliated medical groups include 42 physicians and five nurse practitioners. FemPartners also includes the largest integrated women's health center in the nation, with five types of labs, an assisted reproduction center, and a bone density center. "You have to have someone who knows how to run an imaging center and knows the FDA rules, or knows how to run a CLIA-certified lab," she added.

If physicians find that the practice management organization isn't providing the business balance promised, the company won't be able to go forward for long.

COMMUNICATION

In interviews about leadership skills, the word "communication" surfaces again and again. "You need to be able to communicate at all levels of the organization, from the lowest to the highest," explains Robert Boyle, who has led several physician organizations in California and Texas. "You also need to communicate all the way through the health system, not only in your group but with the leadership of providers and health plans in the community."

Boyle, who was president of the Medical Group Management Association in 1997, says that leaders of physician organizations must impart to physicians an understanding of why they need each other. "If physicians don't believe it's necessary to be interdependent with other physicians in the practice management organization, they're eventually going to conclude that they're better off on their own. It's up to physician leaders to reinforce with physicians the needs that hold them together." Those needs might include capital, the ability to contract effectively with managed care, or the power to negotiate with area health systems.

Physician organizations have chronic communication problems. Few practice management organizations would say they have mastered this area. When the left hand doesn't know what the right hand is doing, it's bound to cause problems, hurt feelings, and financial missteps.

Here are three communication strategies to keep in mind.

- *A communication effort that works well with one constituency might transfer well to another.* Publicly-held companies typically host call-in telephone conferences with investment analysts after announcing earnings, to give them a chance to ask questions about the quarter and get a feel for how the operations might look in subsequent quarters. Hospital companies sometimes hold similar calls with their administrators, but that practice hasn't typically been done at practice management organizations. That's not the case at Physician Reliance Network, however, where John Casey, Chairman and CEO, hosts similar telephone conferences with physicians each time the company announces quarterly earnings results. In a recent call, "We talked about what was going on with the stock and the company," Casey said. "We've had a good response from physicians about it." While publicly held companies obviously want to ensure that they communicate openly with Wall Street, the same should be true with respect to communicating with their physicians who have such a strong stake in the company's current and future operations.

- *Communication in the midst of chaos will win points.* Communications frequently break down during mergers. Practice management companies will go through numerous mergers and acquisitions as they grow and expand, and CEOs can't let communications slide during these busy times.

  In 1997, Michael Fiore was recruited by venture capital backers to run GMS Dental Group, a private dental management company. Four months into that job, he recommended a merger with Gentle Dental, which had just gone public. The merger took place in late 1997, and Fiore was tapped to lead the new company. Things were chaotic, as they always are with mergers—executives were dealing with budgets for the next year, and top managers had to sort out how the two companies, which were of nearly equal size, would achieve the necessary synchronization. Within a week after the merger, Fiore announced his new management team. Then, he made sure that the seven-member team stayed in the loop. Every Monday morning, they meet to discuss business issues. Corporate and regional offices were tied through video conferencing. That type of communication takes time, but pays off in management productivity.

- *Differentiation begins at the top.* When the stock market turned sour for practice management companies, each began to chant the mantra: "But we're different!" No one wanted to be painted with the same brush as the practice management companies who were struggling with restructurings, or even worse, bankruptcy. Gentle Dental's Fiore views his business as being more similar to retail healthcare services, such as plastic surgery and vision care, than the physician practice management business. "All of our presentations are peppered with examples of how our business is different from the physician practice management business," Fiore said.

Although the practice management industry is enduring tremendous turmoil, one key constituency doesn't really care—the patients. Unless a practice can differentiate itself in terms of service or quality, the patient won't care how traumatic the business model is; they'll move on to another provider.

WHO ARE THESE GUYS?

Leaders generally draw on their own experiences. That's why it can be helpful to look at the types of executives that are leading the publicly traded practice management companies. Most came from other healthcare companies. The top executives of physician practice management organizations have led hospital chains like Hospital Corp. of America and American Medical International, out-patient companies like Surgical Care Affiliates, and managed care companies like Magellan and PCA. A few have come from other physician practice management organizations such as American Oncology Resources and Physicians Resource Group. On the dental side, nearly half of the companies have chairpersons who had most recently been in private practice or led other dental groups. Interestingly, in both groups there are several individuals who went straight from investment banking into practice management companies. That demonstrates that wisdom in the ways of Wall Street is a valued asset when it comes to selling stock.

Physician Reliance's John Casey came from a publicly traded hospital company, American Medical International, where he had been president and chief operating officer. When he joined Physician Reliance in 1997, the company had stubbed its toe with some analysts because it hadn't met earnings expectations and had a large accounts receivables balance that had to be written off. Casey brought the attributes of having run a large healthcare company and knowing how to talk and walk with the investor community.

Although he had worked with physicians as a former hospital administrator in Memphis, Tenn., he related that running a physician company requires more sensitivity in working with physicians. "You have a deeper relationship with the physicians because everything you do influences their income and their pocketbook," Casey said. At Physician Reliance, physician compensation is derived from a split of the earnings from their local practice. If expenses rise, the physicians' compensation pool isn't as large; conversely, if earnings rise, both Physician Reliance and the physicians benefit.

With very few exceptions, publicly traded practice management companies employed CFOs who had held that job at other publicly traded companies. For example, Physician Reliance's CFO was treasurer of AMI when Casey led that organization. Some of the physician practice management CFOs may not necessarily be healthcare company execs, though. In the public companies, an understanding of the Securities and Exchange Commission requirements and the know-how to work with Wall Street analysts are givens with the job as a practice management CFO.

COMPENSATION

Leading a practice management company can be one of the most lucrative jobs in physician leadership, according to a survey by Cejka & Co. and the American College of Physician Executives. physician practice management executives had a mean compensation of $279,668 in 1997, compared to a mean of $209,104 for all physician executives. Practice management physician leadership topped all other categories (Table 10–1).

In addition to cash compensation, practice management companies have been effective in using Wall Street vehicles that motivate managers through stock options. Not surprisingly, top executives have a stake in the company's stock price. On average, chairpersons of physician practice management companies owned 10% of their companies. The percentages varied widely, however, from as little as 2% at PhyCor to as much as 49% at Coastal Physicians Group.

Among CEOs, the percentage of ownership was slightly lower at 8%. However, that percentage was skewed downward by two practice management

T A B L E 10–1

Physician Executives' Compensation

Rank	Organization Type	Mean Compensation
1	Practice management company	$279,688
2	Single specialty group	$265,782
3	Foundation	$222,886
4	Physician-hospital organization	$219,610
5	Multispecialty group	$218,750
6	Management services organization	$217,811
7	Health system headquarters	$217,745
8	Hospital	$214,530
9	Hospital management company	$209,777
10	Industry	$209,553
11	Consulting firm	$207,955
12	Pharmaceutical company	$207,830
13	Academic health center	$200,066
14	Independent practice association	$199,781
15	Other	$198,361
16	Health plan/HMO/PPO	$191,802
17	Insurance company	$184,713
18	Government	$130,567

Source: Ceika & Co/American College.

companies that had brought on new presidents in 1998 whose stock ownership was less than 1% (Figure 10–2).

The average percentage ownership among company presidents was even lower—6%. In that group, six of the 30 physician practice management companies had presidents who had less than 1% ownership.

Only three physician practice management companies provided chief financial officers with stock representing more than 1%. All three individuals came to physician practice management companies from either investment banks or other publicly traded companies. Obviously, stock ownership was a negotiating point in hiring those individuals.

Among dental practice management companies, the figures were fairly similar. Each of the 13 companies had chairpersons with equity stakes, the average being 10%. The range was somewhat narrower, with the lowest being 1.8% at Pentegra Dental Group and the highest being 21.7% at Dental Care Alliance.

Among dental CEOs, the average ownership was similar, and among dental presidents, it was just slightly higher at 10.9%. In the dental ranks, two CEOs owned less than 1% and two presidents owned less than 1%.

FIGURE 10–2

Top Executives Likely to Own at Least 1% Equity in Practice
Management Firms

- Chairman—87.5% own stock
- Chief executive officer—93% own stock
- President—80% own stock
- Chief financial officer—10% own stock

The effect of stock ownership on the top executives of practice management companies can be positive for shareholders. Investors often like to see significant ownership by managers and boards to ensure that these executives "feel their pain" in the stock market. In fact, compensation agreements are sometimes structured in a way to award bonuses if the company's stock reaches certain dollar levels. In addition, top executives usually are granted stock options, which are awarded based on performance. Options have an exercise price, which is commonly—but not always—the market price at the time the option is awarded. This gives the executive an incentive to improve the company's performance under the reasoning that the stock market will reward that performance and the stock price will rise. The difference between the exercise price and the price the stock sells (after the option vests) is profit for the executive exercising the option. On the other hand, if the stock price falls, the options then are considered "under water," and are worthless to the executive.

In 1998, many practice management executives saw their options sink under water, rendering this important incentive moot. However, boards have the option of repricing options. Although it may be unpopular with shareholders, several healthcare companies have in the past repriced options for top executives. Practice management boards, too, may succumb to the demands of executives to reprice their options, particularly if these executives can convince the board that the company's falling share price was out of their control. Repricing options also may be a way of retaining top talent. Again, as the industry encountered trouble times, recruiting executives for these companies became more and more of a challenge.

This close tie between the top executives and the stock market can have a negative effect, however, if it predisposes the executive toward focusing on short-term rather than long-term performance. The stock market is not a patient master and is prone to reward short-term performance. CEOs with short-term contracts, usually in the range of one to three years, may not see the value in building the expensive infrastructure necessary to operate a complex organization.

However, stock options can be a way for a start-up organization to recruit new people. "We have some great people and we can attract them from traditional healthcare employers because we can offer options and an entrepreneurial environment," said FemPartners' Spakevicius. FemPartners has the best of both worlds as a private company that can offer stock options. By staying private, the company can build the infrastructure that it needs to support an integrated women's health company.

The women's health practice management company is led by a husband and wife team. Spakevicius led a large OB/GYN practice in Houston, and her husband, William Altman, the company's executive vice president of business development, came from a venture capital firm. The two met while consultants at McKinsey & Company. The husband and wife team at FemPartners isn't that unusual. Many physician organizations are small businesses, and it's not uncommon to see family relationships. For some reason, the dental practice management companies have a plethora of family relationships in their executive ranks. We've already mentioned the Castles, the father and son team at Castle Dental. Other examples include the following.

- Birner Medical Management is led by two Birner brothers, one an investment banker and the other a dentist.
- A husband and wife, one a former university professor and the other a former insurance executive, lead CompDent Corp.
- Terek, Adam, and Tim Diasti are all brothers from Nebraska who manage Coast Dental Services, Tampa. The trio collectively own one-third of the company.
- Orthodontic Centers of America's chairman, president and CEO Gasper Lazzara, Jr., DDS, works with his brother-in-law, Michael Johnsen, the chief operating officer.

STRUCTURING CORPORATE BOARDS

Fem Partners has a five-person board that includes both Spakevicius and Altman, two representatives from the company's venture capital backers and a physician representative who is president of a 26-member physician group, the organization's largest. In the future, they hope to add two outside directors, a physician with national credentials, and an industry expert. At that point, three of the seven board members will be physicians. (One of the venture capital representatives happens to be a neurosurgeon.) As much as anything, the composition of practice management boards is multi-faceted subject. Some lean toward more clinical leadership, others toward business leaders.

Practice management companies in 1998 showed a wide variation on physician and dental practice management boards (Figure 10–3). Of 30 physician practice management companies, board size ranged from four to 12, and the number of physician directors on the boards ranged from none to five. On average, the practice management boards had 34% physician representation. Of the 30 boards, 10 had physicians as chairpersons. In some cases, physician chairpersons were

FIGURE 10–3

Practice Management Board Committees

Most common
- Audit
- Compensation
- Stock options/stock plan administration
- Executive

Other committees
- Acquisition

less likely to have several physicians on the board, perhaps feeling they needed additional business expertise. All but three of those physician chairpersons held another top post at the company, either president or CEO, or both.

Dental practice management companies tend to have lower percentages of dentists or orthodontists on their boards. Of 13 dental practice management company boards, 26% had dentist or orthodontist directors. Four of the companies had dentists or orthodontists as chairperson and two of those chairpersons held additional top posts at the company. Interestingly, six of the dental practice management companies had only one dentist or orthodontist on the board and one company had none.

Ideally, a practice management board will have a mix of individuals who will help guide the company through a myriad of challenges. Gentle Dental is unique in that it has two practice management executives on its board: Wayne Posey, president and CEO of ProMedco, a multispecialty practice management based in Fort Worth, Texas, and Paul Keckley, vice president of strategic development for PhyCor. Two other dental practice management firms also have practice management executives on their boards: American Dental Partners has a PhyCor executive, Derrill Reeves—a co-founder who directs its development efforts. Castle Dental has Emmett Moore, formerly president and CEO of Physician Resource Group.

"It made a tremendous amount of sense to find people who had taken start-up companies and grown them," said Gentle Dental's Fiore. Fiore, who formerly was chief operating officer of Los Angeles-based Salick Health Care and president of its cancer centers subsidiary, joined GMS in 1997 when the company had $18 million in annual revenues. It merged with Gentle Dental in November 1997 and by late 1998, the company had $120 million in annual revenues. "The physician practice management companies are a road map for us," Fiore said. They deal with many of the same regulatory issues, accounting issues, and investment analysts." The shared knowledge will help Gentle, which in 1998 was still in its first year as a public company.

Gentle's board is among the largest for practice management companies—13 members—with three members being dentists. That is primarily a function of the mergers the company has gone through during 1998. Most of the dental practice management company boards have between five and seven members.

Board composition hinges on several factors. Financing is probably the foremost. Venture capital investors typically take a seat on the board. For example, one physician practice management organization has a seven-member board in which four directors are elected by shareholders and Series A preferred shareholders, while the other three are elected by the Series B preferred shareholders. Sometimes, the leaders of the company's founding group practices also have board seats.

Physician organizations usually start small and their boards often are comprised only of physicians. However, one nonphysician executive who led a cardiovascular physician organization recommended that companies seek directors from outside the organization when revenues exceed $20 million. At that point, the company is large enough that it needs help beyond the day-to-day business, he pointed out. The board will start to assist with strategic planning and capitalization issues, he noted. Outside directors also can help support a nonphysician CEO, he said. "My job was a very lonely job," he commented, adding that as a nonphysician, "you're not part of the fraternity."

The key is getting the board to work together as a unit for the good of the organization. Robert Yeager, president and CEO of OrthoLink, said his board—half physicians, half nonphysicians—has been through an evolutionary process during its first couple of years of operation. Initially, "the doctors wanted to say everything and the business people wanted to say everything. Everything got said, but nothing got heard. Then, the board members realized, 'I know a lot, but I don't know everything.'" Yeager said. Board meetings are different now. "We listen," Yeager said, saying directors had to develop a trust for each others' judgment. "The physicians now are very comfortable with the intentions of the business people."

HANDLING LEADERSHIP CHANGES

Physician leaders must consider their eventual demise, which may be coming sooner rather than later, given the state of the industry. "Leaders need to be protected," said Boyle. "You need to have a strong severance package because when the day is done, it will never be the physicians that take accountability for their mistakes." The ax will fall instead on the CEO, he noted.

Boyle knows about the short tenure physician group leaders have. After 20 years of working in and for hospitals and clinics in northern California, Boyle was recruited to head a Dallas area group of specialists that was forming and wanted to raise venture capital. Boyle had run complex integrated health systems in northern California, one of the most competitive markets in the country. He knew and understood risk-based managed care contracting and the politics of large multi-specialty group practices.

Boyle worked for six months, finding the right venture partner. Then, when the venture partner agreed to put in $7 million, it came with strings. The venture firm wanted a CEO who had experience in taking a company public—a credential that Boyle lacked. So, Boyle was out.

AN EXPERT'S PERSPECTIVE: GRANT WICKLUND, PARTNER, HEIDRICK & STRUGGLES

Grant Wicklund, a partner in one of the nation's largest executive search companies, understands the balancing act of those who manage practice management firms and other physician organizations. He doesn't mince words about how leaders are viewed in these organizations and what they must do to command respect.

As an example, he says that when he's interviewing physicians to be CEO of a physician organization, "one of my first questions to the board is, "Are you going to allow them to practice medicine?"" Wicklund said. "If they say, 'No,' I tell them that I think they're making a mistake. Physicians have little to no respect for other physicians who stop practicing medicine." By keeping one foot in the clinical world, a physician CEO can balance the organization's need to garner physicians' respect while he's making the tough business decisions the company needs. In fact, "A lot of physicians will respect the MBA non-doctor more than the MBA doctor that might be viewed as a traitor," he added.

Wicklund has seen the leadership struggles of physician organizations. While some physicians have successfully led practice management companies, it's a tough job. "It's harder for physicians to be leaders because they inevitably have torn loyalties. They feel the doctors' pain, but they have to answer to the business people, the shareholders. They have to be consummate politicians in working with the physicians, but they're walking on eggshells all the time. It's hard to keep their compass oriented."

Regardless of whether the practice management organization's leader is a physician or not, Wicklund underlines the need for strong communication skills. "What a lot of them don't understand is that physicians are basically scientists. You can't hold their attention unless you have empirical evidence for what you want them to do. You can't just keep selling them."

Wicklund noted that many practice management organizations fail to integrate physician leaders into the governance structure. Wicklund likens it to hospital leadership structures. "The smart hospital CEOs have a lot of physician leadership. It may be painful at first, but you have to let these guys into the bosom of the business. It's easy to limit the number of physicians you include on the board because it's a lot less hassle. You have to educate them and it's not a quick process. But, without bringing physicians into the fold, you're not going to have long-term success."

Wicklund said that in addition to being communicators, physician organization leaders must have another trait: "They must have the ability to introduce appropriate discipline and sustain it."

The tenure of physician organization executives isn't long, and Wicklund advises CEOs and other top executives to have contracts of one year, possibly two. In the first year, the only reason to terminate for cause should be fraud or moral turpitude. Although he's seen cases in which executives had three-year contracts, he believes that's too long.

For many start-up physician organizations, the average tenure of the first-year CEO is one year, Wicklund said. Not uncommonly, the CEO is fired by the board in the first year. Then, the board hires somebody else and "finds out the first executive was doing the right thing. They're always sorry about it." For those types of organizations, some of which hope to transition into practice management organizations, the power struggle is even more problematic for physicians.

Leaders also need to know what issues to leave for physicians to sort out. The key one is compensation, Wicklund said. "You need absolutely empirical evidence so the doctors can manage their own compensation," he said. For example, let physicians explain to each other how their compensation is determined. If there are performance-based benchmarks, the physician can say, "Joe was out of line in this, so everybody else didn't make as much this month." Wicklund noted that if the nonphysician CEO does the explaining, physicians tend to be resentful. "The physicians may try to get you (the CEO) to go see Joe and tell him he's screwing up. But the smart guys won't do it. They'll force the physicians to manage themselves on compensation issues," he added.

Or, bring in a good compensation consultant, Wicklund suggested. "They'll have the programs and the data, and can take the heat while the CEO can stay more neutral," he said.

PricewaterhouseCoopers Tips for Practice Leadership

- Clearly communicate the vision and interdependency of the organization.
- Breed physician and dentist leadership within the ranks early and often.
- Recognize the particular skills of each leader and don't overload leaders with responsibilities they can't handle.
- Make sure the composition of the organization's board reflects where the organization is heading, not its past.
- Set a tone of trust. Physicians must learn to trust each other and that culture of trust starts at the top.

11

CHAPTER

Raising Private Capital

Sandy Lutz

William Hanlon III

Raising capital is a necessary evil that can seem easy or impossible, depending on one's perspective.

For example, when Steven Cooley, MD was executive vice president of EmCare, a Dallas-based emergency physicians company, start-up capital for a new practice management company found him. A small group of individuals, described by Cooley as "venture angels," hired a headhunter to find someone to lead a physician practice management company in electrophysiology. The headhunter called Cooley, who was itching to start his own practice management firm and liked the idea of leading one in cardiology. In August 1997, Cooley founded US Cardiovascular with $1 million in start-up capital already supplied.

Bruce Broussard was running Regency Health Services when it was bought out in October 1997 by Sun Healthcare. Smith Management, a venture capital firm in New York, had owned 25% of Regency, and approached Broussard about creating a Smith-financed practice management company.

Given carte blanche with respect to specialty, Broussard selected the dental business. "It's a $45 billion market and fragmented, with one- or two-person practices representing 85% of the industry," he explained. In early 1998, Broussard founded Harbor Dental in Atlanta with $20 million from Smith.

As these and dozens of other stories illustrate, connections and credentials can be handy short cuts to raising capital. However, these individuals raised capital in the heady days of practice management firms. The capital-raising climate darkened considerably in 1998 as the public equity markets closed to most practice management companies. That heightened the need for these companies to raise private capital.

WHAT ATTRACTS A CAPITAL PARTNER

Raising capital is a necessity for physician management organizations, no matter what their stage of development. However, some companies have demonstrated an ability to raise capital much more easily than others. Here are some characteristics that capital partners—public and private—have attributed to management organizations that they deemed "desirable" or "attractive."

Experienced Management Team

Some practice management organizations attract money like flies—capital partners offer checks, regardless of whether or not there's a business plan. Others must fly their CEOs all over the country, making PowerPoint presentations to legions of venture capital firms and investment banks in hopes of raising money. The difference often lies in the experience level of the CEO.

CEOs with extensive healthcare experience are permitted short cuts on the road to raising capital. One example is Larry House, the founder and former CEO of MedPartners. MedPartners started in 1993 with an initial capital infusion from HealthSouth Corp. and the leadership of House, HealthSouth's chief operating officer. Only 18 month after buying its first practice, MedPartners raised $61 million in an initial public offering.

Another example is R. Dale Ross, the CEO of American Oncology Resources (AOR), who shepherded a home healthcare firm through an IPO and later a buyout in the 1980s. PhyMatrix raised $115 million in its 1995 IPO on the strength of its chairman, Abraham Gosman, who had produced outstanding shareholder returns in the long-term care business. Physician Reliance Network was founded by the leader of a large oncology network that had already demonstrated an ability to grow and manage practices. Both OccuSystems (now part of Concentra) and Physician Resource Group were led by former executives at Medical Care International, at one time the nation's largest surgery center chain. However, the ability to raise capital doesn't ensure operational success as witnessed by MedPartners' and PhyMatrix's exits from the business in 1998 and 1999.

None of these name-brand CEOs had specific experience in physician management companies because so few existed at the time. However, as the industry has expanded, physician organizations and the head-hunters they hire now search for executives with prior physician management experience.

One example is Steven Cooley, MD, the former executive vice president at EmCare who was tapped to lead US Cardiovascular. EmCare, one of the industry's most successful physician management companies in terms of stockholder value, had gone public in December 1994 at $11 per share and sold out three years later with a 350% price appreciation over the offering price. Cooley, an ER physician, had headed EmCare's ER practice management subsidiary since 1992 and prior to that, had been with two other ER companies.

With the highly publicized stumbles of many practice management organizations, capital sources also are looking for bench depth beyond the CEO level.

- The *chief operating officer* needs to have a resume that is compatible with that of the CEO and boasts similar credentials—lots of physician contacts and possibly experience in negotiating managed care contracts.

- Also crucial to the management team is a *chief financial officer* who has had experience in financial reporting and initial public offerings. Where a lot of practice management organizations fall down is putting someone in the CFO slot who has experience in running a physician group or clinic, but not with a practice management organization or other healthcare company that has been through an IPO.

- Another successful component is a dynamic lead physician, sometimes known as a *"physician champion."* This person may be the company's CEO or chairman. His credentials add credibility to the practice management organization and reassure investors that physicians will find this company "friendly" to them. This also augments the physician/management relationship, because physicians often are the best individuals to interact with other physicians on contentious issues.

Of course, in addition to picking the right leadership team, the practice management organization must demonstrate that its members can work together effectively.

Infrastructure Issues

Venture capital firms, private equity firms and investment banks are demanding "buy and build" strategies from their investment candidates. In other words, practice management organizations seeking capital had better be able to demonstrate that they can buy practices, integrate them successfully, build them up, and run them profitably.

Capital providers will be on the lookout for the following.

- Core founding practices with name recognition, even if that name recognition is local. These are practices that have run profitably for five to 10 years and are likely to continue doing so. Although it's beneficial to have the number crunchers who can demonstrate the financial viability for physicians, testimonials from physicians themselves can support the premise the model will make sense to their colleagues.

- A satisfied physician "champion" who can discuss the advantages of the practice management organization and how it has been able to support his or her practice.

- Information on the practice management organization's information systems infrastructure. This includes the type of computer system the practice management organization uses, how well it works, how quickly physicians are moved on to a centralized system, and whether legacy systems are allowed to remain in operation. A centralized system isn't a necessity, and many practice management companies haven't yet moved to one.

- Adequate reserves for medical expenses incurred but not reported. Management organizations whose practices will be generating revenues from capitation contracts need to be looking at their future capital needs. Currently, most states aren't requiring practice management organizations to have reserves like insurance companies. However, "it's just a matter of time before the state insurance regulators require practice management companies that take capitation to have reserves. That changes the equation for capital requirements," noted Texas Pacific's Jonathon Coslet. Currently, California is the only state with that type of requirement for practice management organizations.

- Front line managers with experience in running a physicians' office. These are the managers who will deal with the physicians day in and day out. Too often, practice management organizations have hired individuals who have worked in a management services organization for a hospital system, but have little experience interacting with physicians.

- Experienced ancillary managers. If a new practice management organization plans to tout the fact that they will generate additional revenue from ancillaries, they need to be prepared to introduce their capital backers to the managers who will run those ancillary centers. If it's a radiology practice management organization, who will be setting up the imaging centers? If it's an orthopedic practice management organization, who will be opening and operating the occupational rehab centers?

- Brand-name financial backers. Larry Marsh of Salomon looks closely at companies' financial backers, such as venture capital funds that he knows. "Certain backers don't necessarily guarantee success, but you'll have a greater feeling of confidence in the business. It certainly doesn't guarantee that they'll meet their numbers forever, but it can help them get off the ground."

Ability to Demonstrate Returns

To raise sufficient capital, a practice management organization must be able to tell its story using the terms the financial community knows best—terms like *growth, earnings,* and *return on invested capital.* In fact, such measures will be an important arbiter for whether the industry continues to garner the capital at the rate it has seen during the past few years.

To many would-be investors, the key guarantors for success are growth and consistency in earnings. Therefore, the ability to show year-to-year growth in revenues and consistent earnings should be a primary goal.

However, it's also important to understand how the financial community approaches those measures, because different analysts have different approaches. Fore example, in his February 1998 report, H&Q's Lunbeck compared practice management companies' overall shareholder returns, determined as the difference between their current price and their IPO price. In SBC Warburg Dillon Read's report dated March 1998, analyst Jim Lane compares practice management organizations using after-tax cash earnings. As opposed to the traditional earnings per share number, this amount minimizes the impact of intangible assets and their related amortization—which are a significant balance sheet and expense item for most practice management organizations—and thus, levels the playing field for comparative purposes.

SOURCES OF PRIVATE CAPITAL

Like most new businesses, fledgling practice management organizations need money—and lots of it. That money will be spent to hire managers, find office space, buy furniture and computers, provide working capital for the start-up period, and acquire physician practices.

New practice management companies soon learn that raising capital is a journey. It usually begins with seed money from a venture capital firm or another private source. Once those funds are in place, the company may then pursue some form of debt financing to leverage the equity raised (Table 11–1).

Alternatively, a practice management company may accept interim financing from private equity funds or healthcare vendors interested in investing in physician practices. Some private funds won't fund start-ups; they only consider businesses that have reached a predetermined revenue run rate.

T A B L E   11–1

Venture Investing in Practice Management (Figures in Millions)

	Figures in Millions			
	1995	1996	1997	1998
No. of deals	6	25	43	50
Average size	$10.0	$8.4	$7.3	$5.9
Total invested	$60	$211	$314	$294.4

Source: PricewaterhouseCoopers.

Another option for a practice management firm is a private placement in which individuals purchase debt or equity through an offering arranged by an investment banker.

A private placement is an issue of securities that are exempt from SEC registration because they are offered to "sophisticated investors" rather than to the general public. Private placements are a means to raising capital that is less expensive than venture capital and is quicker and less complicated than an IPO (because the offering doesn't have to be registered with the SEC). However, some restrictions do apply (for example, a maximum of 35 individual investors, all of whom must be accredited with a high net worth and annual income).

Venture Capital

The venture capital (VC) process is one of the most traveled finance roads for practice management organizations.

B O X   11–1

INSIDE VENTURE CAPITAL: CORDOVA CAPITAL, ATLANTA

"There's a lot of money chasing good deals," said John Runningen, a partner with Cordova Capital, an Atlanta-based venture capital firm. "Physicians are the only ones that have direct control of healthcare costs. Everybody else has indirect control. This allows the physician organization to assume risk and the associated rewards. But to do this profitably, physician organizations must be able to spread those costs over a larger base." Runningen knows the healthcare business from several sides. Prior to joining Cordova, he was CFO of a healthcare company. Then he spent ten years as a healthcare analyst, most recently as senior healthcare analyst at Robinson-Humphrey Co., Atlanta.

He joined Cordova in 1997, where he works with the company's Enhanced Appreciation Fund to originate, monitor and manage its healthcare portfolio. The nearly $100 million fund can leverage its private capital on a three-to-one basis, which allows Cordova more flexibility in tailoring its investments to the needs of the investee.

Cordova has been active in the physician organization sector since 1997, with investments in three private practice management companies. Even though practice management investments were starting to fall out of favor with many firms at that time, Cordova saw promise in the sector. After announcing two investments, "we started getting calls from every deal on the street," Runningen said.

In autumn 1997, Cordova put $2 million into Rehab Associates, a Montgomery, Ala.–based rehabilitation firm that operates clinics in the

In 1997, investments in practice management organizations represented about one-fourth of the $1.2 billion invested in healthcare service companies overall, according to a survey by PricewaterhouseCoopers. That year, 43 private practice management firms received $314 million in venture capital, up from $211 million in 1996 and $60 million in 1995.

As the amount of practice management funding has increased, so has the number of willing investors. Ninety venture capital firms invested in practice management organizations in 1997, according to the PwC survey. This means that practice management organizations have an audience of listeners who are familiar with their business.

Venture capital firms provide capital for start-up or early stage companies. They are willing to take on higher-than-average risk in exchange for the chance at higher-than-average returns. Because all ventures are speculative, VC firms will receive no returns from some of their projects, and thus expect high returns from the ones that succeed (Box 11–1).

Inside Venture Capital: Cordova Capital, Atlanta Concluded

Southeast, and $1 million into United Emergency Services, Durham, NC. United Emergency operates hospital emergency rooms on a contract basis in underserved rural and suburban markets in the Southeast.

Later in 1997, Cordova took part in a second round of venture capital funding for U.S. Orthopedics, a Little Rock, Ark.–based physician organization. Cordova put up $1.9 million of a $5 million funding, joining Piper Jaffray Ventures (a branch of Piper Jaffray investment bank) and Kitty Hawk Capital, Charlotte, NC. Cordova took just two weeks to decide to participate. Kitty Hawk had supplied the first round of funding in U.S. Orthopedic and done much of the due diligence; Piper Ventures was the co-investor and offered even more due diligence back-up.

At that point, several publicly-traded physician organizations were reporting problems in operations and write-downs in goodwill. Runningen saw the impact. "Almost overnight, all the physician organizations we were looking at were adopting facilities-based models," Runningen said. For example, in addition to managing the practices of orthopedic surgeons, US Orthopedic owns and operates facilities such as ambulatory surgery centers and other diagnostic centers.

Runningen says he gets involved when portfolio companies need to have access to Cordova's existing contacts. For example, two of the companies in Cordova's portfolio are working together in moving a sports rehab business from one to another. By spinning off the business, one of the physician organizations will realize an additional $300,000 in cash flow annually. That cash flow could be leveraged into additional credit line of $1 million, Runningen pointed out.

Frequently, the capital they deploy comes from university endowment funds, pension funds, corporations, financial institutions, not-for-profit foundations, and foreign investors. Often these organizations will devote about 5% of their portfolio assets to invest in riskier ventures that tend to pay higher returns.

The venture firm will usually take shares of stock in the company in return for capital supplied. If the company is successful and is sold or goes public, substantial profits can be realized. For example, TA Associates, a Boston-based venture capital firm, paid $10 million to purchase 20% of Physician Reliance Network, a Dallas-based oncology practice management firm, in 1993. When Physician Reliance went public the following year, TA's $10 million investment was worth $45 million, a 350% return.

To realize those kinds of returns, the VC firm can't leave things to chance. Instead, venture capital managers usually work with their portfolio companies to ensure that the organization is meeting the right people and making the right moves.

It is an active, not passive, role. Jonathan Goldstein, a principal with TA Associates, said practice management organizations often take "half our effort, but a smaller percentage of dollars." This is due partly to the nature of the practice management business. Larry Marsh, the practice management analyst at Salomon Smith Barney, says, "It's a real challenge in this industry to balance the needs of investors with the needs of physicians and with the requirements of payors and regulators."

Another reason that practice management organizations initially require more time than money is the shift in mind-set that is often required of investee companies. Most business decisions in the solo or group practice setting are motivated by tax or retirement planning considerations. In a very small practice, the physician may even be running both his practice and his personal life out of the same checkbook. Goldstein explains, "You're taking a very smart group of people [who have been entrepreneurs] and attempting to implement a business culture. Not all medical groups are able to make that transition." Further, he notes that "You have to reorient top executives to think like shareholders, not employees. They have to want to retain earnings, not distribute everything to the doctors in the form of salary and bonus."

Usually, the VC firm's strategy is to focus management's attention on developing a track record and earnings growth to support an IPO or lucrative sale to another company within a few years. Most firms will establish a schedule of regular board meetings and financial reporting deadlines, enabling them to keep close tabs on their investment. Some may work with the practice management organization to alter or broaden the business plan. Often, they will add directors to the company's board.

This close interaction requires trust from both parties. "The most important question is, can you trust them? Are they going to be there in good times and bad times?" said Harbor Dental's Broussard. "You're bound to trip up a few times. Are they going to shoot you out of the water when you do?"

For example, Harbor Dental's plan calls for acquiring 25 dental practices in the first 12 months of operation. Its investors need to be patient, Broussard noted, because "it doesn't always spin the first time."

The degree and manner of involvement varies among firms. John Runningen, a partner with Cordova Capital in Atlanta, says he talks to the CEOs of Cordova's portfolio practice management organizations two to three times a week. "Where we get involved is when portfolio companies need to have access to our existing contacts," he said. VC firm executives often have valuable connections to other finance and legal experts to whom a practice management organization may not have otherwise have access. It's a small world in healthcare, and that platitude can ring particularly true with the introductions that a venture capital partner makes for his or her portfolio companies.

For example, the Sprout Group, an active funder of practice management start-ups, is affiliated with Donaldson, Lufkin & Jenrette, a large New York investment bank. In 1997, Sprout funded five practice management organizations—First Physician Care, Total Physician Services, NeuroSource, Genus Aesthetic Medical Dental, and Physician Solutions. When it's time for those practice management organizations to do a private placement, merger, or IPO, it's likely that they'll have an inside track with DLJ. This provides a valuable short-cut for them.

The time from funding to a sale or IPO can range from 12 months to five years or longer. However, most venture firms look at an 18- to 36-month window. Giving fewer than 12 months puts too much pressure on the practice management organization to grow the company before it has put the necessary infrastructure in place. Much longer than three to five years lowers the realizable returns.

How Much Funding Is Available?

The amounts offered by venture firms can range from less than $1 million to upwards of $50 million, depending on the firm's investment goals. Expected returns typically begin at 30%.

Some VC firms invest small amounts, between $1 million and $5 million. "If we invest $1 million, we're looking for a 6 to 10 times return (i.e., $6 to $10 million) on our investment," says Runningen. "That's doable on a smaller investment. However, those types of returns are much more difficult to realize on a larger investment, say $50 million," he noted.

On the other hand, TA Associates, with $2 billion under management, typically likes to invest $10 million, although its practice management organization investments have ranged from $5 million to $17 million. To date, TA has invested

$63 million in seven practice management organizations, three of which have gone public: Physician Reliance Network, Sheridan Healthcare, and Monarch Dental Corp.

How Expensive Is It?

VC funding is regarded as an expensive form of capital. The clock starts ticking as soon as the practice management organization has the commitment. Venture capital firms may charge a commitment fee, which is usually 1% to 3% of the total amount invested. The firm also may charge interest or expect a dividend on the amount invested. For example, on a $30 million round of funding, the venture firm may charge one fee on the entire line and another fee on the amount that has been drawn down. There may be other costs as well: for example, directors appointed by the VC firm may draw a nominal salary.

How Deals Are Structured

Typically, the venture capital firm will exchange funding for preferred stock, convertible preferred stock, notes, or warrants to purchase stock. The preferred stock will convert to common stock when the practice management organization goes public. Often, the date of the public offering is anticipated and the conversion date will coincide with that offering. In addition, the notes often will be repaid when the company goes public.

If the company does not go public by the conversion date of the preferred stock, the stock in many instances may convert into a larger stake in the practice management organization, giving the VC shareholders more control over the company's future.

Dividing the Pie

One of the most difficult issues is determining how much equity these venture capital firms receive in exchange for their investment. Here's a common scenario: Two executives, one a physician "champion" (who may or may not maintain an active practice), the other a businessman with crucial ties to possible lender and equity sources, decide to form a practice management organization. Some physician friends verbally agree to join when the time comes.

After several months of research, the two executives devise an ownership structure for the nascent practice management organization and line up venture capital financing. Obviously, the physicians will want a piece of the action—equity in the new venture. Problem is, so do the financing sources. They'll want equity in exchange for their cash. The question is, how to split up the equity fairly?

Capital backers will want to strike a balance that has incentives for growth. For a pure start-up with no revenues, a common formula is for the practice management organization's founders to receive roughly 20% in equity and options. The venture capital investors receive preferred stock and the practices receive equity in some combination based on asset valuation.

Venture "Angels"

US Cardiovascular obtained its initial financing through "venture angels" —a "friendly" source of start-up funds. CEO Steven Cooley describes "venture angels" as wealthy individuals who want to provide seed capital to fund promising business ideas.

The company came about when a physician was discussing with a friend an idea for a practice management organization that would focus on electrophysiologists—the electricians of the heart. His friend happened to be the CEO of one of the nation's largest cardiovascular device companies. The CEO suggested talking to a couple of business friends of his in the Minneapolis/ St. Paul area who were interested in being "venture angels," putting their money to work in new business ventures.

Together, the founders and ultimately a total of about a dozen "angels" put up $1.3 million to get the Dallas-based company started. The first use of the funds was hiring a headhunter to find the CEO (Cooley). The rest of the money was used to hire other managers, rent office space, acquire computers, and provide enough start-up cash for the first several months of the business.

Private Equity Funds

Private equity companies, which usually invest larger sums than venture capital firms, are another financing option. However, these types of firms typically invest in established businesses, preferring spin-offs to start-ups.

For example, in 1997 three private equity firms—Texas Pacific Group, Bain Capital, and Hellman & Friedman—together put up more than $100 million to back the spin-off of Vivra Specialty Partners, the practice management division of the kidney-dialysis chain Vivra. The spin-off happened when Vivra was acquired by Gambro, a European firm. Vivra's CEO wanted to stay with the practice management spin-off, which already had built up $200 million in annual revenues, but expand it to include specialty practices in cardiology, orthopedics, obstetrics/gynecology, and allergy, then builds local networks of other physicians. The networks then go to payors and negotiate capitated carve-out packages.

Some private equity companies are reluctant to invest in healthcare because they don't understand the business. Texas Pacific's Coslet said practice management organizations represent a "complicated niche." "Your customers (insurance companies) are so much larger than you," he said, adding that "your suppliers (physicians) are entrepreneurial, independent people." What's more, most practice management organizations are unprepared for taking risk because they don't have underwriting or medical management skills.

Bank Financing

When the equity markets dried up in mid-1998, many practice management companies turned to lines of credit from banks. In a sense, this type of financing added rationality to practice management companies. Lines of credit usually curbed overly exuberant acquisition plans, the kind that have typified practice management companies. Banks usually require approval of acquisitions over a certain dollar amount and/or a certain number of acquisitions during a specific time frame. That ensures that the borrower isn't getting too far ahead of itself in absorbing acquisitions. Unfortunately, those curbs don't exist the equity markets, which reward growth.

All along the way, financing from banks or other lending institutions is typically needed to bridge the gap where cash equity falls short of working capital needs. Not only is it needed, but it is more so desired by the physician organization and the equity investors, as this form of cash capital neither dilutes equity ownership nor costs the physician organization as much. Thus, the physician organizations' and equity investors' first attempt is to increase the return on equity by leveraging the company with bank debt.

However, banks have a much more conservative investment strategy in mind than the venture capitalists and private equity funds, and require more stringent operating covenants/parameters and monitoring in exchange for accepting a lower return. Therefore, banks will typically get involved later in the game, after the viability of the startup physician organization's operating strategy (including MSA structure, healthcare niche, acquisition strategy, ancillary growth strategy, etc.) has begun to solidify and after the cash flows from operations have become positive. As a risk-return payoff for getting involved earlier in the game, banks will increase their pricing and fees and may often require equity warrants.

Of these operating covenants/parameters, banks, first of all, will typically take a perfected lien in the physician organization's tangible assets (namely, A/R and equipment) and intangible assets (namely, the MSAs and trade names), as well as the tangible assets of the physician organization's affiliated practices (namely A/R, if not already assigned to the physician organization in the MSA). Secondly, banks will typically take much greater comfort in (and subsequently ensure the maintenance of) a strong physician organization capital structure—one supported by sizable and meaningful cash equity investments by outside parties, such as, venture capital firms and private equity funds—as a means of ensuring that the appropriate corrective actions would be taken by an "at-risk" party should the physician organization trip hurdles in their evolution. Finally, banks will typically include a "laundry list" of other operating and financial covenants/parameters to ensure that the physician organization is operating according to the strategy that the physician organization management purported to the bank when it originally obtained the bank financing.

Bank financing typically takes the form of revolving lines of credit, term loans, acquisition lines of credit, equipment lines of credit, and letters of credit facilities, and is used to fund acquisitions, to refinance existing debt, to fund capital expenditures, and for general working capital needs.

Critical factors of physician organizations are the experience level of the management team (in both physician organizations and in the specific medical specialty), the structure and wording of their MSAs, the stability of earnings, the amount of cash flow and balance sheet leverage, and the viability of the organization's operating strategy (including their ability to add and demonstrate value to the affiliated physicians and to exhibit smart growth) weigh heavily on the ultimate pricing and structure of a bank credit facility. As expected, a physician organization with a strong management team, a proven history of stable operating results and low leverage will have ready access to the debt markets and will receive favorable pricing and structure terms. Conversely, physician organizations that cannot demonstrate a record of predictable cash flows or have high management turnover will have more difficulty raising capital from commercial lenders. These physician organizations may have to sweeten the returns to lenders in the form of warrants and/or higher interest rates and closing fees, and will have more restrictive covenants and terms.

Since most physician organizations do not have large asset bases, debt facilities are based on the sustainable cash flows of the physician organization and are usually structured as cash flow revolving lines of credit based on a multiple of debt to EBITDA (earnings before interest, taxes, depreciation and amortization) or "cash flow." In today's market, that multiple will most likely range from 3.0x to 3.75x for senior debt and 4.0x to 6.0x for total debt. Physician organizations with high capital equipment requirements may have access to equipment lines and lease agreements.

For example, Fleet Capital provided a $25 million revolving senior credit facility to OMNA Medical Partners, a physician organization specializing in neuromusculoskeletal care. Proceeds from the cash flow-oriented credit facility were used to pay down existing debt, to fund future acquisitions, to support ancillary business development, and to provide working capital for ongoing operations. Earlier in the year, Fleet provided a $7 million senior credit facility to NeuroSource, Inc., a physician organization focusing on neurosurgical care. The asset-oriented credit facility was structured as a $5 million revolver and a $2 million equipment line.

Joint Ventures with Hospitals

Practice management companies are turning to hospitals to build large capital projects, such as specialty hospitals, and in many cases finding ready partners. The predilection of physicians to go into business with local hospitals will hinge on the level of trust between the facility and its physicians in the community. However, such an arrangement can lessen the capital cost to the physician organization.

Retained Earnings

This is a foreign concept to many physician groups who "zero out" profits by paying year-end bonuses to physicians. However, the short-term pain of holding back profits may become a necessary evil in a tight credit market. After all, most businesses hold back a portion of earnings each year to fund growth and development, or simply have a safety net. Historically, physicians have had no incentive to retain earnings and pay taxes on undistributed income. Accordingly, physicians have typically paid out all of their earnings at the end of the year to avoid taxation on those funds. However, if a physician group truly wants to control its own destiny and turn its back on outside investors, the only way to finance that growth will be through retained earnings. What's more, having a sizable retained earnings pool will enhance a practice's ability to borrow if it wants to do that later.

Retaining between 5% and 10% of earnings is a way for physician groups to invest in their own operations and not have to rely as much on outside funding.

Medical Supply/Manufacturing Companies

At CareSelect, a Dallas-based multi-specialty physician organization, early investors included Beverly Enterprises, the nation's largest nursing home chain, and Biomet, a manufacturer of orthopedic surgery and reconstructive devices (Box 11–2). These two capital partners were interested because CareSelect's earliest physicians included orthopedic surgeons. "They wanted to know the needs of the these physician groups, particularly the orthopedic surgeons," noted Tom Erickson, CareSelect's president and CEO.

In some cases, medical manufacturers are starting their own physician organizations. Two recent examples are Fonar Corp., a Melville, N.Y.–based imaging manufacturer, and Prime Medical Services, an Austin, Texas–based lithotripter services firm.[1]

Generally, this type of capital is less expensive and less restrictive than traditional venture capital. Private investors from related industries may not be focused on the physician organization as an investment in the profit-making sense. Rather, they focus on the physician organization's potential use as an in-house testing ground for new products and processes.

---

[1] More Outsiders Buy PM Companies, Healthcare Practice Management News, September 1997.

BOX 11-2

ONE PHYSICIAN ORGANIZATION SHUNS VENTURE CAPITAL

Although its top executive is a former venture capitalist, Dallas-based CareSelect has shunned VC money, preferring instead to find other sources of private capital. President and CEO Tom Erickson believes venture capital prompts practice management companies to rush their strategies. Because VC investors often want to see a 36- to 48-month return on their investment through an eventual IPO, the focus may rest on building the company only through acquisitions. In the meantime, the physician organization may not build the infrastructure needed to sustain the company long-term, he noted.

Erickson characterizes the modus operandi of some VC firms as, "Get it up, get it out and wait 180 days before you sell out and go on to the next investment." His philosophy is that strategic development takes time and expertise to implement. "If you look at how [a physician organization is] financed, you can tell what they're going to do," added Jim Sillman, MD, an orthopedist and CareSelect's board chairman.

CareSelect was founded in 1994 as a super-IPA. The company brought together 12 independent practice associations with about 600 physicians and 200 other therapists. The original seed money for the MSO was $1.75 million and was raised from the physicians themselves. Another $1.5 million was raised in a second round. In addition, CareSelect received funding from other healthcare companies, including Beverly Enterprises, the nation's largest nursing home chain, and Biomet, a manufacturer of orthopedic surgery and reconstructive devices.

Four years later, the company has developed into a physician organization that intends to be multispecialty as it builds networks in select Southwest markets. It is 82% physician owned and finances growth with a $25 million credit facility.

The board originally was all physicians, but was expanded to bring in representatives of other constituencies—the employer and the payor. The five-member board now consists of Dr. Sillman; Steve Johnston, MD, managing partner of Texas Cardiology; CEO Erickson, and two outside directors, Patricia Nazemetz, director of human resource practice at Xerox Corp., and Marshall Rozzi, president and CEO of United Healthcare of Illinois.

The outsiders were added to the board to bring other perspectives, but "we want to keep it a doctor company," Erickson said.

With annual revenues of about $79 million, CareSelect has 29 corporate staff members whose jobs are to bring value to the physician practices that are paying them a 15% management fee on pre-tax income.

CareSelect managers say that in addition to having the clinical responsibility, they want physicians to have the financial responsibility to effect change in the company. To borrow a phrase from *All the President's Men*, Erickson preaches, "Follow the Money." It's good advice. Ownership issues derive from the simple formula of who put in how much money (Table 11-2).

TABLE 11-2

PricewaterhouseCoopers Venture Capital Survey

First Three Quarters of 1998		
Healthcare Services Company	Service	Total ($000s)
Uro Therapies	Urology PPM	40,000
InteCardia	Cardiology PPM	18,000
Telesis Medical Management	PPM	15,000
Women's Health USA	OB/GYN PPM	15,000
Consolident	Dental PPM	10,000
Genus Aesthetic Medical & Dental	PPM	9,750
Professional Dental Associates	Dental PPM	8,500
Physician Health Corp.	PPM	8,400
MainStreet Dental Management	Dental management company	8,000
U.S. Physicians	PPM	7,700
U.S. Orthopedics	Orthopedic PPM	7,200
OMS of America	Plastic surgery PPM	6,500
Pathology Partners	Pathology PPM	6,069
Oncology Affiliates	Cancer PPM	6,000
InPatient Consultants	Hospitalists PPM	5,854
Heritage Health Systems	Develops IPAs	5,600
NeuroSource	Neurology PPM	5,043
Dyntec	Dental PPM	5,000
U.S. Pathology Labs	Pathology PPM	4,885
Community Physicians Network	PPM	4,500
Quantum Dental Network	Dental PPM	4,000
UniPhy Healthcare	PPM	4,000
ICUSA Inc.	ICU PPM	3,400
DentalCo	Dental PPM	3,000
NovaMed EyeCare	Ophthalmology PPM	3,000
Osler Health	Primary care PPM	1,766
Hospitalists	Hospitalists PPM	1,750
OMNA Medical Partners	Orthopedic PPM	1,750
Pathmakers	Behavioral health PPM	1,750
Omnia Inc.	Women's health	1,554
Cove Healthcare	Hospitalists PPM	1,000
First Physician Care	PPM	1,000
Princeps	Radiology PPM	1,000
Sedona Healthcare Group	Primary care PPM	638
Accountable Oncology Associates	Oncology PPM	500
Dental Care Partners	Dental PPM	100
Total		**227,209**

Other Points to Ponder

There are other variables that practice management companies should take into consideration before wading into a relationship with a capital partner, including the following.

- From whom? Physician executives need to consider the strategic direction of the company before accepting capital from private or public sources. If the practice management company's majority owner is interested simply in consolidation, the physicians who trade their practices for stock may find themselves with a series of different companies in succeeding years as mergers dominate the company's direction.

- How much? The amount of capital needed by a practice management firm will hinge on its growth plan and infrastructure needs. Another consideration is the $75 million equity threshold in the Stark "safe harbors" for fraud and abuse. Some physician organizations have attempted to reach a total equity value of $75 million in order to be within that anti-kickback harbor.

- How often? The physician organization's executive team should decide whether to raise the money in one lump sum or stages over a period of years. The disadvantage to raising capital in stages—on an as-needed basis—is that the CEO, CFO, and managers end up spending a lot of their time simply raising capital. That takes time away from operating the company, recruiting physicians, making acquisitions and developing the company.

  However, for a physician organization that is expanding through acquisition, the benefits to raising capital through rounds may more than offset the disadvantages. Here's why: When an investor buys into a privately-owned physician organization, a value will be established for the private equity shares he or she is buying. As each subsequent round of capital is raised, the value of the stock rises. That's because the business probably has expanded since the first round, and that growth is reflected the increased value of the private equity shares. For example, if the investor receives 5 million shares valued at 25 cents each for the first round of funding, the next round of capital may raise that value to 50 cents per share. If the physician organization had instead raised a lot of cash in one lump sum, the value of the private shares may have started out at 25 cents and stayed there.

  A stock with a rising valuation can be helpful in many ways. For example, the practice management company can use its equity as currency to buy physician practices. If the share price increases, the company won't need to issue as many shares to make acquisitions. Stock also is often used as a sweetener to recruiting executives to a start-up practice management company.

PricewaterhouseCoopers Tips for Raising Private Capital

- Build relationships with a variety of capital sources to ensure making the best choices.
- Begin positioning your company early with audited financial statements and a well-documented and conservative business plan.
- Make sure your investors know the risks inherent in physician organizations.
- Ensure that your business has a sustainable return and isn't acquisition dependent.
- Be conservative on acquisition projections; deals always take longer than expected.

12

CHAPTER

Raising Capital from the Public Markets

Sandy Lutz

Mel Hope

Most new businesses suffer from undercapitalization. That wasn't necessarily true for practice management companies, which attracted at least $3 billion in publicly raised capital during the 1990s.

Dr. Steven Scott's Coastal Physician Group raised $60 million in one of the first physician management initial public offerings. At the time, Coastal was a contract management company remaking itself into a physician practice management firm. Coastal managed hospital emergency departments, and as part of that, managed the practices of emergency physicians.

Three other physician firms also went public that year, although two were regarded more as managed care companies than physician companies. Pacific Physician Services, which would later be bought by MedPartners, raised $16.4 million, and PHP Healthcare raised $20.3 million. The last, Medaphis Corp., raised $28.1 million. Altogether, these four firms raised $125 million in equity capital.

The number of offerings and capital raised increased each succeeding year, with the biggest single-year jump occurring in 1995 when 15 physician companies raised equity capital of more than $700 million (Figure 12–1).

In 1996, the amount of equity capital raised ballooned to $820 million. That summer, price/earnings (P/E) multiples for practice management organizations peaked in the high-flying mid-60s. Subsequently, those ratios—which measure the price of a company's stock in relation to its earnings, and are an indicator of

FIGURE 12–1

Equity Issues by Physician Groups Peaked in 1996 (Dollars in Millions)

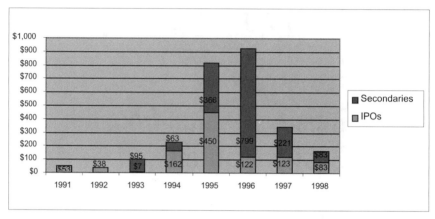

Source: Salomon Smith Barney.

market demand for the stock—fell hard when a handful of recognizable names in the industry failed to meet analysts' earnings expectations.

The industry lost $5 billion in market capitalization during the next year, and in 1997 new practice management companies raised $70 million less than they did the previous year. That represented the first drop in raising public equity capital since the industry began. Of the total new capital raised in 1997—about $750 million, according to BancAmerica Robertson Stephens—nearly half was aimed at dental practice management companies, a sector that is even more fragmented, and seemingly equally primed for consolidation, than physician practices.

By 1998, industry P/Es had dropped to the 20s and some were much lower. Since P/E often mirrors perceived future growth rates, it was clear that investors were viewing these stocks' prospects less enthusiastically. It's also interesting to note that as the industry's market cap expanded, the P/E ratio dropped. Obviously, the P/E of the few high flyers from three years before was diluted by the less successful companies.

"PRACTICE MANAGEMENT COMPANIES: THE MONEY PIT" (HEADLINE IN THE JUNE 20, 1997, ISSUE OF *HOSPITALS & HEALTH NETWORKS*)

This headline from a popular trade journal summed up one attitude toward practice management organizations. To understand the wave of capital behind practice management organizations, one must understand how and why Wall Street backs fledgling industries.

"Money flows to opportunity," says Larry Marsh, director of equity research for practice management organizations at Salomon Smith Barney. "Most everything in healthcare is influenced by the physician. Putting capital behind that means of production is compelling. It has captured the investment community's fancy." Judging by the tomes written by Wall Street analysts, practice management companies could be one of the nation's most closely scrutinized and analyzed service industries. Dozens of analysts follow the 40-plus publicly traded practice management companies. In 1997 and 1998, at least four major Wall Street firms issued reports of between 100 and 300 pages on the practice management organization industry. Dozens of other investment banks also published their own heavyweight analyses.

PhyCor, probably the industry's most closely watched stock, had at one time the attention of 35 healthcare analysts. On the dental side, Orthodontic Centers of America was the most watched, with coverage by 11 analysts.

The sheer number of analysts following these companies fuels interest in them. Analysts are talking about these stocks almost daily to their firms' salespeople and to money managers, keeping them apprised of what's going on in the sector. By and large, the tone of analysts' comments will be positive because they are "sell-side" analysts, and most will have "buy" ratings on the stock. As "sell-side" analysts, their job is to generate trades from the "buy-side" analysts at mutual funds and other institutional investors.

All this watchfulness over such a small industry may seem a bit out of sync. For example, General Electric, which generates more profits than any other American company, garners the attention of just 13 analysts. When asked why such small companies would get so much attention compared to a giant like GE, Saloman's Marsh, said, "GE can be its own bank. Whatever it wants to do, it can generate the cash itself." Practice management organizations, on the other hand, must raise cash from external sources. "In the great capitalist fashion, interest follows capital opportunity," Marsh said. "People said, 'Wow! This industry is going to have to raise billions of dollars. Let's help them.'"

Analysts have, of late, become fairly choosy about the practice management organizations to which they'll devote time and energy. For example, Robert Lunbeck, Jr., senior healthcare analyst for Hambrecht & Quist, was following only three practice management organizations in early 1998. His February 1998 report on the industry, aptly titled Better Shop Around, "is not a sweeping endorsement of the industry," he cautioned. He expected to broaden his list somewhat, but said he's only interested in a handful of names.

GOING PUBLIC

Going public is big step that can transform the fabric and destiny of a physician or dentist company. Before making that step, executives should weigh the pros and cons of such a move (See Box 12–1). Gary Cage, CEO of Monarch Dental, has some advice. Cage has participated in taking two practice management companies public: EmCare in 1993 and Monarch in 1997. Monarch was founded by a Dallas-area dentist who opened his first office in 1983 and expanded by opening a new office each year. After a $15 million venture capital infusion in 1996, the company was in a position to go public and hired Cage as a seasoned veteran who could take it through the process. Cage joined the company in March 1996 and Monarch went public in July 1997, a journey that would have taken much longer if Cage hadn't known the ropes.

Cage has this list of "dos" and "don'ts" for companies before they go public.

B O X   12–1

PROS AND CONS OF GOING PUBLIC

Here's a brief summary of some of the pros and cons of an initial public offering.

Pros

- Provides cash that doesn't need to be repaid as debt. The IPO generates immediate cash and once a company is publicly traded, it can go back to the market with secondary offerings to raise additional capital.

- Brings visibility and prestige. Public companies are better known and carry a patina of having successfully survived the scrutiny of government regulators, bankers, and other audiences.

- Adds market value. The value of public companies tends to be higher than that of comparable private companies because of increased liquidity, available information, and a readily ascertainable value.

- Provides a currency. The newly traded stock can be used as currency to buy physician practices, reward and recruit executives, and merge with or strike alliances with other companies. The ability to use stock as currency facilitates merger and acquisition activity, which can help the company grow faster.

- Offers an exit strategy. Financial backers will want an exit strategy in which they can cash out of this enterprise and invest their money in something else. An IPO allows them to do it.

Cons

- Expense. The cost of going public will be between 5% and 7% of the total proceeds. In addition to the up-front cost, the process will take

DO

- Build the strongest infrastructure you can afford.
- Relentlessly build reserves so you can have the strongest balance sheet possible. Too many companies focus on strong historical earnings to make their companies look good. However, they'd be better off building reserves to strengthen the balance. View this is a "free kick" as if playing a game of soccer. Your company's share price will be based on future earnings, not historical results.
- Retain lawyers and accountants who have specific experience with practice management organizations and the SEC. Don't buy these

time away from other initiatives. Executives must spend months with investment bankers and institutions to position the stock. Once public, the cost of being a public company continues as reports to the investing public must be continually generated. In addition, the company will have to pay directors and purchase directors and officers liability insurance.

- Loss of privacy. A public company is always in the public light, opening its activities to the scrutiny of investors, the media, the SEC and the public. Not only must the company file quarterly financial reports, but it must make disclosures on competitive contracts, salaries, the sale of stock by key executives, the cost of significant acquisitions, and other business moves. The company's strategy is an open book. As a private company, practice management companies don't have to disclose such information to the world, which includes their competitors. In addition, there are certain restrictions on insider sales of stock that aren't there for private companies.

- Loss of control. A public company must manage its business to reward shareholders. That mind-set may be difficult for physicians to adjust to. Physician practices are accustomed to distributing the profits among their partners. This intrusion is a necessary evil and one that is difficult to control. For example, a practice management company could be taken over by another company with the financial wherewithal to buy a majority interest. If another company has the capital to buy the practice management's outstanding stock, the whole direction of the company could shift very quickly. Future executive bonuses may take the form of stock-based incentives, making compensation dependent on the fate of the stock market.

services based on relative fee estimates. You're better off paying more for experience.

DON'T

- Go public until you're ready.
- Rely on future acquisitions to sustain earnings results. The market will accord your company a higher multiple for same-store earnings.
- Underestimate the complexity and cost of integrating acquisitions when projecting future earnings results.

In addition, practice management companies may have to go through a thought conversion process. Their private company will be thrown to the whims of Wall Street and their finances, strategy and personnel moves will become fodder for analysts, shareholders, and the media.

The Registration Process

At some point, a practice management organization may decide it is ready to go from being "private" to being public. This means that a portion of the company's capital stock (which up to this point has been privately owned) will be made available for purchase by the investing public. To do this, the shares must be registered with the SEC in a rigorous process known as "going public." The reason for the rigorousness is that once the stock is registered, it becomes, in effect, a private form of currency that can be used to effect certain corporate transactions, such as acquisitions.

The process of going public is complicated and expensive, and involves many steps (Figure 12–2).

Selecting the Underwriter

When it's time to go public, a practice management organization markets itself to various investment banks to determine which one will lead the effort to sell its stock. The lead underwriter assumes the risk of buying the newly registered stock from the practice management organization and reselling it to the public, either directly or through dealers. This commitment is made by a contract called the underwriting agreement. The underwriting agreement will usually not be executed until after the road show is completed and the registration statement is declared effective by the SEC, but its form is generally agreed to early on.

An underwriter can make or break an offering. On its shoulders rests the ability to start off on the right foot with institutional investors, get the best price for the shares, and establish a strong rapport on Wall Street. When selecting an underwriter, consider the following about the investment bank.

FIGURE 12-2

IPO Timeline

Week 1: Begin writing registration statement.

Week 2: Begin due diligence and circulate first draft of registration statement.

Week 4: Circulate second draft of registration document. Work with underwriter to develop road show presentation and begin selecting syndicate.

Week 5: File registration statement with SEC and begin talking to syndicate members. Lead underwriter meets with sales force managers to talk about the company.

Week 6: Underwriter begins to invite syndicate members.

Weeks 9–11: Receive comments from SEC and refile registration statement. Underwriter circulates "red herring" (preliminary prospectus) and meets with sales force to talk about marketing the offering.

Week 10–12: Road show begins followed by pricing, final prospectus, and offering.

Source: Salomon Smith Barney.

- Track record with similar offerings
- Commitment to healthcare services research, particularly in practice management
- Ability to coordinate a road show that matches the company with investors who would have a particular interest in this niche of healthcare
- Capacity to stabilize pricing in the stock after the offering

The investment bank selected will work with the practice management organization to plan details of the issue and prepare the registration materials to be filed with the SEC. The investment bank also selects the other investment banks that will be part of a "syndicate" to help spread the financial risk and ensure good distribution of the stock once the deal is completed. The syndicate may involve two to five additional underwriters and as many as 20 regional investment banks. It also may include retail distribution.

In selecting an investment bank, a practice management organization must also consider how the stock will be supported after an offering. Some brokerage houses underwrite stock offerings, but may not have research analysts dedicated to physician or dental management companies.

Without a strong, reputable analyst covering the company, a practice management stock could languish because the large institutions won't be aware of the stock and won't buy it. On the other hand, the more analysts that follow the stock, the more expectations there are to manage, which can be problematic and time-consuming for a CEO and CFO (as we shall see later).

"Any major firm can get your deal done," noted Monarch's CEO Cage. He explained that practice management companies need to choose a bank based on the quality of an investment bank's on-going research, its after-market trading capabilities, and its savvy in the mergers and acquisitions deal flow. In addition, he said that practice management companies should consider their importance to the investment bank. "Can you get their attention if you need to?" Cage asked.

Filing the Registration Statement

The SEC has three types of registration statements that can be used for practice management organization IPOs. Form S-1 is by far the most comprehensive (and most commonly used). "Small business issuers" may wish to use Form SB-1 or SB-2; this will be discussed later.

The registration statement serves two potentially conflicting purposes. The prospectus has embedded within it is, in effect, a sales brochure that should present the best possible image of the company. However, because the interests of the investing public must also be protected, the prospectus must include complete and fair disclosure of all important aspects of the company, including the less favorable ones.

One of the most important sections of the prospectus is the "risk factors." For practice management organizations, it tends to be voluminous. When American Physician Partners, a Dallas-based radiology practice management organization, went public in November 1997, its prospectus included 11 pages of risk factors. Because practice management organizations are a new industry, there is quite a bit of uncertainty associated with them. For example, many practice management organizations require their physicians to sign noncompete agreements; however, the enforceability of these covenants has, for the most part, yet to be tested. In addition, fraud and abuse statutes on self-referral, corporate practice of medicine laws, and fee-splitting laws also pose issues with respect to the potential legality of practice management organization arrangements.

Although it may seem that the risk factors section would scare off potential investors, the value of disclosing as much as possible is incalculable. If the price of the practice management organization's stock collapses, opportunistic lawyers and shareholders may file lawsuits, claiming they were not informed of certain risks inherent in the stock. A thorough "risk factors" section may provide a hedge of protection against such expensive and time-consuming suits.

The prospectus also must describe what the company plans to do with the capital raised through offering. This "use of proceeds" section in a prospectus typically mentions repaying debt. Often, that debt is the notes held by the private equity and venture capital sources.

After the registration statement has been prepared and all of the exhibits assembled, the financial printer will "EDGARize" the document (discussed later) and transmit it electronically to the SEC.

The SEC Comment Period

Once the practice management organization has filed the registration statement, the waiting or "cooling-off" period begins. Technically, the cooling-off period extends from the time that the registration statement is filed until it is declared effective by the SEC. The SEC mandates a cooling-off period of at least 20 days; as a practical matter, it will take much longer than that for the SEC to process a new registration statement.

The SEC review will involve a team of government attorneys and accountants, and in some cases, industry specialists. After the examiners have reviewed the registration statement, they provide the company with a letter containing the SEC's comments. This is usually received about a month after filing. It's not unusual to receive 100 or more comments on its registration statement. Because the industry is still so new and the accounting rules are still evolving, the SEC is more diligent about scrutinizing the details, and must consider some issues on a case-by-case basis. However, the SEC does not pass judgment on whether the stock is a good investment or even whether the information is accurate, only that the statement contains full and fair disclosures that will allow potential investors to make informed decisions.

It's unusual for a practice management organization's registration statement to be cleared after just one round with the SEC. As a result, multiple amendments may be required, which can delay the transaction significantly (or sometimes, stop it altogether).

The Road Show

Toward the end of the cooling-off period, the underwriters and selling group can use a preliminary version of the prospectus (called the "red herring") to undertake a road show to cities like New York, Boston, San Francisco, and Atlanta over a two-week period. During the road show, top executives from the company, along with the underwriters and selling group, tell the company's story to potential buyers such as institutional investors, portfolio managers, and other securities dealers in an effort to build interest in the stock. The road show includes one-on-one meetings with institutions that may make large purchases of the stock. It also will include lunch and dinner meetings with groups of fund managers and institutional sales forces. The level of interest determined during the road show will be important to stock pricing decisions. The underwriters will be "building the order book," sizing up the level of interest in the offering. Indications are placed in the order book, which will help determine pricing of the offering.

Pricing

Once the issue is declared effective by the SEC—meaning the stock can be sold to the public—the company and the underwriters will complete negotiations as to the price at which the securities will be sold.

Although there is no standard formula, certain factors are always considered in the valuation process. Market conditions at the time the IPO is undertaken constitute the prime consideration for pricing. Prices and price/earnings ratios of established practice management firms will also come into play as will the aftermarket performance of similar IPOs. If similar practice management organizations are trading at a P/E of 12, for example, it's going to be difficult to price a new issue at a P/E of 30. P/E doubles as a perceived growth rate. When the shares are marketed by underwriter, the P/E and its comparison to its growth rate will be an important selling point. If the practice management company is selling at a P/E of 20 and its annual earnings growth rate is 30, it's trading at a 33% discount to its growth rate. The price also will reflect the "indications of interest" generated as a result of the road show—in other words, how strong the perceived demand for the stock is.

When AOR went public in 1995, market excitement about practice management was high. As a result of that excitement, practice management companies generally were trading at multiples in the 40s and 50s. AOR's offering was priced at $10.50 per share, and opened the first day of trading at $14. Interest was strong, the offer was over-subscribed, and AOR raised $114 million.

However, by 1998, "indications of interest" were becoming harder to find, and the window seemed to be closing on equity offerings for physician and dental companies. When the proposed PhyCor-MedPartners megamerger fell apart in late 1997, the subsequent fallout cooled investor interest in practice management companies. That in turn affected nearly a dozen similar companies that were in some stage of the SEC registration process. Some chose to delay their IPOs until they could get better pricing. Others forged ahead, only to find that the actual offering price was 10% to 40% lower than originally expected.

As the market cap for practice management organizations collapsed, the IPO window slammed shut. In fact, health services stocks as a whole drew a chill from Wall Street. Only 5% of the 1998 IPOs were in healthcare through September, according to Securities Data Corp., while healthcare companies in registration represented 11% of the backlog.

Executing the Underwriting Agreement

Finally, the company and underwriters will execute the underwriting agreement. This process will involve negotiating the price at which the securities will be sold (as explained above) along with the discounts and commissions to be retained by the underwriters as compensation for their services.

The underwriter assumes the risk of buying the newly-registered stock from the practice management organization and reselling it to the public, either directly or through dealers. The underwriter purchases the stock from the practice management organization at a negotiated discount, which is called the "underwriting spread." That "spread" is how the underwriter is compensated for the time and money it has invested in assisting with preparation of the prospectus, assembling the syndicate, managing the road show, and myriad other responsibilities.

Here's how it works. If the offering price is $10 and the underwriting spread is $1, the practice management organization receives proceeds of $9 per share. If the offering involved 1 million shares, the spread would be $1 million; on 2 million shares, $2 million, and go up from there. Usually, the spread averages about 7%.

The allocation of the spread among the lead underwriter or "syndicate manager," the syndicate, and the selling group varies. Of the $1 spread, the manager's fee is usually 10% to 20%, the underwriting fee is usually 20% to 30%, and the selling group's portion (called the concession) is 50% to 60%.[1]

Closing

Once the underwriting agreement has been executed, trading in the company's stock may begin. The closing of an IPO—at which the practice management organization delivers the securities to the underwriter in return for the proceeds from the offering—generally occurs five to seven business days after trading begins.

IMPORTANT IPO CONSIDERATIONS

Selecting an Underwriter

As discussed earlier, selecting an investment bank involves a number of determinants. If the investment bank is too small, it may not have a big enough syndicate of institutions and investors available to buy the stock. If the bank is too large, a small practice management organization may get lost in the shuffle and not receive the devotion it wants to its deal.

---

[1]Dearborn Financial Publishing, General Securities Representative, 9th ed.

Costs of an IPO

An IPO is an incredibly costly proposition; if it fails, the company will have incurred staggering costs on which no return will be realized. By far the largest cost associated with an IPO is the underwriter's fee, as we have already discussed. Other costs for an IPO include the following.

- Legal fees. These can range from $100,000 to $200,000, but for large offerings the cost can be $500,000 or more.
- Accounting fees. Again, this can range from $50,000 to $100,000 for smaller offerings, but may be much more for larger offerings.
- Road show. After registration and prior to the effective date, the practice management organization's management team and its investment bankers present the company's story to potential investors. Management organizations need to realize that this is taking time away from operating the company because the road show can last several weeks and keep executives on the road continuously.
- Printing and engraving costs. These range from $50,000 to $250,000 for the registration statement, prospectus, stock certificates, and other documents.
- Other costs. Covered here are such expenses as the costs of retaining a transfer agent, application fees payable to the relevant stock exchange or quotation service, and the filing fees paid to the SEC, the NASD, and various state securities administrators.

Because these costs can vary widely, it's a good idea to keep close tabs on how the money is being spent. For example, financial printers market heavily to attorneys, who decide which vendors to recommend to aspiring registrants. The printer they recommend may not be the least expensive, just the most generous to their referral sources.

Financial printers have electronic connections to EDGAR, the Electronic Data Gathering, Analysis and Retrieval system of the SEC. Most publicly held companies already file their documents electronically with the SEC, and as of October 1998, all publicly held companies must do so. Typically, companies provide their documents on disk to the financial printer, which has software to transmit them to EDGAR. Some larger companies have installed the software in-house, thus bypassing the need for the financial printer.

A few smaller practice management organizations have taken advantage of a short-cut to an IPO for small businesses. Certain small businesses can file Form SB-1 or SB-2. The SB-1 is a simplified and abbreviated form for businesses that are issuing $10 million or less in securities in any 12-month period. The SB-2 puts no limit on the offering size. The annual revenues and value of the public float stock of small business issuers cannot exceed $25 million annually.

Management organizations might want to mention these alternatives to their attorneys and consultants. Such filings are less expensive and aren't likely to generate the legal and accounting fees of a full-blown IPO. Because of that, they may be a good deal for the practice management company, but less lucrative for their advisers.

SEC Planning Considerations

Once a decision to go public is made, the practice management organization must ensure that it's prepared from a financial standpoint. It must have audited financial statements and advisers who are aware of the issues particular to practice management (for example, amortization and goodwill).

Recently, the SEC moved to impose a 25-year ceiling on amortization of practice management companies' long-lived intangible assets. Normally, such intangibles have been amortized over their contractual terms of 30–40 years. When the amortization period is shortened, the company's earnings per share likely will be lowered. Practice management organizations need to figure this into their financial models so that there won't be any surprises when it's time to go public.

Another issue is "contingent consideration." Often practice management firms have bought physician practice assets for a lump sum—usually a combination of cash, notes and stock. However, many add a sweetener to the deal: If the practice achieves a certain level of profits or cash flow, the physician receives a bonus. Sometimes this is structured in a way that makes it an incentive to ensure that physicians continue at their previous levels of production.

Depending on how it is structured, contingent consideration arrangements may be considered salary rather than part of the acquisition price. In such cases, they can't be considered part of goodwill and amortized over future periods. If the SEC requires reclassification of contingent consideration to salary expense, this could be a jolt to the income statement because it will lower EPS.

In general, if the practice management organization has any unusual accounting or disclosure issues, it's wise to ask for a preliminary SEC clearance before filing. This could save time and printing expense.

LIFE AS A PUBLIC COMPANY: KEEPING THE GROWTH MACHINE GOING

Congratulations—you survived your IPO! This marks the beginning of a new—and different—future for the practice management organization. The changes go right to the core of the organization and how it does business. For example, there are new constituents to deal with. It will seem like analysts and brokers are constantly on the phone seeking information. Dealing with Wall Street will bring about a new set of rules and expectations to deal with. What's more, it will change the way the practice management organization is run, because now the impetus is to balance the long-term needs of the company against Wall Street's short-term expectations for earnings and growth.

Communicating with Analysts

Once a practice management organization goes public, the role of its CEO and CFO change very quickly. One of the most difficult changes is learning to respond to all of the company's new constituents, particularly the analysts and investors. Research coverage is critical to a company's continuing success in the financial markets after an IPO, and research analysts who follow a company will be making frequent requests for information. In fact, most practice management organization execs find that the amount of information they are expected to provide, and the number of conference calls and meetings they must have with analysts, is much greater than they ever expected. As the practice management organization grows larger, it may be able to relegate some of those duties to an investor relations director, but that won't completely relieve the burdens placed on the CEO and CFO.

One reason healthcare analysts spend much of their time visiting and calling practice management companies is to ensure that their quarterly earnings estimates—the numbers by which public companies live and die—are reasonable. Sell-side analysts are expected to be experts about the companies they follow, and a big part of their job is to forecast companies sales, earnings, and other key financial measures of growth.

An analyst's track record of success or failure in forecasting correctly translates into increased (or decreased) revenues from stock trades for the investment bank for which the analyst works. As discussed earlier, money managers and institutional investors usually buy and sell stock through brokerage houses, like everyone else. Generally, they choose to trade with the banks whose analysts bring them the best ideas, analyses, and recommendations. In the case of large money funds like Fidelity, for example, portfolio managers will vote quarterly or semiannually for their favorite analysts. This signals their trading desks to pay those investment banks by making a certain amount of trades through the brokerage houses for which those analysts work.

Missed estimates reflect poorly on the analysts who make them. The worst thing for an analyst is to be caught by surprise by negative developments in a company he or she is following, because that can erode the confidence that portfolio managers and other investors have in that analyst. In turn, that will affect the amount of revenue the investment bank earns trading for those investors.

Analysts' ability to accurately forecast growth and earnings is dependent in large measure on the quality of information they receive from the companies they follow. Therefore, once a company is publicly traded, its CEO and CFO must ensure that analysts are fed a steady stream of information, both to ensure good relationships (and therefore, current research coverage) and to ensure that the analyst has access to appropriate information about the company.

Managing Wall Street's Expectations

Once public, a practice management company will be expected to play by a whole new set of rules. Earnings per share is the great financial measuring stick against which all publicly traded companies are measured. Practice management company executives quickly learn to keep that financial measuring stick in mind at all times.

Here's why: The price of a public company's stock indicates how that company is being perceived by the market. The more an investor is willing to pay today (relative to current earnings), the greater will be the expectation for future earnings, and the more pressure that is put on the company to perform. This is true of all public companies, but seems more pronounced in the practice management industry because of its basic premise. "The premise of this business is to empower physicians," says Salomon's Larry Marsh. "You're backing the change engine for a trillion-dollar industry that's one of the few cottage industries left. People say, 'Holy smokes, we can really change things.' Sometimes, the hope becomes disjointed from reality."

On Wall Street, perceptions sometimes get ahead of reality. Even though investors and analysts may realize that a company (or industry) is overvalued, they will go along for the ride as long as there are profits to be made. But as soon as they see the foundation crumbling even a little, they often will drop the "buy" recommendation or sell the stock, causing the share prices (and with them, the company's market worth) to decrease more than a fair valuation would suggest.

Wall Street is particularly ruthless when companies do not meet expectations for revenue and earnings growth. If a company reports 10 cents per share when the analysts predicted 11 cents, that makes the company look bad. A penny may not seem like much, but it can cost a company millions of dollars. When AOR missed estimates by 1 cent in the second quarter of 1996, the company lost half its market value.

CEOs may criticize analysts who downgrade stock for not meeting expectations, but analysts argue that the company is well aware of those expectations. Analysts' estimates are available at the touch of a button through services such as First Call. If the company doesn't agree with the expectations, its CEO or CFO can voice those concerns. "I keep an eye on consensus numbers," noted Fred Pounds, AOR's chief financial officer. "If we think people are way out of line, I'll say something to them." If they're aware of them, but fail to meet them, there's something wrong.

What or who drives the market's expectations? Analysts are a key driver, due to the central role they play in the investment process. Much of their influence is derived from advising institutions with investment responsibilities for billions of dollars—investors that can take such big positions in a stock that, in effect, they can establish its price. Often, a powerful analyst can move a stock price up or down, depending on what he or she is telling the Street about a company. Simply put, if analysts paint the company as a growth company, it can command a higher P/E ratio. Perceived growth is used to justify high P/Es; a perceived stall will do the opposite.

A big part of an analyst's job is to forecast companies' sales, earnings, and other key financial measures of growth for a company. Analysts keep a watchful eye on each others' earnings expectations and don't want to be too far off the consensus without a very good reason. One advantage of having several analysts follow the stock is that they keep each others' expectations in check. Sometimes, if only two or three analysts are following—and subsequently, touting—a stock, earnings projections can get overheated.

H&Q's Lunbeck acknowledged that there's "enormous pressure" placed on analysts by practice management executives to pump up their company to get investors' attention. Naturally, the executives will tend to be optimistic about their company. It's the analyst's job to temper those expectations. "Management's job (in describing company prospects) is, at a minimum, to be sincere," said Lunbeck. "They may be wrong, but they must at least be sincere."

This highlights another significant driver of expectations—the company itself. Physician company CEOs and CFOs soon come to understand just how much their interaction with analysts can affect the financial community's evaluation of the company—specifically, as it is reflected in their stock price. As a result, executive management must walk a fine line. They must be careful not to make unrealistic promises about a company's earnings growth (for legal as well as economic reasons). However, if they downplay the company's prospects too much, the stock price will suffer, as money managers buy the stock of companies who promise to have more potential.

The point is to help keep investors' and analysts' expectations at realistic levels. Although CEOs often fault analysts for hyping the market too much, Marsh said that the executives themselves bear some of the blame. As investors see the momentum shift to companies that are making a lot of acquisitions, that manifests itself in higher stock prices. "The market will reward that growth with a higher P/E multiple for every dollar of earnings that you show," Marsh said. "There's a temptation to tell the market you are going to grow at a higher rate because of the benefits of that expectation," he added.

The higher the P/E multiple, the cheaper the capital, enabling a management company to make more acquisitions for less money. If a fast-growing practice management company is buying physician practices primarily with stock, the number of shares outstanding will increase each quarter. That could be good if the practice management company doesn't want to spend a lot of cash on acquisitions.

However, the down side is that if those practices aren't bringing a comparable amount of earnings to the company, earnings per share won't keep up with the growth in total shares. That means that growth may lag behind expectations and—you've got it—share prices tumble.

A timely, consistent flow of information to keep everyone fully informed in making recommendations and buy/sell/hold decisions is probably the best way to manage the expectations of everyone interested in the company. The company must also give the analyst comfort that there won't be any surprises down the road. Companies that know their earnings are going to be less than the market expects are wise to get the information out a few weeks early, before the actual results are reported.

When AOR executives realized the company would miss earnings estimates in 1996, the company preannounced the miss so that analysts could reset their expectations, said CFO Pounds. Market disappointment will most likely cause the price to fall, but the overall drop may not be as steep as when the market is hit with the reported results by surprise. The preannouncement can cushion the fall and also help a company build a case in the event of a shareholder lawsuit.

Balancing Short-Term and Long-Term Objectives

Executives of newly public management companies also quickly learn that stock prices have an effect on far-reaching business decisions. Decisions begin to be framed by their effect on short term earnings—in particular, what impact the decision would have on the quarterly earnings number—rather than what's in the company's best interest long-term. Sometimes it's difficult separating what you should do for the business and what you should do based on the marketplace. Long-term prosperity may be jeopardized by shareholder emphasis on short-term results.

It can be easy for practice management firms to get caught up in analysts' expectations and stray from their own strategy of building the company block by block. "We need to look at Wall Street as a finance source," says Ross of AOR. "Other than that, you need to focus on your business and not get too caught up with stock performance."

One way in which Wall Street's excessive expectations for a company's growth might influence management is that the company will be pressured to grow quickly through affiliations and acquisitions. "PPMs are in the business of selling services to groups. To attract groups, they need to be as attractive as possible," says Salomon's Larry Marsh. "One way you can be seen as attractive is by demonstrating a lot of momentum. The faster you grow, the more sense of momentum, and the more attractive you may seem to the groups you're trying to attract," he added.

A practice management executive says, "It's a delicate balance. We have to pay attention to managing these practices to generate the earnings that will sustain us in the long haul. On the other hand, we are under intense pressure to grow faster than we can internally. The only way to do that is through acquiring new practices. If we focus too much on acquisitions, we don't take care of our existing practices. At the same time, if we don't grow rapidly, investors aren't interested in our stock."[2]

"That conflict is the reality of this business," Marsh said.

Problems also may arise if those acquisitions are dilutive to earnings per share. As we said earlier, if a fast-growing practice management company is buying physician practices primarily with stock, the number of shares outstanding will increase each quarter. That could be good if the practice management company doesn't want to spend a lot of cash on acquisitions. However, the downside is that if those practices aren't bringing a comparable amount of earnings to the company, earnings per share won't keep up with the growth in total shares. That means growth may lag behind expectations.

"Growth is good, but growth has its dangers," Pounds said, noting that practice management organizations should be aware that when they're making acquisitions at breakneck pace, the operational consequences of those deals may not show up until twelve months later, causing the company to miss earnings. In AOR's case, the company had wanted to make $150 million in acquisitions in 1995. Just prior to filing the IPO, one large medical group wanted to join. That pushed AOR's acquisition volume higher than expected. Integrating those practices into the AOR model was difficult and showed in the results one year later, when AOR's stock tumbled from $20 per share to $8 as a result of missed earnings.

Rapid growth can have a waterfall effect on strategic decisions in other areas. When a practice management organization is growing fast, it's building higher and higher hurdles over which it needs to improve earnings the next year. The company must look for new strategic avenues to keep the growth machine going. Sometimes those decisions aren't made in the same way as they would have been if made in an entirely long-term mind-set.

From his earlier days at EmCare, US Cardiovascular's Cooley knows only too well the pressures involved in clearing those hurdles. Growth expectations typically are expressed in the form of percentages. The smaller you start, the bigger your growth percentages will be and the faster you will appear to grow. "To show a 20% growth rate in 1992, we needed to earn $10 million in additional revenues. But by 1997, we needed $50 million in additional revenues" to keep that same pace, Cooley said. The pressure gets tougher as a market becomes more mature because, in a maturing market, there are fewer places to go for growth. Although EmCare was making more acquisitions in big-city markets—its primary focus—than ever before, they weren't enough to drive 20% growth. "A lot of our time and energy went into deciding what we were going to do the get the next $50 million in," Cooley said.

---

[2]*Capitalizing Medical Groups*, p. 288.

EmCare made a strategic decision to stay within its niche of emergency medicine, but broaden into smaller geographic markets and to increase its acquisition pace. The company bought another emergency medicine firm that was providing services to small hospitals in smaller markets. That was totally outside EmCare's previous strategy of big-city markets. "It represented a dramatic change in our business mix," Cooley said.

Its close competitor, Coastal Physicians, sought growth in a different direction—managing primary care practices. The decision prompted Coastal's near demise as it struggled with those practices and the capitated contracts that were subsequently part of them.

Wall Street also drives the wagon (or at least holds the reins) when a company is considering ways in which it might raise additional capital. If the practice management organization raises capital through the sales of additional stock, this would dilute earnings per share. That's why publicly-held practice management companies often turn to other capital sources, such as bank debt or publicly traded bonds. The decision on bonds versus stock may rest on a company's debt-to-equity ratio. More debt translates into more leverage, increasing that ratio.

PREDICTORS FOR THE FUTURE

There's quite a challenge involved in balancing the shorter-term time horizon of investors' expectations for the practice management industry against the industry's need to change physicians' behavior and practice patterns.

It's a catch-22. Management companies' ability to meet earnings and growth expectations will be an important arbiter for whether the industry continues to garner the capital it has received during the past several years. However, too much focus on earnings and growth detracts from management's ability to pay attention to how the business is being operated.

Thomas Hodapp, an analyst with BancAmerica Robertson Stephens, qualified his buy ratings on practice management stocks in a December 1997 report by saying, "Investors remain skeptical of PPM companies' ability to produce earnings greater than their cost of capital—a view that appears justified to us in most cases, gauging by analysis of returns." However, he went on to predict that "the industry is just entering a second major stage that will be characterized by accelerating internal growth and escalating returns on invested capital into the next decade."

From an operational perspective, established practice management organizations in 1998 needed to shift their focus away from acquisitions and over to integration and positioning for managed care. However, investors—who jump in and out of stocks daily—are unlikely to reward practice management organizations for "doing the right thing" operationally, focusing on internal improvements rather than the acquisition of medical groups. As a result, if investors are not satisfied with the earnings and growth rates associated with this shift in emphasis, then equity funding for practice management organizations dries up, as it did in the fall of 1998. "There are people who truly understand the vision, but if they think the stock is not going to go up, they won't buy it," AOR's Ross noted.

AN EXPERT'S PERSPECTIVE: LAWRENCE C. MARSH, CFA, DIRECTOR OF EQUITY RESEARCH IN PHYSICIAN PRACTICE MANAGEMENT FOR SALOMON SMITH BARNEY, NEW YORK

Less money up front to physicians, smaller management fees, and a slower momentum of physicians aligning with practice management organizations. That was the consensus in the summer of 1998 for the practice management industry from Larry Marsh, director of equity research in physician practice management for Salomon Smith Barney.

Salomon Smith Barney has been one of the most active investment banks in raising capital for and trading practice management stocks. The New York–based investment bank has helped raise $4 billion for 35 practice management companies since 1990. In addition, the firm has been involved in 14 M&A transactions valued at $5 billion since 1990. In March 1997, its research department set the tone for its commitment to practice management organizations by issuing a mammoth tome of nearly 300 pages, titled "Of Minds and Men—Changing Behavior in the New Physician Enterprise." The report's lead author was Marsh, who had joined Salomon the previous year from another investment bank, Wheat First Butcher Singer in Richmond, Va. Marsh, who has followed healthcare stocks since 1987, had covered two of the earliest practice management organizations, Coastal Physicians and PhyCor, while at Wheat First. In 1996, Institutional Investor tapped him for its All-American Team for regional and boutique firms, a recognition that investment analysts covet.

Marsh's clients primarily are money managers and institutional investors. Money managers pay investment banks like Salomon by trading stocks through them. They generally choose to trade with the banks whose analysts bring them the best ideas, analyses and recommendations. Marsh's job is to get—and keep—his clients interested in trading practice management stocks. He certainly has succeeded. In 1997, Salomon handled 23% of all of the trades in practice management stocks, more than any other investment bank. By focusing on this sector of healthcare, Marsh brings value by selecting the practice management organizations that he believes have the best prospects for making money for investors. Further, once Salomon gets involved in raising capital through an IPO for a physician company, Marsh typically will support the stock by initiating coverage of it and following it. This is one of the most significant services an investment bank can provide, as it can be crucial to maintaining investor interest.

Marsh makes recommendations on practice management stocks based on his own screening process. "Investors want to see a track record. Second, they want some feeling of predictability, they want to feel that the earnings are sustainable. Third, they want a return on their investment." His screening process takes into consideration a practice management firm's infrastructure, operations, dependency on acquisitions, dependency on external capital, management philosophy, how long the company has operated separately, the company's track record, and what sort of culture the management is trying to build. In his 1997 report, Marsh also introduced a new practice management index that highlighted "best of class" models: PhyCor, Pediatrix, EmCare, MedCath, MedPartners and Physician Resource Group (Table 12–11).

"The volatility we sometimes see in the stock market is investors' best guess of what's going to happen in the future," he said. "It's not so much a reaction to the quarter just ended, as it is to what's ahead. With practice management organizations, some of the volatility is a reaction of investors trying to determine how profitable this industry is really going to be. Will it be very successful, moderately successful, or not successful? There is an enormous opportunity, but the models are going to have to evolve from what's currently out there."

The economic equation is changing and physicians going forward are likely to receive less up front, Marsh believes. He thinks that most practice management organizations will adopt the new model that PhyCor put into place in the spring of 1998, under which they will pay physicians less up front for their practices, and charge a lower management fee on the back end. "The dynamics of paying groups large amounts of money up front are going to have to change. There's too much going out initially and not enough sustaining these companies," he said. (Other problems Marsh sees are in Figure 12–3.)

FIGURE 12–3

Marsh Sees These Problems at Many Practice Management Organizations

- Creating a lot of volume without building an infrastructure.
- Making unreasonable predictions about acquisitions. "The reality is, the selling cycle is very long and the complexity is high."
- Physician groups competing with their customers (HMOs and other managed-care payors).
- Assuming that if you have operations in multiple market, the model is transferable. "Scattered resources makes management more challenging, not less challenging."
- Rushing to market. "The longer the incubation process the better."

As an example of practice management organizations paying too much on the front end, Marsh noted the charges that MedPartners took for 1997. The company took a $522 million charge for impairment of goodwill and $82.4 million to write down of other assets. "In plain English, they paid 50 percent too much for some of the groups they acquired," Marsh said. "I'm not saying all PPMs have overpaid by 50 percent, but this is an example of one that did."

Another factor impacting how much practice management organizations are willing to pay up front is goodwill. The SEC has begun to enforce a ceiling of 25 years as an appropriate amortization period for goodwill. Most practice management organizations had instead been amortizing goodwill or capitalized MSA costs over the term of the management agreements, which was usually 30–40 years. Because there's a shorter period over which to amortize these upfront costs, the bigger payments will impact earnings per share more directly.

T A B L E   12–1

Salomon Smith Barney Price Management Index

	1995	1996	1997	1998
Advanced Health	NA	NA	69.3%	−89.0%
American Dental Partners	NA	NA	NA	−4.2%
American Oncology Resources	73.7%	−57.8%	56.1%	9.0
AmeriPath	NA	NA	−4.2%	−47.4%
Coastal Physician	−49.8%	−74.1%	−74.9%	−43.2%
EmCare	71.4%	−3.1%	60.2%	NA
FPA Medical	53.1%	138.7%	−16.7%	−99.3%
InPhynet Medical Management	84.6%	−25.0%	37.5%	NA
MedCath	40.0%	−23.8%	−5.4%	25.6%
MedPartners	97.0%	−37.1%	7.9%	−76.5%
Monarch Dental	NA	NA	1.9%	−69.6%
OccuSystems	24.0%	35.0%	0.5%	NA
Pediatrix Medical	28.7%	34.5%	15.5%	40.2%
PhyCor	202.6%	−15.8%	−4.8%	−74.8%
PhyMatrix		−26.0%	10.5%	−88.9%
Physician Reliance Network	109.2%	−61.0%	34.7%	25.8%
Physicians Resource Group	40.7%	−11.3%	−73.0%	−78.9%
ProMedCo	NA	NA	11.1%	50.0%
Specialty Care Network	NA	NA	70.4%	−90.8%
Sheridan Healthcare	−4.9%	−51.5%	155.3%	−44.1%
Group Average	**59.3%**	**−12.7%**	**13.8%**	**−45.5%**

PricewaterhouseCoopers Tips for Public Companies

- Consistently manage expectations of investors and analysts.
- Don't overpromise.
- Don't go public until you're sure the company can produce predictable quarterly results.
- Have a management team in place and working together long before the going-public process begins.
- Obtain professional advice from accounting and legal experts who understand the practice management industry.

13
CHAPTER

The Bar is Raised for a New Generation of Management Companies

Sandy Lutz

Spring of 1998. An ominous cloud began settling over the physician practice management arena. Most practice management stocks began a long slide toward 52-week lows; some hit bottom at half their valuations of two years before.

The pages of trade journals are full of stories of disgruntled doctors, executives and investors, and this coverage spills over to the newspaper business pages. Once-high hopes have been dashed. "In terms of comparables, it's a dead niche," said Sarah Garvin, president of Atlanta-based Physician Health Corp.

Garvin's firm had filed for an initial public offering (IPO) in late 1997, but four days into a spring 1998 road show with potential investors, the deal was called off due in large part to the falling stock prices for physician companies. As a multispecialty practice management firm, Physician Health's IPO would rely on "comps" from companies like FPA Medical, PhyCor, and MedPartners. Those companies' stock prices all plunged from the winter of 1997 and spring of 1998 as they took charges for massive write-offs, closed practices, and labored through restructurings.

Just a few years ago, practice management companies were attracting investors and physicians like flies to honey. Expectations were so high that companies with no operating history at all were raising millions of dollars in initial public offerings. Then, almost like dominoes, physician practice management companies toppled. Many had too much capital and too little management control. Bad publicity about the industry in publications like the *Wall Street Journal* began to take its toll as well. "Doctors and the stock market are not blind," said Larry English, a former top Cigna executive, who now is running a practice management start-up, Aesthetic Medical Management. "People have recognized that not all practice management companies add value."

By mid-1998, practice management companies had raised less than $200 million in equity offerings compared to $1 billion during all of 1997.

A LITTLE HISTORY OF PRACTICE MANAGEMENT COMPANIES

The practice management industry is young, having started about a decade ago. As with any new industry, a shake-out ensued after a few years. Some of the early practice management organizations are still around, and a few have been bought out. Unfortunately, few have done consistently well and others clearly will not survive the shake-out.

PhyCor's Joe Hutts has ridden the industry roller-coaster the farthest, experiencing its dizzying heights as the company climbed to $1.5 billion in annual revenues, and its spirit-flattening lows as its share price was cut by three-fourths in less than a year. "It would be an understatement to say that in the last year we have experienced a turbulent series of events," Hutts said, obviously referring to the industry's multi-million-dollar write-offs, plummeting stock price, lawsuits from disgruntled physicians, and loss of confidence on Wall Street.

When PhyCor was the sector's reigning champion, the financial engine behind practice management was nearly unstoppable. Future promise is what buoys the stock market. Many PPMs were valued on their emerging worth, rather than their current or historical returns. The climate was ideal. A booming stock market, a fragmented segment, an aging population that required more of the product (healthcare services), and low interest rates. What could go wrong?

Overpaying for practices and a failure to focus on operations sunk the PPM ships.

When some PPM stocks hit a downdraft, it sucked down the others as well. During 1998, the market value of practice management stocks dropped 75% as company after company reported write-offs and restructuring charges. Early sellers held to the cockroach theory of investing—if you've seen one problem, there are many more to come. And, they were right. When problems hit the PPM industry, investors who were indiscriminate in buying in were just as cavalier about selling out. They got out—fast. While the buildup in PPM market caps had been strong but steady, the pullback was rapid, prompting shareholder class action suits and an almost total freeze on new equity capital.

Let's look at some of the pioneers.

Coastal Physician Group

Founded in 1977, the firm initially managed hospital emergency departments by providing the emergency physician services component. By 1995, only about half the company's $1 billion in revenues stemmed from hospitals, but its future was believed to be in operating primary care physicians groups that could contract for risk. Recognized as one of the first PPMs, Coastal began to see some of the first cracks in its veneer in 1995. Stock analysts began citing fundamental operating problems stemming from contracts in Florida with Humana.

Caremark

The Illinois-based company was spun off of the giant hospital supply firm, Baxter International. Initially regarded as a home infusion therapy business, Caremark expanded into the physician practice management business and became one of the largest pharmacy benefit managers in the U.S., with annual revenues of $1.1 billion. Caremark's PPM revenues were small but growing—from $190 million in 1994 to about a half-billion-dollars in 1995. Its next frontier was touted as disease state management.

EmCare

Like Coastal, EmCare sprung from the growing business of efficiently operating hospital emergency departments. In a few cases, EmCare had expanded into primary care clinics, but its bread-and-butter remained in the emergency venue. Between 1991 and 1995, the Dallas-based firm tripled its revenues. In 1997, it was purchased by Laidlaw, a Canadian-based firm that had bought several ambulance chains and wanted to further expand into the emergency services area.

FPA Medical Management

In 1995, its first year as a public company, FPA's stock price doubled and its future looked bright. The company's southern California roots made it look prescient as managed care was sweeping from west to east across the United States. FPA's business model was slightly different from other PPMs in that its strength was in managing IPAs as opposed to operating physician practices. At one point, Oxford Health Plans purchased a 5% stake in the burgeoning firm. Then, the fortunes of both Oxford and FPA came crashing down. In 1998, FPA filed for bankruptcy reorganization after years of overpaying for physician groups and signing unprofitable managed care contracts.

InPhyNet

A physician-led company that provided physicians' services to hospitals, managed care companies, and correctional facilities.

PhyCor

The Nashville-based company was well on its way to being a premiere "pure play" in practice management. In 1995, it was making several acquisitions, but not at a breakneck pace.

Pacific Physician Services

Although it managed physician practices, the company was truly a managed care firm, generating about 80% of its revenues from capitated contracts.

Looking at the list, it's clear that this industry was built on the experiences of a handful of multispecialty models or those that derived most of their revenue from hospital contracts. Before these types of companies could prove any modicum of success, a new wave followed. Of the early PPMs, three (Caremark, Pacific Physician Services, and InPhyNet) were bought by MedPartners, and one was bought by Laidlaw. Conditions worsened for Coastal as the company's managed care losses deepened.

We must point out, however, that EmCare was regarded by shareholders as a success. EmCare delivered an annualized return of 55%, the highest among 25 PPMs, according to Hambrecht & Quist's February 1998 report on PPMs. EmCare was purchased for $400 million by Laidlaw Inc., a Canadian firm with annual revenue of more than $4 billion, in September 1997.

However, a closer look reveals that EmCare was something of an anomaly among today's PPMs and it would be precarious to use its success as a yardstick for other physician companies. The company was founded in 1992 as a contract management firm to hospital emergency departments. Increasingly during the 1980s, hospitals began to realize the financial advantages of contracting out emergency medical services to outside vendors such as EmCare. By the time EmCare went public in 1994, this specialty had some 20 years of experience in aggregating emergency medicine physician practices. No practice management niche can match that track record.

PPM advocates should interpret EmCare's success cautiously because the company had the advantage of building on an industry that had spent nearly two decades consolidating.

On the opposite side of the fence was the ill-fated Physicians Resource Group. An ophthalmology PPM based in Dallas, the company's stock fell from a high of $34 in the second quarter of 1996 to just under $1 at the end of 1998.

The tumble occurred after the company failed to meet earnings expectations, wrote off $28 million to close some practices, and fired its founding CEO.
By November 1998, the company's stock languished at about $1, well below its
$13 IPO price. The company was facing numerous lawsuits from its own physi-
cians and shareholders and had to deal with a cash flow crunch when physicians
stopped paying their management fees.

However, critics would say that Physicians Resource was structured on
toothpicks, making its future performance insecure at best. The company was
what many describe as a "poof." It rolled up several ophthalmology and optom-
etry practices, but the company hadn't operated them as a group prior to the
public offering.

Essentially, the company went from non-existence to a 4% share of the $30
billion eye services market overnight. Yet, its lack of a track record in operations
clearly hurt. What's more, as the company continued to acquire practices, it
lacked the infrastructure to bring value to them.

PRG collected a 35% management fee on operating profits, but had problems
collecting those monies. By the end of 1997, affiliates owed PRG $64 million.

The problems endemic in too much growth are plentiful among today's
PPMs. "You can't have the impact on a group if you're constantly traveling from
time zone to time zone," says Thomas Erickson, CEO of CareSelect, a Dallas-
based PPM that has focused on the Southwest market. He notes that CareSelect
has operations, managed care, ancillary, and information systems specialists who
spend time in the practices weekly. Taking a quick flight to Oklahoma City or
elsewhere in Texas increases the amount of time those people can spend helping
the practices. If they were constantly flying off to California or Miami, the company couldn't serve its physicians as effectively, Erickson believes.

Three dental practice management companies completed IPOs in 1998, but
the well dried up for physicians. Only BMJ Medical Management went public,
completing an offering begun in the fall of 1997. The Florida-based firm had hoped
for a pricing in the $10 to $11 range, but ended up with $7. In addition, just two sec-
ondary offerings made it to the Street. ProMedCo, a Fort Worth, Texas–based multispecialty firm, raised $63 million and Physicians' Specialty Corp., an Atlanta-
based firm, raised $15 million. Physicians' Specialty, which manages ear, nose and
throat physicians, ran into problems within months, though, and by the end of 1998
was restructuring and trying to sell some of its practices back to the physicians.

In the wake of the failures or near-failures, expectations are higher among
all of practice management's constituents. The Securities and Exchange
Commission is holding practice management companies to stricter financial reporting standards, Wall Street is forecasting lower earnings growth, and physicians themselves are questioning whether the model is workable.

Wall Street is taking a breather on practice management companies in general, and that may allow some of them to focus on operations rather than quick

growth. That is probably a good thing. The downside is that these firms will lack the easy access to capital they once enjoyed. It will be tougher, and maybe impossible, for some practice management companies to go public in 1999. Can they afford to pay for their capital by borrowing through banks instead of getting it free from Wall Street? They'll have to.

When children have hard times, parents tell them: "This will build character." Perhaps the same will be true for practice management firms. They'll emerge stronger and smarter, but they'll have to overcome growing skepticism and cynicism to do so.

PHYSICIAN CYNICISM

When practice management companies grew too fast, some physicians felt they were on a moving sidewalk to disaster. In fact, the proliferation of management organizations, health systems, and practice associations knocking on physicians' doors has created what some have termed "deal fatigue" in physicians.

One physician describes how he got on that sidewalk, then felt he couldn't bail out as the practice management company swelled larger and larger. Here's his story.

The physician, who declined to be identified, joined a California medical group in the late 1970s. "For 10 years, we grew like crazy," he said. The physicians were equal partners and the clinic's profits were divided among them each month, based on production.

By the late '80s, various physician groups had nearly carved up the entire local market. "The easy growth days were gone," he said. "We felt we were really at a crossroads." The group, which had by then grown to 30 physicians, started to contemplate three options: remaining independent, joining a local hospital system, or joining an even larger clinic. It was a choice faced by hundreds of clinics in the late 1980s and 1990s.

After much debate and soul-searching about the future of medicine, the physician's group decided to join a larger clinic, which was going through a series of such mergers. At this juncture, growth felt good. Physicians were happy and financially successful. "The future seemed unlimited," this physician said. "We were putting aside money into an equity pool and it was growing very fast. It seemed we had unlocked the key to the medical future," he noted. Unlike many physician groups, this one had planned ahead. It was building retained earnings, setting aside a percentage of profits each year. That made the organization attractive to potential investors.

Yet, big changes were on the horizon. Physicians began hearing rumors that clinic founders were thinking of liquidating their ownership stakes. Investment bankers began sitting in on most of the group's management meetings, and talk of an initial public offering surfaced. To get ready for an offering, management was told that profits would need to rise; to accomplish this, 15 physicians would have to be laid off. Consultants were brought in to analyze which physicians would be cut and offer them outplacement services. The process took months and "was analyzed to death," the physician recalled.

Yet, the hoped-for IPO never took place. Instead, the clinic decided to sell out to a large publicly traded practice management firm. It was a financial bonanza for many of the physicians, whose equity interests converted into publicly traded shares. Nearly 100 became instant millionaires, on paper at least. "It seemed too good to be true," one physician said.

Yet, the growth streak became addictive as the company set a goal of expanding at a 40% annual clip. Physicians weren't sure how this was going to be accomplished, but it soon became clear: The growth would come from acquisitions. Despite the doubts of insiders and outsiders, the acquisitions kept mounting. "Everybody was saying, 'This is too much too fast.'" the physician recalled.

Yet, in the trenches, physicians and managers had no choice but to try to make the deals work. Soon, it meant cutting physicians and other workers to achieve the earnings growth projections. "There was no analysis—it was just slash, slash, slash," the physician said. This was in stark contrast to the layoffs of the physicians he had previously witnessed at the large group practice. No consultants, no outplacement—just good-bye.

"Things really went crazy when we tried to integrate overlapping groups," the physician said. Making matters worse, managers hadn't seen any financial reports for nearly a year. "Everybody was making decisions in the dark," the physician said. Clinics were closed and physicians were laid off "without any really good numbers to justify it. All that did was anger the patients and the employees," he added.

When the company needed to recruit more physicians, there were few financial incentives to entice them. While the group was private, physicians who wanted to join traded their assets for a percentage of the practice. Once they were under the publicly traded corporate umbrella, new physicians simply became employees. The incentive to work for a percentage of the overall profits was gone. Even the savings from capitated contracts flowed to the corporation, not the physicians. "People perceived us as a sick company. Within the company, people became passive-aggressive. They would drag their heels about everything because they were so mad at the leadership," he added.

What this physician witnessed firsthand was the dark side of publicly traded practice management whose growth strategy ran amok. He advises physician organizations to stay "small enough so you can control all the variables." When growth runs ahead of operations, the results can be disastrous. Corporate management loses touch with the front line physicians and providers, and operations turn down a slippery slope.

It's easy for physicians to feel like pawns in the merger and acquisition fever of practice management companies. As with any partnership and business relationship, there are certain expectations by both parties that are sometimes not fully understood. As a result, strained relationships develop after the deal is finalized. Physicians need to focus on key business issues to help them determine if their relationship with the practice management company is a good fit, and if the practice management company can meet their objectives.

Practice management companies must also remember that the physicians are their customers as well as their business partners. Both parties must have a thorough understanding of each others' expectations. Unfortunately for physicians, all the due diligence in the world may not matter if the practice management company sells out to another firm. That's when integration problems inevitably arise. However, it's nearly impossible for physicians to guard against that possibility. Some have contracts that contain change-of-control clauses that allow buy-outs if the company changes hands. That could be problematic for companies hoping to do IPOs. "You're not going to be able to go public with that," cautions John Allen, vice president of development for Corda, a Houston, Texas-based cardiology practice management firm. "The company has to have the ability to transfer assets as a right of ownership."

Dental Practice Management Company Failure Rate Not as High

Dental practice management firms have encountered a little less skepticism because the failures haven't been as frequent or dramatic. "The dental business is less complicated and less regulated," said Joseph Frank, president and chief executive officer of Valley Forge Dental, now part of Monarch Dental Associates. In early 1998, First New England Dental Centers filed for Chapter 11 bankruptcy. The Malden, Mass.–based company had once hoped to go public. After three years, the company operated nearly 30 dental offices in New England. The company had "acquired practices at too quick a clip, and consistently found itself short of cash," said the *Boston Business Journal*.[1] As the case wound its way through bankruptcy court, some dentists tried to buy back their practices and about 150 unpaid wage complaints were filed with the attorney general's office, the Journal reported.

QUESTIONS FOR PHYSICIANS

How do physicians and their organizations avoid such disasters? Here's a PricewaterhouseCoopers checklist for physicians or dentists who are weighing the pros and cons of being acquired by a practice management company to ponder.

---

[1] Salemi, T. (1998). Creditors go after Lakian's dental firm. *Boston Business Journal,* May 4.

Management Structure

- Is the company the right size for the physician or the physician group?
- Does the company offer the services that will meet the physicians' needs—comprehensive in-office ancillary services, clinical research opportunities, and medical facility development?
- Does the company offer access to referral networks within the specialties the physician or physician group needs?
- What types of management resources are available to support the physician? What is the company's track record for providing management services to its physicians?
- What type of human resource support does the company have for employees?
- What is the financial accounting expertise of the company? What methodology of financial reporting is in place, since physician practices have traditionally operated using the cash basis of accounting?
- Does the company retain competent legal counsel with respect to antitrust issues?

Information Systems Technology

- Does the company offer state-of-the-art information systems that can provide good data for entering into risk contracts?
- What is the company's information system conversion plan for integrating new practices into its network? Are experienced individuals responsible for the conversion, and is there a set time frame for the physician practice to be online?
- Is training and education on the new systems provided to physicians and their staffs? Is there a designated information systems specialist who will be supporting the practice's information technology needs?
- What is the company's plan for system upgrades? How will the practice's operations be affected when upgrades are installed or changes made to the system applications?
- What management reporting is in place to provide practice data to the physicians, and is this data transmitted electronically or manually? What educational process is in place to train physicians on analyzing the data and using it as a tool for monitoring the financial and operational performance of the practice?

Financial Performance

- What billing procedures are in place for the entire revenue cycle—registration, insurance verification, charge capture, coding procedures, claims processing, accounts receivable management, collections?

- What is the company's history on aging accounts receivables by payors within the physician's market area? The days in receivable is a good evaluation tool to assess collection efforts.
- What services are included in the management fee? Are these services performed by qualified individuals who are experienced in human resource management, billing and collections, physician credentialing, and managed care contracting?
- How does the company manage overhead? Is there a set overhead percentage based on the physician specialty? What degree of control does the physician have in managing this overhead or making decisions to affect overhead and practice cost structure?
- How does the company communicate with physicians on financial issues and practice standards for improving financial performance? How often does this communication take place, and how accessible are the company's executives when these issues come up?
- How is physician productivity monitored? What benchmarking data is used? How does this data affect an individual physician's compensation?
- What compensation model does the organization use, and who makes compensation decisions?
- Is the company planning on staying private or does it plan to go public?

Operating Performance

- What is the company's process for physician credentialing to managed care organizations? Does the company have existing provider contracts in the practice's geographic area? What has been their timing for adding physicians to the network?
- Does the company use guidelines for staffing ratios by job position within the individual physician practice? Who is responsible for determining the practice's staffing needs? How much can the physician participate in determining staffing needs?
- What salary structure and benefits are in place for nonphysician personnel?
- Does the company have job descriptions by staff position?
- Does the company have a compliance program in place? What is the company's policy with respect to monitoring physician coding procedures and billing claims? Are there experienced coding specialists who provide training, education, and quality control assistance to physicians or staff?
- What is the company's philosophy on growth through acquisitions?

Marketing

- Does the company understand the healthcare climate in the practice's local market, and can it help the physicians adapt to that environment?
- What are the firm's marketing plans for growing the practice? Is it an overall corporate marketing plan or is it specific to each practice?
- What is the company's reputation nationally and locally? How have they served other physicians in their network?
- What relationships does the company have with managed care organizations within the area? Does the company have the ability to expand those?
- What referral patterns have been put in place by the company? Does the physician group or physician have the ability to refer outside the network?

INVESTOR SKEPTICISM

"I've significantly tempered my own expectations for the PPM industry," said Larry Marsh, director of PPM equity research for Salomon Smith Barney, in mid-1998. "I once said 20% to 25% (of physicians) would be in some sort of affiliation in five years compared with 8% at the time. However, now I believe the growth will be slower, more like 12% to 15% will be affiliated."

He also believes the practice management organizations forming now will have a tougher time than the early pioneers. "The SEC is making it more challenging to become a public company," he said, noting new accounting restrictions on writing off intangible assets, which make up the bulk of most physician organizations' assets. "Plus, investors are more educated now. They're more apt to look at things like track record and infrastructure," Marsh added.

Not surprisingly, analysts who had cast a jaundiced eye toward the industry are getting more attention. "To demonstrate our grasp of the obvious, we would like to point out that the PPM sector has been a difficult place for investors to make money," stated a May 1998 report by Raymond James & Associates. The St. Petersburg, Fla.–based firm recommended only five of the 40-plus practice management company stocks that are publicly traded. All are single-specialty practice management organizations in the high-revenue areas of oncology and orthopedics.

One reason investors have struggled with understanding the practice management niche is because of the apples-to-oranges comparisons among practice management companies with different management fee models and amortization schedules. Raymond James' healthcare analyst John Ransom stated that traditional Wall Street measurements have severe shortfalls with practice management companies. For example, price/earnings ratios are irrelevant because earnings per share "is subject to so much manipulation and distortion," he said. Another traditional measurement—return on assets—also is changeable depending on the inclusion of goodwill.

Ransom instead uses return on total capital and after-tax cash flow return on total equity as measuring sticks. Return on total capital is fully-taxed earnings before interest, taxes, depreciation and amortization (EBITDA) divided by debt and equity plus charge-offs. After-tax cash flow return on total equity is net income plus depreciation and amortization divided by book equity and charge-offs. Both of these measures take into account the charge-offs that have proliferated among practice management companies recently, and which can artificially inflate return on equity. He also believes that this ratio shows how well the practice management company is investing its cash. His final measuring stick is cost of equity spread, which shows whether after-tax cash flow returns on equity are covering the cost of equity.

Yet, not all of Wall Street has been willing to invest the time necessary to analyze the financial structure of an industry in turmoil. That prompted one practice management firm, MedCath, to take itself out of the public eye in 1998. The 10-year-old cardiac services provider, which raised $32 million in a 1994 public offering, agreed to taken private by two investment powerhouses—Kohlberg Kravis Roberts & Co. and Welsh Carson Anderson & Stowe—for $240 million in 1998.

During its tenure as a public company, MedCath saw its stock reach a high of $43 per share and a low of $7 per share. Company executives got frustrated dealing with Wall Street's short-term outlook and the impact that was having on the company's stock prices. "Health care analysts don't know how to analyze cash flows, only EPS (earnings per share)," said Steve Puckett, president and CEO of MedCath. "I was growing cash flow by more than 80%," he said. However, EPS dipped when MedCath invested in four new heart hospitals at $50 million a pop. "I couldn't tell the market what our EPS was going to be because I didn't know," MedCath's Puckett said.

What's the lesson for practice management organizations in this? Puckett gave this advice: "You have to remain private until you're big enough." What's big enough? For MedCath, Puckett believes the company must hit a $1 billion revenue run rate before he'll consider going back to the public markets. At that point, the large capital expenditures required for building new hospitals won't have such a dramatic effect on the company's earnings per share.

Despite the sector's turmoil, Puckett believes strongly in MedCath's model of combining cardiac specialists with heart hospitals. He predicts that at least 25% of this heart specialty will turn to a practice management organization and that other specialties will turn to this model as well.

A smaller cardiology practice management company, Corda, is also looking toward heart hospitals and realizes that the market dictates building a sustainable model. "At the end of the day, we have to be able to deliver same-store growth," Corda's John Allen said. Once Corda builds critical mass in a practice, it can add profitable ancillary services such as cath labs and nuclear cameras, he said.

Corda manages 35 physicians in northern Virginia, New Orleans, Phoenix, Tucson, and Las Vegas. Corda focuses on expansion through growing its presence in targeted local markets, rather than expanding to new markets "Rather than 300 physicians in 30 markets, we'd rather affiliate with 500 physicians in 10 markets," Allen said.

Despite the fact that some investors are turning away from practice management companies, Physician Health's Garvin still senses "a lot of interest out there for consolidation." Her company, which is estimated to generate $100 million in 1998 revenues, now partners with more than 170 physicians. It also manages networks of 4,000 physicians in its key markets, including Orlando, Fla.; Cincinnati; Dallas/Fort Worth; Atlanta; and St. Louis.

Garvin's philosophy reflects that of many in the practice management business today—a practice management organization must be ancillary driven. "We don't buy practices that don't have significant ancillaries. You can't make money simply owning physician practices," she said.

For example, Physician Health owns and manages a bone marrow transplant center, outpatient surgery centers, oncology and cardiovascular centers, a sleep lab, and is in the process of developing other ancillaries including birthing centers.

Ancillaries also are a key focus for Aesthetic Medical Management, a Connecticut-based practice management organization that focuses on plastic surgery, a specialty in which physicians have traditionally practiced in groups of one or two. Aesthetic helps change the mix of a physician's patients from reconstructive surgery to plastic surgery in professional centers as they brand and market more elective healthcare treatments. The company looks for younger physicians who need capital to expand. Since its start in Florida, Aesthetic has expanded into Texas, Illinois, California, New York, and New Jersey.

AMMI brings capital to the practices by building aesthetic surgery centers, which cost between $1 million and $1.5 million and offer a wide range of services. The model center has two surgery suites and includes two to four board-certified plastic surgeons, one or two cosmetic dermatologists, and subspecialists such as ocular and facial plastic surgeons. The centers also provide a full range of profitable ancillary services, including collagen implants, laser hair removal, chemical peels and other noninvasive treatments. In addition, the company is developing its own line of skin care products. A fully mature center will generate about $10 million per year in revenues, of which 20% will stem from ancillaries.

With all that AMMI is doing to put more money in its physicians' pockets, English believes they'll stick around long after their five-year employment agreements have run out. It's up to a practice management organization to deliver value and help physicians make more money, he said. The ability to keep physicians past the five-year contract period is a true test for practice management companies as the industry matures. If investors and regulators see physicians bailing out of these companies as soon as their employment agreements expire, they'll ask pointed questions about the life of the assets the practice management company is acquiring.

AN EXPERT'S PERSPECTIVE: WAYNE POSEY, PRESIDENT AND CEO OF PROMEDCO, FORT WORTH, TEXAS

Amid the skepticism and gloom surrounding publicly traded physician practice management companies in mid-1998, one company actually succeeded in raising $72 million in a secondary offering.

ProMedCo is an anomaly among publicly held multispecialty companies. Wayne Posey, its founder and chief executive officer, is a former Hospital Affiliates executive, and, as most healthcare veterans know, his colleagues have led many healthcare companies during the past decade.

Posey went into consulting after Affiliates Hospital was bought by Hospital Corp. of America, and by the early 1990s was almost completely absorbed in consulting assignments with physician groups. Posey saw a need for a national physician management company back in 1992. After extracting himself from the busy life of consulting, Posey talked to two other former Affiliates executives, Dick Ragsdale and Thomas Chaney, about the idea in mid-1994. The idea became a company, ProMedCo, in December 1994.

Two years after its 1997 IPO, ProMedCo has grown to an annual revenue run rate of $275 million in 1998. It manages the practices of 440 physicians and 100 physician extenders and has 540 physicians affiliated through IPAs.

Because of his experience in growing a hospital company, Posey knows the delicate balance required between promoting growth and developing infrastructure. "You don't want to have too much infrastructure before you have the revenues, but you don't want to have the revenues without the infrastructure," he said. "This is not a science. It's instinct." Yet, it's an instinct that many practice management companies have lacked.

Just a year earlier, the newly public ProMedCo was an underdog competing with giants like MedPartners and PhyCor for acquisitions. By early 1998, ProMedCo was considered a leading practice management organization. "Our pipeline is the largest its ever been," Posey said. Even so, "most people—even some sophisticated investors—lump all practice management companies together," Posey said.

As the company was forming, Posey became a student of practice management companies. A cabinet in his office contains several volumes of documents that contain the details of PhyCor's first 17 physician deals. "I read every word of them," Posey said. "PhyCor's economic model was the best one out there. It aligned the physicians' interests to the bottom line rather than the top line." In adapting the PhyCor model to ProMedCo, however, Posey added a twist: a second fee structure for managed care revenues. Surpluses from managed care contracts are split with the physicians; ProMedCo takes between 25% and 50%. This benefits ProMedCo in that it doesn't have to go back and restructure its physician agreements when managed care contracts come up.

CAPITALIZATION

In some respects, Posey took a contrarian approach to building a multispecialty company. During a time when dozens of start-up practice management companies were being showered with millions of dollars, ProMedCo turned its back on venture capital money. "We started out with our own money, and we got to the IPO stage spending less than $5 million," Posey said.

"We talked to lots of venture capitalists and told them we only needed $5 million. They told us, 'We think you need $25 to $30 million and we'll take 65% of your company for that,'" Posey recalled. Posey and his partners just said no.

Although venture capital firms may have viewed ProMedCo's capital requirements as unrealistically low, Posey believes some of the early practice management firms were overcapitalized, leading them to seek growth for growth's sake. One reason ProMedCo needed so little cash was that its pre-IPO physician groups took 85% of their purchase consideration in stock, rather than cash. "We didn't tell them they had to take stock," Posey explained. "They wanted to."

In December 1995, Posey and his partners decided to say "yes" to Bessemer Venture Partners. ProMedCo accepted a $3 million stake from Bessemer, because the venture firm's strong reputation would carry weight with physicians and the investment banking community. However, the investment was a passive one. In an unusual move, Bessemer didn't even take a seat on ProMedCo's board.

Market Focus

ProMedCo is the only practice management organization company that has exclusively targeted secondary markets in areas of low managed care penetration, typically those with less than 500,000 residents. Its markets include Pittsfield, Mass.; Corpus Christi, Texas; Reno, Nev.; and Naples, Fla.

Specifically, Posey and his staff look for markets where they can purchase a large medical group that has strong market share and negotiating strength with the two or three hospitals in town. The company prefers markets that have more than one hospital. Because these markets have little managed care, ProMedCo can work with physicians before they've developed significant relationships with managed care payors. Since its contracts with the physician groups already address how those revenues will be split, the company isn't scrambling to figure out the percentages later.

For example, Promedco's second deal was with Abilene (Texas) Diagnostic Clinic. The group had 23 physicians when ProMedCo acquired it in December 1995. It has since grown to 39. The next largest physician group in Abilene had five pediatricians—a substantial drop off from Promedco's aggregation. "When we affiliate with a group, we usually are or quickly become the dominant group in the market. That creates momentum for us and causes other physicians to start coming to us. That momentum makes it easier for us to grow these groups than if we were targeting urban markets," Posey said.

Although practice management companies usually manage groups in urban, suburban and secondary markets, Posey believes that targeting the secondary niche exclusively will benefit the company and give it plenty of room for expansion. His research shows there are more than 1,200 secondary markets, which contain about half of the country's total population and generate more than $50 billion in physician revenues.

"We focus first on the market, then on the physician group," said Posey, who added that his company has turned down many deals in markets where it didn't want to be.

Interestingly, two successful hospital companies have similarly targeted secondary markets: Universal Health Services and Quorum Health Group. In a somewhat different aspect, Health Management Associates, another publicly held hospital chain, has been successful in targeting rural and suburban markets where managed care penetration is low.

Raising the Bar

While PPMs generally are being forced to go to a 25-year amortization period, ProMedCo completed its IPO and secondary using a 30-year schedule. The SEC "accepted the fact that our exclusive focus is on these secondary markets and that competition is less out there. This justifies a longer life for intangible assets." In May 1998, ProMedCo completed a secondary offering, and was able to keep the 30-year amortization. The SEC "posed no challenges about it," Posey said.

Posey agrees that the bar has been raised for practice management companies going public. For example, when ProMedCo went public in March 1997, it had a revenue run rate of $70 million. In contrast, in 1994 FPA Medical Management went public with $14 million in annual revenues.

He believes it would be nearly impossible for a practice management firm with similarly small revenues to go public in today's environment. Investors want to see more scale and operating history before they invest.

Another change: "Physicians are asking different, and more pointed questions," Posey said. The most frequent question: "Are you going to stay disciplined?" So many practice management companies have changed course, which sometimes resulted in chaos. Posey said physicians want to know if ProMedCo is going to stick with its strategy of secondary markets and primary-care focus. About 60% of ProMedCo's physicians are in primary care. Although some practice management companies started with similar ratios, they eventually became top-heavy with specialists. "Every single deal we have done is precisely on strategy from when we started the company," he said.

Physicians who are considering joining ProMedCo typically do a lot of homework, which benefits both parties. "It's rare that a physician group that is affiliating with us doesn't talk to every single physician group we've got," Posey said.

For every group that ProMedCo has managed for more than a year, it has been able to grow the practice such that it more than pays for the management fee within a year. "We don't promise that, nor do we expect that will occur with every group," Posey added. "However, we do tell physicians that within about two years, we'll be able to achieve that." Therefore, what is delivered exceeds expectations rather than falls short of them.

Although ProMedCo initially based its fee model on the PhyCor model, it didn't follow PhyCor's lead in 1998 when PhyCor changed its model to reduce the amount paid to physicians up front in exchange for a lower management fee. From the beginning, the company has been flexible in offering a lower management fee with a lower consideration if the physicians are interested in that. However, "physicians are still more driven by the level of consideration than a lower management fee," he said. The range of ProMedCo's fees is 15% to 20%.

PricewaterhouseCoopers Tips for Conforming to Higher Standards

- Ensure that the practice management company's resources are more concentrated on building and operating practices more than on acquiring new ones.
- Make sure physicians due their homework, asking the right questions in the due diligence period so expectations won't go awry.
- Recalibrate growth and integration goals. It always takes longer to integrate practices than you think.
- Look at longer time frames for raising capital.

14

CHAPTER

Turnarounds, Unforced Errors, and Lessons Learned

Sandy Lutz

The theory seemed so simple. Bring economies of scale to a $250 billion fragmented industry. Shift power to physicians, who are increasingly at the mercy of larger health plans and health systems. Capitalize them, manage them, and help them concentrate on practicing medicine by relieving them of administrative tasks.

Yet, there's never a simple answer in healthcare. The intertwined relationships and constituencies necessitate complex solutions. The industry still desires competent practice management, but has suffered from a debilitating series of unforced errors.

No magic bullet exists to cure troubled practice management companies. However, a pattern of what happens to them has already begun to emerge.

TURNAROUND STRATEGIES

When the wheels came off their racing cars, practice management companies attempted a host of quick fixes and long-term strategies to ease their woes. Among them are the following.

Quick Fixes

- *Close down underperforming clinics.* Managers decide on a satisfactory level of revenue, profits, and patient volume for each clinic. Then, they

close down those that don't measure up. This strategy can backfire if
the management company has capitation contracts to deliver care to
enrollees who will be disappointed when they find that their doctor isn't
in business anymore.

- Sell practices back to the physicians. If physicians are unhappy, this
  may be a fine solution for all. However, the question is: Sell them
  back at what price? After all, the practices aren't doing as well
  as when they were purchased. (We addressed this situation in
  Chapter 9.) If the company is publicly traded and is selling back
  practices that were paid for in stock, the company would buy back the
  stock, decreasing the number of shares outstanding and hopefully
  increasing earnings per share. That's the upside. The downside is that
  the company will have to take on more debt to buy back those shares
  if it doesn't have the cash reserves to pay for them. What about the
  consideration paid to the doctors? Forcing physicians to pay back that
  consideration may be a problematic and litigious process. If the
  practices were not performing as expected, whose fault was it? The
  physicians may claim it was the management company; the
  management company may claim the opposite. What is a fair value
  for both sides to get out?

- Ax management. Management turnover has been rife in practice
  management companies and physician groups in general. At some
  venture capital (VC) portfolio companies, VC executives have taken
  over and attempted to raise additional capital from either existing
  shareholders or affiliated physicians and dentists. Interim venture
  management is usually a stop-gap measure to ensure the firm's
  investment is secure before putting a new management team in place.

- Bring in new investors. When a practice management company runs out
  of money, it immediately looks for more. One solution is to add more
  investors. That comes at a price, however. New investors dilute the
  ownership stakes of the current investors—often physicians—who then
  feel more detached from the company's operations.

Long-Term Changes

- Restructure management fees. More often than not, this means
  lowering fees in exchange for a lower level of services. Although this
  may seem like a minor change, it can change the profitability and
  desirability of the company going forward. It also means that the
  company must renegotiate all management services agreements, an
  expensive and time-consuming task.

- Adopt new business venues. With shrinking margins in practice management, some companies have looked at ways to diversify. For example, one physician practice management company selected the red-hot niche of Internet commerce. In late 1998, Specialty Care Network, a physician practice management company, launched HealthCareReportCards.com, an Internet site that functions as a hospital rating service.[1] The company is positioning itself as a healthcare information company.

- Focus on just one aspect of the physicians' business. In 1998, PhyMatrix announced it was going to divest most of its physician practices to concentrate on its site management organization (SMO), which oversees research offices that perform clinical trials for new drugs. West Palm Beach, Fla.–based PhyMatrix ventured into the SMO business in 1997 when it purchased Clinical Studies, a Rhode Island–based company that manages sites directing drug studies.[2] Drug companies are farming out more and more business to site management organizations as a way to speed up development of new medicines. PhyMatrix's clinical research company had 34 research-only sites, including an inpatient center in Fort Lauderdale, and reported $25 million in revenues in 1997. The company conducted 129 trials in 1997.[3]

- Buy back stock. Practice management companies can repurchase the shares on the open market or in private transactions with large holders of the shares. Obviously, this is a financial fix that applies only to the publicly traded practice management firms. It is almost always a popular strategy with Wall Street. Typically, practice management companies buy back their shares when the price falls too low. What's too low? That's a difficult question; it hinges on market conditions, future growth prospects, book value of the shares, and numerous other factors.

  Wall Street likes stock buybacks because that means fewer shares will be outstanding. Fewer shares translates into a higher earnings per share because the company is spreading its earnings over smaller holdings. So, if a practice management company reported earnings of 10 cents per share in the first quarter of 1998 and 12 cents in the first quarter of 1999, that would amount to a 20% earnings growth rate.

---

[1] "HealthCareReportCards.com Receives Incredible 1.6 Million-Plus Hits in First Week on the Internet!" Nov. 2, *PRNewswire*.

[2] Chandler, M. (1998). West Palm Beach, Fla., Physician Management Firm May Sell Practices. *Miami Herald*, Aug. 8.

[3] Ibid.

Depending on how many shares were repurchased, part or all of that growth rate may be attributable to the fact that fewer shares were outstanding in 1999.

Practice management companies considering stock buybacks must take a long-term view of the stock market and have a thorough understanding of their own company's life cycle. If they believe they have a strategy that works, and their shares are being oversold because of other companies' problems or a misstep, it's smart to follow the dictum of buy low, sell high. For example, in 1996, American Oncology Resources announced a stock buyback of 3 million shares. They saw an opportunity to buy back the stock for under $10 a share and issue it later at a much higher value. The stock did rebound, making investors happy.

- Sell physician groups. In numerous areas, physicians have left the equity-model practice management company and run straight into the embrace of local hospitals. Although much has been written about the losses incurred by hospitals buying physician practices, those losses were mitigated by additional revenues generated by the hospital. When a multispecialty group is purchased by a hospital, the hospital gains the loyalty of those physicians to admit patients to its inpatient and outpatient services. Those revenues may or may not be carefully calculated and analyzed. In fact, the hospital may not calculate them at all for fear of being accused of buying admissions, a violation of Medicare's anti-kickback regulations.

Still, some say that hospitals cannot sustain losses in their physician practices indefinitely. For some not-for-profit organizations, the financial drain is affecting their bond ratings, and many hospital systems are divesting practices. "I think (local hospitals) are going to be offloading them. Give it about another five years. You'll see more and more physician practices spun out of hospital orbits," said Greg Harbaugh, chairman of Houston Harbaugh, a Pittsburgh law firm, and an expert in healthcare law.[4] Harbaugh was referring to the expensive strategy formerly used by Pittsburgh hospitals, of buying physician practices.

Although some hospitals are selling their practices, others continue to buy in select instances. In late 1997, a not-for-profit foundation was created by Santa Rosa Memorial Hospital in northern California to buy the largest group of primary care physicians in the area.

---

[4] (1998). A defensive blunder: Hospitals, Highmark face hefty losses from their medical practice purchases," *Pittsburgh Business Journal,* April 20.

"Now a patient's records will be immediately available anywhere—in x-ray, surgery, intensive care or the doctor's office," said Robert Fish, CEO of Memorial. "Nobody has to go looking. It's those kinds of efficiencies that will improve care."[5] The purchase of the 38-physician group by the hospital's foundation is expected to help the hospital with managed care contracts by allowing them to offer an integrated network.

THE CONSEQUENCES OF FAILURE

When a practice management company begins to spiral down, developments can quickly turn from bad to worse. Bad things beget bad things. At some point, it may be too hard to turn the ship around because problems will accelerate. Those problems include the following.

- Mounting legal expenses. Lawsuits from physicians, shareholders, and payors complicate the day-to-day operations of practice management firms.
- Fights over assets. When things fall apart, physicians often discover that their practice management companies' finances are far from simple. They may have complex debt and equity entanglements—in the tens of millions of dollars—with banks, investors, and individual doctors.
- Cash flow problems. This is a vicious cycle that can take on a life of its own. When physicians get disgruntled, they may stop paying their management fees. With less cash coming in, the management company can't fund expansion for the physicians or do some of the services it promised. This makes the physicians more disgruntled, who in turn withhold more cash. At some point, the practice management company may have little redress except to sue the practices themselves.
- Loss of health plan contracts. If health plans believe that a physician group is financially shaky and may not be able to live up to its contract, they may drop those groups sooner rather than later.
- Physician unionization. Physician empowerment, an underlying theme in practice management formation, is fueling another trend as well— unionization. At a recent practice management conference in Nashville, representatives from four physician unions all agreed on one thing: Their membership is increasing, and the calls from interested physicians keep coming in.

---

[5] "Memorial, Doctors Group Join Nonprofit; Deal Affects 38 Physicians," Santa Rosa (Calif.) Press Democrat Santa Rosa, Nov. 27, 1997.

As more physicians become employees of practice management organizations or health systems, the specter of unionization grows stronger. Many physicians say they feel powerless against large managed care organizations that dictate the terms and reimbursement levels to them. In addition, about 43% of physicians are now employees of a corporation, institution, or government agency, according to the American Medical Association.[6]

- Uphill struggles. No longer the darlings of Wall Street, publicly traded practice management companies have become, in some respects, the black eye of the healthcare industry. Although other physicians organizations have struggled as well, the spectacular failures of some practice management organizations have alienated many physicians. Consider the bankruptcy of FPA Medical Management, which at its height employed 7,900 physicians. After emerging from bankruptcy, FPA estimated that number would drop to just 349. Meanwhile, 13,000 of FPA's creditors were physicians.[7] Such highly publicized failures will scare away physicians, investors, and management talent away for years to come.

LEARNING FROM OTHERS

Mark Wagar, chairman, president, and CEO of American Physician Partners, says the secret to turning around troubled physician companies is "measuring the pace at which you can create change. There's no question you can improve both the financial operational performance and the service operation performance of medical organizations and physician groups."

In January 1995, Wagar was tapped to be chief operating officer of Mullikin Medical Group in southern California. He basically was hired with one goal in mind: Turn the struggling group around and get it into financial shape for an initial public offering. Wall Street was lapping at the heels of Mullikin and several other premier physician groups that seemed to be on the cutting edge of this emerging sector. Mullikin had many of the desirable elements in place: a recognized name, a long track record, and medical management programs that enabled it to take global capitation as a true integrated delivery system. Because the group also owned a hospital, physicians could financially benefit from its ability to cut inpatient days.

Mullikin lacked one prime attribute, however: profits. The group was losing money.

---

[6] "Physicians, Unions and Anti-trust," presentation to American Health Lawyers Association by Ed Hirshfeld, vice president, Health Law, American Medical Association, June 28, 1998.

[7] Cook, B. (1998). Go Figure: Behind the numbers of FPA's bankruptcy filing. *Modern Physicians*, November.

After 45 days on the job, Wagar walked into founder Walter Mullikin's office and told him and Mullikin president John McDonald the practice was worth $400 to $500 million—possibly even $600 to $800 million—but changes needed to be made. "You need to be *here*," he told them, indicating a specific level of pretax profit. Mullikin gave him the green light.

"I sat down with the information and said here's where we're at and here's where we need to be. What are the important things we need out of these changes, not just performance changes. How can we make sure the key service and medical management goals continued to improve," Wagar said.

Wagar said the key to getting financial improvements he needed was showing the physicians that they were also making patient care improvements. For example, to expand access and attract additional enrollees, clinic hours were expanded. The group also set patient service benchmarks.

With a two-pronged approach to operational change—improving both financial and patient service benchmarks—the physicians didn't feel as though "we were just doing this for the money."

Wagar stressed that this was the key to Mullikin's turnaround. When physicians believe they are only making improvements to increase profits for the company, the motivation won't be nearly as high as when they believe that the changes are also increasing the quality of care they can provide to their patients. "We're going to go after dollars, but we're going to be balanced about how we use the dollars we've found," Wagar said.

"[Physicians] can deliver extra financial change if they believe human values are in place. But, you can't be Pollyanna and just pursue the service improvements," Wagar cautioned.

Although the desire to take Mullikin public underlined Wagar's work, he stressed to the physicians that even if they were to stay private, they needed to have a profitable company to go to the bank and borrow money to fund future growth.

Physicians understood and helped lead the change, Wagar said. Part of the change involved cutting some physicians and employees that had been absorbed by numerous mergers. "They had not addressed crunching the infrastructure," he said.

However, Wagar didn't want to touch the medical management model that had made the group so successful. In terms of hospital days per thousand, Mullikin was held up as a model for other integrated delivery systems to emulate.

By the fall of 1995—only nine months after Wagar was hired—Mullikin was showing pretax profits of about 5%.

THINGS TO DO

We know that physician practice management is a necessary and growing business. The failures and struggles of other practice management companies can provide valuable lessons for their colleagues. Out of those failures have emerged some guidelines for what companies need to do in order to succeed.

- Have a strategic plan. Having a strategic plan that is followed by management divides the successful from the unsuccessful practice management organizations. The plan helps the physician organization set goals and establish accountability. Private physician groups will want to set goals for growth and hold back a portion of profits to build a retained earnings base.

  Some clinics schedule one-day strategic planning retreats each year. Those meetings give administrators and physician leaders a chance to make presentations on issues facing the group. At the retreat, physicians can vote on changes that may include recruiting goals, retained earnings percentages, major capital expenditures, and income distribution plans. Subsequently, the clinics schedule monthly update meetings to apprise physicians on how the group is progressing towards its goals.

  Break down the organization into manageable units. "People assume the largest physician offices are the most efficient," said American Physician Partners' Wagar. "What we found (at Mullikin) was the opposite. Some of the largest offices were the least efficient."

  He noted that physician leadership needs to be personal and hands-on. Once an office grows beyond what a physician leader can get his or her arms around, it will become less and less efficient.

  For Wagar, analyzing the efficiencies in physician offices was the fun part of his job at Mullikin. He related reporting on wide variations in staffing to physicians, who invariably brought up ways to justify higher overhead. Then, he would drill deeper into the data to show them surprising conclusions. "We would find smaller offices managing more patients, and the other physicians would say, but what about the quality? So, we'd look at patient satisfaction surveys and find they were higher in some of these small offices where they'd have less support staff."

  Wagar believes the ideal size is between 20 and 25, or less. Go larger than that and efficiencies tend to melt away.

  Another example was offered by A.J. Rosmarin, who was acting CEO of a 15-physician OB/GYN group in Dallas. He said that his group, which operates at three locations, once handled scheduling for all 15 physicians at a centralized location. The scheduling became a source of constant complaints. For example, if a physician had to run out to deliver a baby, the central scheduling office might not be aware of it. "Patients got tired of coming in and finding out the doctor wasn't there," Rosmarin said. So, he decentralized the system and moved the schedulers into each of the three physician office locations.

One interesting data point about small groups. The National CPA Healthcare Advisors Association found that, although small group practices were able to reduce the size of their staffs through the use of practice management software, larger groups were not. The organization reported that its survey found no group of more than 50 physicians that was able to reduce staff size through the use of practice management software. Perhaps these groups began adding other staff, which offset any savings from information technology–induced efficiencies.

- Look outside the industry for talent. Practice management companies have a recruiting challenge. Because of the industry's pocked record of accomplishments, they'll have a difficult time attracting top healthcare executives to their organizations. Good. The industry needs new blood and the insights of leaders who are technologically savvy and aren't of the mind-set that "This is the way we've always done it." Too often, physician executives have not been the best managers, just the ones who volunteered or were assigned the difficult task of managing physicians.

  Unfortunately, young managers in the 1990s have favored the more exciting industries of information systems, telecommunications, and entertainment. The healthcare services industry is viewed as one populated by stodgy, gray-haired executives. This has to change.

- Make physicians feel like owners, not employees. This will require developing leadership, establishing an incentive-based pay system, and creating a governance system that ensures clinical excellence. For reasons that have never been clear, some physician management companies have tried to shield physicians from the financial operations of the business. This almost always backfires. Many management companies and health systems that own practices have been guilty of not communicating the organization's financial status to their physicians. Of course, publicly held companies must disclose financials every quarter. They need to go one step further, however, and include physicians in the development of their financial models. Those models and the expectations they create will determine the company's eventual success.

  Physician leaders must always have a seat at the table for all discussions.

- Pick your battles carefully, especially if the adversary is a strong local hospital system. Healthcare is an ecosystem in which each entity has its own natural enemies. Despite trends toward integration, physician groups have tended to view hospitals and health plans as their natural enemies. These adversarial relationships play out in each local market amid battles over market share and negotiating strength. More than one medical group has won the battle but lost the war with a local hospital system. It takes a very large medical group to match the financial resources of even an average-sized hospital system.

Sometimes, instead of fighting, partnering with a recognized market leader is a better way to go rather than battling. For example, MedCath has agreements with two hospital systems—Franciscan Health System of Ohio Valley in Dayton, and St. Joseph Healthcare System in Albuquerque—to build heart hospitals.

- Structure executive compensation to ensure long-term operational success. Some practice management companies have been roundly criticized for their multi-million-dollar payouts to former executives. Unfortunately, corporate incentive plans are often structured to reward executives for mergers by allowing them to vest enormous quantities of stock options when a company is sold. When the personal inducements to sell out are so appealing, executives will spend their time working toward that end rather than building a company that will endure into the next several decades.

   In addition, some compensation programs award bonuses to CEOs for completing mergers or for earnings-per-share growth. Again, this tends to focus executives on quick earnings hits, rather than long-term value creation. Incentives that are built around value creation, however, can sway executives to maximize existing operations rather than deploy capital on acquisitions. The investment made in infrastructure may not come to fruition for two to three years. You can't blame executives for steering their companies in a way that maximizes their own compensation.

- Take time to breathe. Remember the "Breathing Lessons" analogy in Chapter 2? Don't forget to breathe, digest, and assess. Trees won't grow to the sky. Eventually, the branches must flower and roots take hold. The same is true with a business, especially a complex one such as healthcare.

- Be prepared to differentiate your business. Look into the future and you'll see a time when payors will have the data to judge physician groups based on quality and cost. Only a handful of physicians have brand equity. The rest are viewed as commodities and will see their fees driven lower and lower if they lack the market clout to force payors to pay more. For the foreseeable future, physician groups will lack the clout possessed by large payor and hospital systems. That means they'll be on the short end of the negotiating stick unless they get their costs down or demonstrate why their services are worth higher fees than those of other groups.

- Be frugal in paying for acquisitions. In 1998, PhyCor changed its acquisition strategy. It decided to start paying physicians less on the front end in acquisition price, and take out less on the back end in a management fee. At an October 1998 conference, PhyCor's CEO, Joseph Hutts, summed up the company's experience this way: "We paid a fair amount of proceeds to physicians and they appreciated that." He paused before continuing, "Over the weekend." That drew a chuckle from the crowd.

   For years, PhyCor was the poster child of the practice management industry. Hutts had often opined that PhyCor made the business look too easy, prompting dozens to follow down the multispecialty road to fame and profits. When the breath got knocked out of the company in 1998 with write-offs and restructurings, investors interpreted it as a signal of defeat in the strategy that PhyCor had so carefully molded and so many others had meticulously followed.

   PhyCor's new model, however, may be the wave of the future, prompting other practice management firms to follow its lead.

- Don't let Wall Street steer management's attention from running the business. In public practice management companies, CEOs and CFOs are often on a whirlwind of trips to market the stock. Such activity requires management's day-to-day attention and can cripple an organization that's new. Unfortunately, CEOs who are good communicators and good managers are also the ones who are best at marketing the stock. However, that chore should be delegated to investor relations. In addition, the company's stock price should not be used as an indicator of whether the company is successful. Many mismanaged companies had great price/earnings (P/E) multiples because no one outside the company realized the problems. Thinking that the company was golden, management expanded more and more without fixing problems inherent in its structure.

- Healthcare is local. The more scattered the dots, the higher the risk in operating an efficient company.

- Study successful mergers. Few healthcare organizations have experience in successfully integrating multiple mergers. Several practice management executives mentioned acquisitions that turned into train wrecks, burning up time and money when the company was running low on both. In the go-go growth stages of these companies, there seemed to be a feeling of merger machismo: "We will make this work. Once these guys are on board, they'll see this wisdom of our ways." There used to be a Saturday morning cartoon called "The Get-along Gang." With a feeling of omnipotence, these mergers took on that optimistic sentiment, that the physicians would become part of the "Get-along Gang" and fall in step.

Unfortunately, some acquirees never had any intention of "getting along," and fought management every step of the way. One executive mentioned a particularly high-priced acquisition that seemed almost doomed from the start. The practice management firm was buying a large, complex physician organization and had to depend on that group's leaders to go forward. However, the acquiree felt like the deal was more of a hostile takeover and was slow to cooperate. The feeling that these executives would "come around" to the acquirer's requests—eventually demands—dragged on for nearly a year.

There comes a time in the life of many medical organizations when they're presented with what looks like the opportunity of a lifetime. They're given the chance to buy an organization two or three times larger than themselves, an acquisition that can transform the organization into a momentum machine. Those opportunities must be weighed carefully because they may be the biggest mistake an organization ever makes.

When Physician Group A buys a much larger Physician Group B, leadership issues can become all-consuming. If the leadership team going forward is not immediately decided, questions will linger, confusion will abound, and resentment will seep into the management ranks. Physician Group A will have to have the cooperation of Physician Group B in order to understand what's going on in that larger organization. That's especially true if Group B has several moving parts, such as laboratories, outpatient centers, third-party billing administrators, or any other divisions that are common to healthcare organizations.

No matter how well planned Group A's management believes the acquisition is, Group B's management may view it as a takeover by a less-experienced management team. And, they may be right. One management company executive described such an acquisition as "trench warfare, an organizational fist fight."

In fact, Group B's management may grow stronger in their united confrontation against Group A.

You can sum up the problems of many practice management companies in the experience of one former practice management executive: "Too many acquisitions with too many assumed changes."

When acquisitions go too fast, there's a tendency to mistake assumptions for facts. "Things may start to go wrong, but won't show up immediately. They'll show up six months or a year later." So, the planned growth of one clinic may have not taken place yet, but it's already figured into the assumptions about the company when planning the next acquisition. Because healthcare reimbursement lags services by weeks or months, problems may not arise during the same period of time. Yet, the optimistic assumptions haven't changed, and may even have taken on a rosier hue. "Three months into the acquisition and we haven't had a hiccup," managers might say. Usually, problems don't show up until a year down the road.

Final PricewaterhouseCoopers Tips for Managing Practices

- Make sure physicians or dentists are willing to share the financial gains of their practice. That sharing will likely mean lower compensation for the physician in the short term.

- Do a reality check. Are these practitioners truly ready to work together for the good of the larger organization?

- Tell physicians that they shouldn't join a practice management company unless they believe that changes are occurring in their marketplace that will lower their future compensation. If a physician believes his or her compensation will increase in the future, why change?

- Understand that the practice management organization may not be physician-centric. The larger an organization becomes, the more likely it will be a company driven by ancillaries, such as inpatient or outpatient facilities, or one that negotiates risk-bearing contracts.

- Make sure physicians find a model that fits their market, specialty, and priorities. Just because a particular model worked in Dallas or Miami doesn't mean it will work everywhere else.

SUMMARY

For two decades, medical care decisions have been driven by an overriding desire to reduce the rate of increase in healthcare spending. Managed care executives, major employers, and the government all worked in tandem to drive "unnecessary costs" out of the system. The result, physicians and other healthcare providers have lost control over decisions regarding their individual patients and the excellent patient/physician relationship we all took for granted has deteriorated.

Today everyone is unhappy with our healthcare system. Patients are upset with their inability to make choices related to their healthcare needs, physicians are upset over their inability to control healthcare decisions without the intrusion of nonphysician executives, and large employers are unhappy because more and more of their workforce are complaining. Many have chosen not to enroll in the healthcare insurance programs they provide. Federal and state legislators are upset because while the rate of growth in healthcare spending has been reduced, it is still high and their constituents are demanding change. As we near the end of the 20th century, healthcare issues have become a top priority of the general public and unfortunately, the national debate is narrowly focused on protecting patients and expanding Medicare coverage.

The time has come to launch a new phase of the healthcare debate. Physician-directed healthcare organizations must lead this debate and we must focus the debate away from patient protections to the single greatest issue, which is the rising number of uninsured in the United States. In 1999, there are more than 43 million individuals without health insurance. This is one and one-half times the total population of Canada. As we address the issues of the uninsured, we must also provide the American public with choice, and we must have policies that re-establish the patient/physician relationship.

Why does the number of uninsured continue to increase? A 1996 study by the University of California at Los Angeles, Center for Health Policy Research reported an increase in the number of uninsured in every size corporation that offered health insurance to its employees. This seven-year increase is due in large measure to two factors: cafeteria plan fringe benefit structures that allow individuals to opt out of buying health insurance in favor of more vacation days, etc., and the shifting of costs from employers to employees. During the seven-year period reported in the study, the employees' cost rose at a rate of three times that of the employers' cost increase.

There is little doubt that if costs continue to be shifted to employees and employers continue to allow individuals to opt out of insurance programs, the number of uninsured in the United States will continue to grow. Two issues, the growing number of uninsured and the growing desire of Americans to have more choice in their care, are going to be the major drivers of change in our healthcare system.

Having this choice has already begun to change our system. Today, most employees with health insurance must go to one of the physicians included in the panel of the insurance company selected by their employer. To make matters worse, most small employers can offer their employees only one insurance plan. The change that has begun has been the addition in most health plans of an "out-of-network" option. Also, Congress has begun to consider having one option for small employers to contract with a health-mart that would provide employees of these employers with the ability to choose insurance plans from a wide variety of options. While the employer would still pay for the premium, the employee would choose the insurance program that best met their needs. They would have many more choices indeed.

Another option under consideration is to give employees a tax deduction for health insurance premiums equal to or greater than that currently enjoyed by their employers. This action would create a very large individual market for health insurance not present in today's markets. Making sure that Americans purchased health insurance would be a major consideration in granting this tax credit and in moving away from an employer-driven system.

So, what would these changes mean for medical groups? First, if we move from an employer-driven healthcare system to an individually driven healthcare system, medical groups with an ability to offer insurance products directly to the people in their community would be in an advantaged position because most individuals care a lot about the system from which they receive their healthcare, but they care little about who finances that care. Giving Americans the option of selecting a care system first and then having this care system provide them with the insurance (either directly or indirectly) they and their families need would go a long way in meeting the demand for choice in the current market. Imagine choosing a care system that then arranges a tax-deductible insurance program that meets your and your family's particular needs. Your choice totally, with no employer involvement.

When you purchase a car, you select the car of your choice and the dealer helps you choose financing that meets your particular needs. Why can't it be the same with healthcare? Your employer doesn't send you to a bank or GMAC and they don't tell you which car you can buy, what color it has to be, and/or where or how fast you can drive it. Healthcare should be no different. To ensure that individuals purchase health insurance, one might have to register annually with the state as part of the state tax return proving that they have purchased health insurance. If they do, they get a state and federal deduction. If they don't they could be taxed based on income with such taxes being contributed to a state insurance fund for the uninsured.

There are several major implications for medical groups, not all attractive. First, medical groups would have to transition from enrolling patients from insurance plans and employers to individual enrollment mechanisms. The increase in marketing and enrollment costs could be enormous. Medical groups would have to embrace and become students of change management. The extent and number of changes the above system would create are mind-boggling and the magnitude of the change alone would require an extensive investment in change management. In order to be partners and leaders in the process, physicians and physician organizations need to be schooled in the basic business principles presented in this book.

Another important change that is coming, irrespective of whether the system changes as significantly as described above, is a move toward purchasing healthcare on value and not on price alone. Outcomes measurement and customer satisfaction measures are common in most medical groups and the American public is becoming aware of the significant variance across medical providers. Patients' increasing awareness and vastly expanding use of the Internet to gain insight into disease management and quality indicators will continue to drive the system toward a clear demonstration of value. Once available, medical groups will be in the position of demonstrating their value to the people they serve. This movement toward purchasing healthcare on value will undoubtedly also drive medical groups toward branding their practice. This has not been done to any large extent to date but will make a difference in the future.

Medical practice groups can expect to see the magnitude and rate of change increase in the coming years. To be competitive, medical groups will have to be players in the healthcare insurance business, and they will have to demonstrate value to patients. Medical groups will also have to invest significantly in their management information systems to manage their core business functions as well as to measure and manage value. While change brings uncertainty, I remain confident that physician-directed multispecialty medical groups will retain their distinct advantage over other forms of healthcare delivery and that they will be successful.

Donald W. Fisher, Ph.D., CAE, is chief executive officer of the Alexandria, Virginia-based American Medical Group Association. AMGA represents more than 230 medical groups and 45,000 physicians dedicated to the delivery and continuous improvement of comprehensive healthcare of the population they serve.

Donald W. Fisher, Ph.D., CAE
Chief Executive Officer,
American Medical Group Association

ABOUT THE AUTHORS

Sandy Lutz is a writer, speaker, and analyst who has followed the healthcare business for more than 12 years. She is a manager in the Dallas office of PricewaterhouseCoopers. Sandy is the author of three other books, *The For-Profit Healthcare Revolution, Columbia/HCA: Healthcare on Overdrive, and Med Inc.: How Consolidation is Transforming Tomorrow's Healthcare System.* Before joining PricewaterhouseCoopers, she was a sell-side healthcare analyst for Rauscher Pierce Refsnes, a Dallas-based investment bank and an industry analyst with MDB Information Network, also in Dallas. Previously, Sandy was Dallas bureau chief for 10 years for *Modern Healthcare* magazine, a weekly trade journal.

OTHER AUTHORS

Frank Cavanaugh is principal-in-charge of the information technology division of the integrated healthcare consulting services practice in Chicago for PricewaterhouseCoopers. He has more than 30 years' experience in the information technology field, including more than 28 years in healthcare information systems. He has extensive experience in the use of automation in healthcare, having worked as a manager of information systems for a hospital group and with three HIS vendors.

Gary Garbrecht is a partner in the managed healthcare industry services group in Los Angeles for PricewaterhouseCoopers. He is the leader of the PricewaterhouseCoopers assurance and business advisory healthcare industry services group for the firm's West region. He has 17 years of experience providing audit and business advisory services to the healthcare industry.

Cynthia Fry is physician practice management leader for the Southeast region for PricewaterhouseCoopers. She is a senior manager in Audit and Business Advisory Services, Senior Manager in Philadelphia. Cynthia has been responsible for the strategic vision, planning, and operational development for a number of diverse medical practices and clinics in her 20 years of experience in healthcare management.

Charles Goldberg is a senior consultant in Global Human Resource Solutions for PricewaterhouseCoopers in Atlanta. He has 16 years of experience in managed care as well as in the development of integrated healthcare organizations. Prior to joining PricewaterhouseCoopers, he was a consultant for five years with another Big Five firm and served in a number of capacities including director of marketing for Kaiser Permanente over an 11-year time period.

Peter Gyorgy is senior manager and functional leader for managed care for the West region in the Audit and Business Advisory Services of the managed health-care industry services group for PricewaterhouseCoopers in Los Angeles. During his 10 years of industry experience, Peter worked for several managed care firms in California, including Health Systems International, Maxicare Health Plans, and Blue Cross of California. Peter has worked in provider relations and con-tracting, network development, sales and marketing, and administration and health plan operations.

Allen Hahn is valuation manager in financial advisory services for PricewaterhouseCoopers in Boston. Prior to PricewaterhouseCoopers, Allen was finance officer at Shawmut Bank and business development officer at Meditrust, a real estate investment trust. Allen provides valuation and transaction advisory services to both publicly traded and early stage physician practice man-agement companies.

William B. Hanlon III is a managing director for Shattuck Hammond Partners, a division of PricewaterhouseCoopers Securities, based in Atlanta and respon-sible for the firm's healthcare investment banking efforts in the Southeast region. For more than 15 years he has provided strategic advisory and investment banking services to healthcare organizations across the country ranging from non-profit institutions to publicly traded and privately owned corporations with an emphasis on medical groups, hospital systems, and practice management com-panies involved in consolidation and restructuring transactions involving physi-cian practices. His experience includes both public and private offerings of debt and equity, partnership, acquisition, and joint venture transactions.

Mel Hope is a partner in the managed healthcare practice for Pricewaterhouse-Coopers in Houston. Mel has more than 14 years of experience with providers of healthcare services. He has advised and participated in public offerings related to practice management companies, assisted with periodic public reporting, designed and performed pre-acquisition due diligence related to physician practices and the development of corporate compliance structures for physician organizations.

Jo Ann Jany is a partner in the financial advisory services group for PricewaterhouseCoopers in New York City. She specializes in forensic ac-counting and investigations, and has performed investigations in matters in-volving healthcare fraud in the payor community, and in the acute care, renal dial-ysis, pharmaceutical, and laboratory industries. Prior to joining PwC in 1990, she served as a special agent for the Federal Bureau of Investigation.

Jane Sarra is a director in the Pittsburgh office of PricewaterhouseCoopers' healthcare regulatory group practice responsible for physician practice management services. Jane has more than 25 years of experience with hospitals, academic medical centers, integrated delivery systems, and physician networks. She has participated in more than 150 practice acquisitions that included due diligence operational analysis, practice integration, and developing compensation and benefit structure for the new physician networks.

INDEX